THE WASHINGTON MANUAL™

Hematology and Oncology

Subspecialty Consult

Third Edition

Editors

Amanda Cashen, MD
Assistant Professor of Medicine
Section of Leukemia and Stem Cell Transplantation
Washington University School of Medicine
St. Louis, Missouri

Brian A. Van Tine, MD, PhD
Assistant Professor of Medicine
Division of Medical Oncology
Washington University School of Medicine
St. Louis, Missouri

Series Editors

Thomas M. De Fer, MD
Former Barnes-Jewish Hospital Internal Medicine Resident
Associate Professor of Internal Medicine
Washington University School of Medicine
St. Louis, Missouri

Katherine E. Henderson, MD
Assistant Professor of Clinical Medicine
Department of Medicine
Division of Medical Education
Washington University School of Medicine
Barnes-Jewish Hospital
St. Louis, Missouri

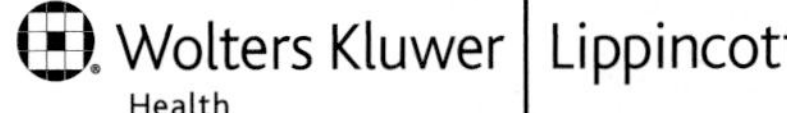

Philadelphia • Baltimore • New York • London
Buenos Aires • Hong Kong • Sydney • Tokyo

Acquisitions Editor: Sonya Seigafuse
Product Manager: Kerry Barrett
Vendor Manager: Bridgett Dougherty
Marketing Manager: Kimberly Schonberger
Manufacturing Manager: Ben Rivera
Design Coordinator: Stephen Druding
Editorial Coordinator: Katie Sharp
Production Service: Aptara, Inc.

Printed in China

Library of Congress Cataloging-in-Publication Data
The Washington manual hematology and oncology subspecialty consult. —
3rd ed. / editors, Amanda Cashen, Brian A. Van Tine.
p. ; cm. — (Washington manual subspecialty consult series)
Hematology and oncology subspecialty consult
Includes bibliographical references and index.
ISBN 978-1-4511-1424-9 (alk. paper) — ISBN 1-4511-1424-9 (alk. paper)
I. Cashen, Amanda. II. Van Tine, Brian A. III. Title: Hematology and oncology subspecialty consult. IV. Series: Washington manual subspecialty consult series.
[DNLM: 1. Hematologic Diseases—Handbooks. 2. Diagnosis, Differential—Handbooks. 3. Drug Therapy—methods—Handbooks. 4. Neoplasms—Handbooks. WH 39]
616.1'5—dc23

2011046133

To purchase additional copies of this book, call our customer service department at (800) 638-3030 or fax orders to (301) 223-2320. International customers should call (301) 223-2300.

Visit Lippincott Williams & Wilkins on the Internet: at LWW.com. Lippincott Williams & Wilkins customer service representatives are available from 8:30 am to 6 pm, EST.

CCS0112

10 9 8 7 6 5 4 3 2 1

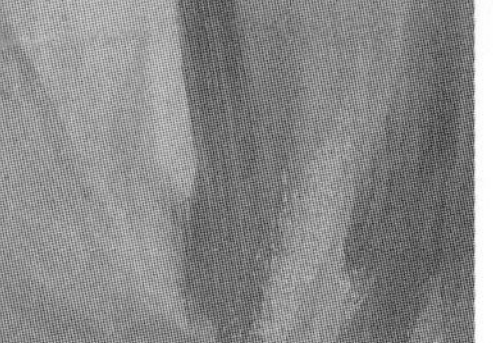

Contributing Authors

George Ansstas, MD
Clinical Fellow
Division of Hematology/Oncology
Washington University School of Medicine
St. Louis, Missouri

Michael Ansstas, MD
Resident Physician
Department of Medicine
Saint Louis University School of Medicine
St. Louis, Missouri

Kristan M. Augustin, PharmD, BCOP
Clinical Pharmacist
BMT/Leukemia
Department of Pharmacy
Barnes-Jewish Hospital
St. Louis, Missouri

Leigh M. Boehmer, PharmD, BCOP
Clinical Pharmacist
Department of Pharmacy
Barnes-Jewish Hospital
St. Louis, Missouri

Sara K. Butler, PharmD, BCOP, BCPS
Clinical Pharmacist
Department of Pharmacy
Barnes-Jewish Hospital
St. Louis, Missouri

Amanda Cashen, MD
Assistant Professor of Medicine
Section of Leukemia and Stem Cell Transplantation
Washington University School of Medicine
St. Louis, Missouri

Yee Hong Chia, MD
Clinical Fellow
Division of Hematology/Oncology
Washington University School of Medicine
St. Louis, Missouri

Kim French, APRN-BC
Division of Hematology
Washington University School of Medicine
St. Louis, Missouri

Armin Ghobadi
Clinical Fellow
Division of Hematology/Oncology
Washington University School of Medicine
St. Louis, Missouri

Andrea R. Hagemann, MD
Assistant Professor
Department of Obstetrics and Gynecology
Washington University School of Medicine
St. Louis, Missouri

Lindsay M. Hladnik, PharmD, BCOP
Clinical Pharmacist
Department of Pharmacy
Barnes-Jewish Hospital
St. Louis, Missouri

Xiaoyi Hu, MD, PhD
Fellow
Division of Hematology/Oncology
Washington University School of Medicine
St. Louis, Missouri

Amie Jackson, MD
Resident
Department of Medicine
Washington University School of Medicine
St. Louis, Missouri

Ronald Jackups, MD
Chief Resident
Laboratory and Genomic Medicine
Washington University School of Medicine
St. Louis, Missouri

Kian-Huat Lim, MD, PhD
Fellow
Medical Oncology
National Cancer Institute/National Institutes of Health
Bethesda, Maryland

Daniel J. Ma, MD
Resident Physician
Department of Radiation Oncology
Washington University School of Medicine
St. Louis, Missouri

Paul Mehan, MD
Fellow
Division of Hematology/Oncology
Washington University School of Medicine
St. Louis, Missouri

Ali McBride, PharmD, BCPS
Clinical Pharmacist
Department of Pharmacy
Barnes-Jewish Hospital
St. Louis, Missouri

Gregory H. Miday, MD
Resident
Department of Medicine
Washington University School of Medicine
St. Louis, Missouri

Gayathri Nagaraj, MD
Fellow
Division of Hematology/Oncology
Washington University School of Medicine
St. Louis, Missouri

Parag J. Parikh, MD
Assistant Professor
Department of Radiology Oncology
Washington University School of Medicine
St. Louis, Missouri

Parvin F. Peddi, MD
Fellow
Division of Hematology/Oncology
Washington University School of Medicine
St. Louis, Missouri

Aruna Rokkam, MD
Fellow
Division of Hematology/Oncology
Washington University School of Medicine
St. Louis, Missouri

Cesar Sanchez, MD
Fellow
Division of Hematology/Oncology
Washington University School of Medicine
St. Louis, Missouri

Kristen M. Sanfilippo, MD
Fellow
Division of Hematology/Oncology
Washington University School of Medicine
St. Louis, Missouri

Brian A. Van Tine, MD, PhD
Assistant Professor of Medicine
Division of Medical Oncology
Washington University School of Medicine
St. Louis, Missouri

Tzu-Fei Wang, MD
Clinical Fellow
Department of Medicine
Division of Hematology/Oncology
Washington University School of Medicine
St. Louis, Missouri

Saiama Waqar, MD
Instructor
Division of Medical Oncology
Washington University School of Medicine
St. Louis, Missouri

Israel Zighelboim, MD
Assistant Professor
Department of Obstetrics and Gynecology
Division of Obstetrics and Gynecology Oncology
Washington University School of Medicine
St. Louis, Missouri

Imran Zoberi, MD
Assistant Professor
Department of Radiation Oncology
Washington University School of Medicine
St. Louis, Missouri

Chairman's Note

It is a pleasure to present the new edition of The *Washington Manual*® Subspecialty Consult Series: *Hematology/Oncology Subspecialty Consult.* This pocket-size book continues to be a primary reference for medical students, interns, residents, and other practitioners who need ready access to practical clinical information to diagnose and treat patients with a wide variety of disorders. Medical knowledge continues to increase at an astounding rate, which creates a challenge for physicians to keep up with the biomedical discoveries, genetic and genomic information, and novel therapeutics that can positively impact patient outcomes. The *Washington Manual* Subspecialty Series addresses this challenge by concisely and practically providing current scientific information for clinicians to aid them in the diagnosis, investigation, and treatment of common medical conditions.

I want to personally thank the authors, which include house officers, fellows, and attendings at Washington University School of Medicine and Barnes-Jewish Hospital. Their commitment to patient care and education is unsurpassed, and their efforts and skill in compiling this manual are evident in the quality of the final product. In particular, I would like to acknowledge our editors, Drs. Amanda Cashen and Brian A. Van Tine, and the series editors, Drs. Katherine Henderson and Tom De Fer, who have worked tirelessly to produce another outstanding edition of this manual. I would also like to thank Dr. Melvin Blanchard, Chief of the Division of Medical Education in the Department of Medicine at Washington University School of Medicine, for his advice and guidance. I believe this Subspecialty Manual will meet its desired goal of providing practical knowledge that can be directly applied at the bedside and in outpatient settings to improve patient care.

Victoria J. Fraser, MD
Dr. J. William Campbell Professor
Interim Chairman of Medicine
Co-Director of the Infectious Disease Division
Washington University School of Medicine

Preface

We are pleased to present the third edition of *The Washington Manual*™ *Hematology and Oncology Subspecialty Consult*. The field of medical oncology continues to advance at a remarkable pace. Every year, new indications are found for existing therapies and new anti-cancer drugs are approved. Staging systems, classifications, and prognostic models are in flux, reflecting the discovery of new biomarkers, changes in treatment algorithms, and the general improvement in patient outcomes. Therapeutic advances have also been made in benign hematology, particularly with the introduction of novel anticoagulants.

This edition has been updated to include new standards in the treatment of malignancies and hematologic disorders, mechanisms of action of new therapeutic agents, and current use of molecular prognostic factors. The information in each chapter is now presented in a consistent format, with important references cited. Our goal is to provide a concise, practical reference for fellows, residents, and medical students rotating on hematology and oncology subspecialty services. Most of the authors are hematology–oncology fellows or internal medicine residents, the physicians who have recent experience with the issues and questions that arise in the course of training in these subspecialties. Primary care practitioners and other health care professionals also will find this manual useful as a quick reference source in hematology and oncology.

As the practice of hematology and oncology continues to evolve, changes in dosing and indications for chemotherapy and targeted therapies will occur, and staging systems will be modified. We recommend a handbook of chemotherapy regimens and an oncology staging manual to complement the information in this book. And of course, clinical judgment is imperative when applying the principles presented here to the care of individual patients.

We appreciate the effort and expertise of everyone who contributed to this edition of the *Hematology and Oncology Subspecialty Consult*. In particular, we would like to thank the authors for their enthusiastic efforts to distill volumes of medical advances into a concise, useable format. We also recognize the faculty in the divisions of hematology, oncology, bone marrow transplantation, radiation oncology, and gynecologic oncology at Washington University for their mentorship and commitment to education.

—A.C. and B.A.V.T.

Contents

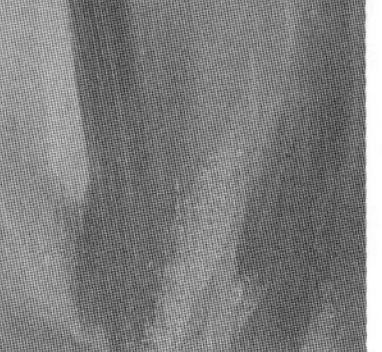

Introduction and Approach to Hematology

1

Parvin F. Peddi

GENERAL PRINCIPLES

Approach to the Hematology Patient

Hematologic diseases are a heterogeneous group of diseases that can have multiple clinical and laboratory manifestations that mimic nonhematologic diseases. History, physical exam, labs, peripheral smear, and bone marrow biopsy are critical in making the correct diagnosis. The diseases can be approached by identifying the primary hematologic component that is affected: RBCs, WBCs, platelets, or the coagulation system. The major abnormalities in hematology are quantitative in nature, with either excessive or deficient production of one of the hematopoietic constituents (e.g., leukemias, anemias). Qualitative abnormalities that can be inherited (e.g., sickle cell disease) or acquired also occur.

DIAGNOSIS

Clinical Presentation

History

The medical history is, of course, the first step in hematology diagnostic assessment. Table 1-1 offers some general questions for evaluation of a hematologic disorder.

Physical Exam

The physical exam is also an important part of the diagnostic process. Along with the history, it can suggest a diagnosis, guide lab testing, and aid in the differential diagnosis. Table 1-2 offers some general physical exam findings that are useful in the hematology patient.

Diagnostic Testing

Laboratories

The clinician should be comfortable using the complete blood count (CBC) and peripheral smear to evaluate patients for possible hematologic disorders. Patients may be referred to a hematologist based on a lab abnormality that is drawn for a reason other than the diagnosis of a primary hematologic disorder. There are certain limiting values in hematology that can help exclude or confirm the need for further testing or warn us of the possibility of potential physiological consequences (see Table 1-3).

- **The Peripheral Smear.** The visual study of peripheral blood is necessary to diagnose hematologic and nonhematologic diseases, for example, thrombotic thrombocytopenic purpura or malaria. In these cases, as in others, automated hematology analyzers are able to provide a large number of data regarding all the blood cells but will not be able to detect subtle anomalies critical in the diagnosis.

TABLE 1-1 PERTINENT HISTORY IN THE HEMATOLOGY PATIENT

Pertinent Medical History	Hematologic Differential Diagnosis
History of present illness	
Recent infections	
Fever, chills, rigors	Leukemias, lymphomas, multiple myeloma
Antibiotic use	Hemolysis
Bleeding	
Hemorrhage, epistaxis, bleeding gums, petechiae, ecchymosis, menorrhagia	Thrombocytopenia, leukemias, coagulation disorder
Hemarthrosis	Clotting factor deficiency
Skin coloration	
Pallor	Anemia
Jaundice	Hemolysis
Dyspnea, chest pain, orthostasis	Anemia
Pica	Iron deficiency
Abdominal fullness, early satiety	Splenomegaly
Alcoholism, poor nutrition, vegetarianism	Megaloblastic anemia
Headache, neurologic deficits	Leukostasis, thrombocytopenia, thrombosis, Waldenström macroglobulinemia
Pruritus	Polycythemia, Hodgkin lymphoma
Medical history	
Prior malignancies, chemotherapy	Secondary malignancies (leukemia), myelodysplasia
HIV risk factors	Anemia, thrombocytopenia
Previous hepatitis	Anemia, cryoglobulinemia
Pregnancy	Anemia, HELLP syndrome
Venous thrombosis	Thrombophilia
Family history	
Bleeding disorders	Hemophilias, von Willebrand disease
Anemia (African American, Mediterranean, Asian)	Hemoglobinopathies

HELLP, hemolysis, elevated liver enzymes, and low platelet count.

Slides for a peripheral smear are typically prepared either by automated methods or by qualified technicians in a specialized laboratory. This step is critical since poorly processed samples can lead to incorrect diagnoses. Smears may be prepared on glass slides or coverslips. Ideally, **blood smears should be prepared from uncoagulated blood** and from a sample collected from a finger stick. In practice, most slides are prepared from blood samples containing anticoagulants and are thus prone to the introduction of morphologic artifacts. Blood smears are normally stained using Wright or May–Grünwald–Giemsa stain.

TABLE 1-2 PHYSICAL EXAM IN THE HEMATOLOGY PATIENT

Pertinent Exam Findings	Hematologic Differential Diagnosis
HEENT	
Conjunctival or mucosal pallor	Anemia
Jaundice	Hemolysis, hyperbilirubinemia
Conjunctival or mucosal petechiae	Thrombocytopenia
Glossitis	Iron deficiency, vitamin B_{12} deficiency
Lymphadenopathy	Lymphoma
Skin/nails	
Pallor	Anemia
Jaundice	Hyperbilirubinemia
Bronze appearance	Hemochromatosis
Spoon nails (koilonychia)	Iron deficiency
Ecchymosis, petechiae	Thrombocytopenia
Erythematous, indurated plaques	Mycosis fungoides
Cardiovascular	
Tachycardia, S4, prominent post-MI	Severe anemia with high-output cardiac failure
Abdominal	
Splenomegaly	Hairy cell or other leukemias, polycythemia, lymphomas
Neurologic	Megaloblastic anemia
Loss of vibratory sense and proprioception (dorsal and lateral columns)	
Musculoskeletal	
Bone pain/tenderness	Multiple myeloma

HEENT, head, ears, eyes, nose, and throat; MI, myocardial infarction.

- **Examination of the Peripheral Smear.** Examination of the smear should proceed systematically and begin under low power to identify a portion of the slide with optimal cellular distribution and staining, which normally corresponds to the thinner edge of the sample. As a general rule, the **analysis starts with RBCs, continues with leukocytes, and finishes with platelets.** Under *low power* (×10 to ×20) it is possible to analyze general characteristics of RBCs to discover, for example, the presence of Rouleaux associated with multiple myeloma, estimate the WBC and platelet counts, and determine the presence of abnormal populations of cells, such as blasts, by scanning over the entire smear. Under *high power* (×100), each of the cell lineages is examined for any abnormalities in number or morphology.
- **Red Blood Cells.** Quantitative analysis of RBCs is difficult on a peripheral smear. Automated analyzers are used to calculate:
  MCHC, the mean cell Hgb concentration, expressed as grams per deciliter;
  MCH, the mean corpuscular Hgb, expressed as picograms; and
  MCV, the mean corpuscular volume, expressed as femtoliters (10^{-15} L).

TABLE 1-3 DECISION LIMITING VALUES FOR COMMON HEMATOLOGIC TESTS

Diagnostic Test	Limiting Value	Comment
Hgb	<5 g/dL	Transfusion indicated even in absence of symptoms
	<10 g/dL	Anemia workup indicated
Hct	>70%	Urgent phlebotomy indicated
Platelet count	<10,000/mm^3	Risk of spontaneous bleeding
	<50,000/mm^3	Risk of bleeding increased with surgery/trauma
	>500,000–1,000,000/mm^3	Risk of thrombosis
	>2,000,000/mm^3	Risk of bleeding
Neutrophil count	<500/mm^3	Greatest risk of infection
Blast count (acute leukemia)	>100,000/mm^3	Risk of leukostasis; urgent treatment indicated
Prothrombin time	<1.5× control	No increased bleeding risk
	>2.5× control	Risk of spontaneous bleeding
Partial prothrombin time	<1.5× control	No increased bleeding risk
	>2.5× control (>90 s)	Risk of spontaneous bleeding
Bleeding time	>20 min	Possible risk of spontaneous bleeding
Antithrombin III	<50% normal level	Risk of spontaneous thrombosis

Qualitative analysis of RBCs should demonstrate uniform round cells with smooth membranes and a pale central area with a round rim of red Hgb. Variations in size are called anisocytosis, and variations in shape, poikilocytosis. The following abnormalities may be observed:

- **Hypochromia** corresponds to a very thin rim of Hgb and a larger central pale area. These red cells are often microcytic and are seen in iron deficiency, thalassemias, and sideroblastic anemia.
- **Microcytosis** (<6 μm): Differential diagnosis includes iron-deficiency anemia, anemia in chronic disease, thalassemias, and sideroblastic anemia. These cells are usually hypochromic and have prominent central pallor.
- **Macrocytosis** (>9 μm in diameter): Differential diagnosis includes liver disease, alcoholism, aplastic anemia, and myelodysplasia. Megaloblastic anemias (B_{12} and folate deficiencies) have macro-ovalocytes (large oval cells). *Reticulocytes* are large immature red cells with polychromatophilia.
- **Schistocytes** (fragmented cells) are caused by mechanical disruption of cells in the microvasculature by fibrin strands or by mechanical prosthetic heart valves. Differential diagnosis includes thrombotic thrombocytopenic purpura/hemolytic uremic syndrome, disseminated intravascular coagulation, hemolysis/elevated liver enzymes/low platelet count (HELLP) syndrome, and malignant hypertension.

- **Acanthocytes** (spiculated cells with irregular projections of varying length) are seen in liver disease.
- **Burr cells** (cells with short, evenly spaced cytoplasmic projections) may be an artifact of slide preparation or found in renal failure and uremia.
- **Bite cells** (cells with a smooth semicircle extracted) are due to spleen phagocytes that have removed Heinz bodies consisting of denatured Hgb. They are found in hemolytic anemia due to glucose-6-phosphate dehydrogenase deficiency.
- **Spherocytes** (round, dense cells with absent central pallor) are seen in immune hemolytic anemia and hereditary spherocytosis.
- **Sickle cells** (sickle-shaped cells) are due to polymerization of Hgb S. They are found in sickle cell disease but not in sickle cell trait.
- **Target cells** (cells with extra Hgb in the center surrounded by a rim of pallor; bull's-eye appearance) are due to an increase in the ratio of cell membrane surface area to Hgb volume within the cell. These have a central spot of Hgb surrounded by a ring of pallor from the redundancy in cell membrane. They are found in liver disease, postsplenectomy, in hemoglobinopathies, and in thalassemia.
- **Teardrop cells/dacryocytes** (teardrop-shaped cells) are found in myelofibrosis and myelophthisic states of marrow infiltration.
- **Ovalocytes** (elliptical cells) are due to the abnormal membrane cytoskeleton found in hereditary elliptocytosis.
- **Polychromatophilia** (blue hue of cytoplasm) is due to the presence of RNA and ribosomes in reticulocytes.
- **Howell–Jolly bodies** (small, single, purple cytoplasmic inclusions) represent nuclear remnant DNA and are found after splenectomy or with functional asplenism.
- **Basophilic stippling** (dark-purple inclusions, usually multiple) arises from precipitated RNA found in lead poisoning and thalassemia.
- **Nucleated red cells** are not normally found in peripheral blood. They appear in hypoxemia and myelofibrosis or other myelophthisic conditions, as well as with severe hemolysis.
- **Heinz bodies** (inclusions seen only on staining with violet crystal) represent denatured Hgb and are found in glucose-6-phosphate dehydrogenase after oxidative stress.
- **Parasites,** including malaria and babesiosis, may be seen within red cells.
- **Rouleaux** (red cell aggregates resembling a stack of coins) is due to the loss of normal electrostatic charge–repelling red cells due to coating with abnormal paraprotein, such as in multiple myeloma.
- **Leukoerythroblastic smear** (teardrop cells, nucleated red cells, and immature white cells) is found in marrow infiltration or fibrosis (myelophthisic conditions).

○ **White Blood Cells.** WBCs normally seen on the peripheral smear include mature granulocytes (neutrophils, eosinophils, and basophils) and mature agranulocytes (lymphocytes and monocytes). Under normal conditions, immature myeloid and lymphoid cells are not seen and their presence is related to conditions such as infections and hematologic neoplasias.

- **Neutrophils.** Neutrophils comprise 55% to 60% of total WBCs (1.8×10^9 to 7.7×10^9/L). They have nuclei containing three or four lobes and granular cytoplasm. The normal size is 10 to 15 μm. Hypersegmented neutrophils contain more than five lobes and are found in megaloblastic anemias. The cytoplasmic granules correspond to enzymes that are used during the acute phase of inflammation. Increased prominence of cytoplasmic granules is indicative of systemic infection or therapy with growth factors and is known as *toxic granulation.* Neutrophils develop from myeloblasts through promyelocyte, myelocyte, metamyelocyte, and band forms and progress to mature neutrophils. Only mature neutrophils and bands are normally found in peripheral blood. Metamyelocytes and myelocytes may be found in pregnancy, infections, and leukemoid reactions. The presence of less mature forms in the peripheral blood is indicative of hematologic malignancy or myelophthisis.

- **Lymphocytes.** Lymphocytes comprise 25% to 35% (1×10^9 to 4.8×10^9/L, or thousands per cubic millimeter) of total WBCs. They contain a dark, clumped nucleus and a scant rim of blue cytoplasm. The differentiation of T and B cells using light microscopy is very difficult. The normal size is 7 to 18 μm. **Atypical (or reactive) lymphocytes** seen in viral infections contain more extensive, malleable cytoplasm that may encompass surrounding red cells.
- **Eosinophils.** Eosinophils comprise 0.5% to 4% of total WBCs (0.2×10^9/L, or thousands per cubic millimeter). These are large cells containing prominent red/orange granules and a bilobed nucleus. The normal size is 10 to 15 μm. Increased numbers are found in parasitic infections and allergic disorders.
- **Monocytes.** Monocytes comprise 4% to 8% of total WBCs (0 to 0.3×10^9/L, or thousands per cubic millimeter). These are the bigger circulating cells with an eccentric U-shaped nucleus. They contain blue cytoplasm and are the precursors of the mononuclear phagocyte system (macrophages, osteoclasts, alveolar macrophages, Kupfer cells, and microglia). The usual size is 12 to 20 μm.
- **Basophils.** Basophils comprise 0.01% to 0.3% of total WBCs (0 to 0.1×10^9/L, or thousands per cubic millimeter). Their cytoplasm contains large dark-blue granules and a bilobed nucleus. They are involved in inflammatory reactions and increased numbers are also seen in chronic myeloid leukemia. As for eosinophils, the normal size is 10 to 15 μm.
- **WBC Abnormalities.** Quantitative anomalies result in leukopenia and leukocytosis. Main causes of leukopenia include bone marrow failure (aplastic anemia), myelophthisis (acute leukemia), drugs (immunosuppressive drugs, propylthiouracil), and hypersplenism (portal hypertension). Main causes of leukocytosis are infection, inflammation, malignancies, and allergic reactions.
  - **Pelger–Huet anomaly** (neutrophils have a bilobed nucleus connected by a thin strand and decreased granulation) is seen in myelodysplastic syndromes.
  - **Hypersegmented neutrophils** (more than four nuclear lobes) are found in megaloblastic anemias (vitamin B_{12} and folate deficiency).
  - **Blast cells** (myeloblasts or lymphoblasts; large cells with large nuclei and prominent nucleoli) are seen in acute leukemia.
  - **Auer rods** (rodlike granules in blast cytoplasm) are pathognomonic for acute myelogenous leukemia, especially acute promyelocytic leukemia (M3).

  - ☐ **Hairy cells** (lymphoid cells with ragged cytoplasm) are seen in hairy cell leukemia.
  - ☐ **Sézary cells** (atypical lymphoid cells with cerebriform nuclei) are seen in cutaneous T cell lymphoma.
- ○ **Platelets.** Platelets appear as small (1- to 2-μm-diameter), purplish cytoplasmic fragments without a nucleus, containing red/blue granules. Derived from bone marrow giant cells called megakaryocytes, they are involved in the cellular mechanisms of primary hemostasis leading to the formation of blood clots. Normal counts are 150,000 to 400,000 per cubic millimeter of peripheral blood. The number of platelets per high-power field multiplied by 20,000 usually estimates the platelet count per microliter. Alternatively, one should find 1 platelet for every 10 to 20 red cells.
  - ■ Numbers of platelets can decrease due to bone marrow disease (myelophthisic bone marrow), consumption (disseminated intravascular coagulation), or drugs. An increase in numbers can be seen in bone marrow overproduction (myeloproliferative syndromes) or in a normal response to massive bleeding. **Pseudo-thrombocytopenia** represents clumping of platelets in blood samples collected in EDTA, resulting in spuriously low platelet counts. This phenomenon can be avoided by using citrate to anticoagulate blood samples sent for blood counts.

Diagnostic Procedures

- **Bone Marrow Evaluation.** For many hematologic diseases that affect the bone marrow, evaluation of the peripheral blood smear does not provide sufficient information, and a direct examination of the bone marrow is required to establish the diagnosis. The bone marrow biopsy can be done at the bedside under local anesthesia alone or in combination with low doses of anxiolytics or opioids. Despite advances in the bone marrow biopsy and aspiration techniques, they are still commonly considered painful procedures, but with expertise, they can be performed safely and with minimal discomfort to the patient.
  - ○ **Indications and Contraindications.** The most common indications for bone marrow evaluation are workup of bone marrow malignancies; staging of marrow involvement by metastatic tumors; assessment of infectious diseases that may involve the bone marrow (i.e., HIV, tuberculosis); determination of marrow damage in patients exposed to radiation, drugs, and chemicals; and workup of metabolic storage diseases. There are a few absolute contraindications for the procedure, including infection, previous radiation therapy at the site of biopsy, and poor patient cooperation. Thrombocytopenia is not a contraindication to bone marrow biopsy, although it may be associated with more procedure-related bleeding. Patients who have a coagulopathy require factor replacement or withholding of anticoagulation to minimize bleeding complications.
  - ○ **Technique.** In adults, the most common places to do the procedure are the posterior and anterior iliac crests. Other potential biopsy sites are the sternum and tibia. The posterior iliac crest is the preferred site, as it allows collection of both aspirate and biopsy specimens and is associated with minimal morbidity or complications. Usually, a *Jamshidi* bone marrow aspiration and biopsy needle is used. Additional aspirate is often obtained for studies such as flow cytometry, cytogenetics, and cultures. In some instances, marrow cannot

be aspirated and only a biopsy is obtained (a "dry tap"). This can be due to the technique or may signal myelofibrosis or previous local radiotherapy. In such cases, touch preparations of the biopsy can be made to allow for a cytologic exam. The biopsy specimen is embedded in a buffered formaldehyde-based fixation for further processing.

- **Complications.** Bleeding at the site of puncture is the most common complication. It is easily controlled with compression, but some thrombocytopenic patients will require platelet transfusions. Other uncommon complications are infections, tumor seeding in the needle track, and needle breakage.
- **Bone Marrow Examination**
  - The examination of the bone marrow aspirate begins under **low power** to obtain an impression of overall cellularity, an initial scan for any abnormal populations of cells or clumps of cells, and an evaluation of the presence or absence of bone marrow spicules. Megakaryocytes are normally seen under low power as large multinucleated cells. The overall cellularity of the marrow is difficult to estimate from the aspirate because of contamination with peripheral blood.
  - The **myeloid-to-erythroid (M:E) ratio** is also determined under low power and is normally 3:1 to 4:1. The ratio is increased in chronic myeloid leukemia due to an increase in granulocyte precursors and is increased in pure red cell aplasia due to a decrease in red cell precursors. The ratio is decreased in hemolytic disorders in which increased erythroid precursors are present or in agranulocytic conditions secondary to chemotherapeutic agents or other drugs.
  - Under **high power,** the aspirate should contain a variety of cells representative of various stages of myeloid and erythroid maturation. Myeloid cells progress from myeloblasts to promyelocytes, myelocytes, metamyelocytes, band forms, and then mature neutrophils. As these cells mature, their nuclear chromatin condenses, with a resultant decrease in the nuclear-to-cytoplasmic ratio. Their cytoplasm gradually develops granules seen in mature neutrophils.
  - **Erythroid precursors** progress from proerythroblasts through varying stages of normoblasts known as *basophilic, chromatophilic,* and *orthochromic.* The nucleus gradually condenses, and the cytoplasm gradually takes on the pinkish hue of Hgb found in mature red cells.
  - **Bone marrow core biopsies** are fixed in a buffered formaldehyde-based solution and then embedded in paraffin or plastic. Biopsies are used to assess the cellularity of the bone marrow and the presence of neoplasias, infections, or fibrosis. Cellularity is estimated by observing the ratio of hematopoietic cells to fat cells. Cellularity is usually 30% to 60% but typically declines with advancing age.
- **Abnormalities in the Bone Marrow Evaluation.** Listed below are some of the more common abnormal findings of the bone marrow.
  - **Acute leukemia:** The presence of >20% blasts in the bone marrow establishes the diagnosis of acute leukemia.
  - **Myelodysplastic syndrome** is a heterogeneous group of diseases characterized by the presence of immature erythroid precursors with loss of synchrony between nuclear and cytoplasmic maturation. Mature myeloid cells have decreased lobes (Pelger–Huet cells). Iron staining may reveal ring sideroblasts with iron granules surrounding the nucleus.

- **Chronic myeloid leukemia:** Findings include a hypercellular marrow with an increased M:E ratio. Myeloblasts represent <5% of cells, with the marrow containing predominantly myelocytes, metamyelocytes, and mature neutrophils.
- **Chronic lymphocytic leukemia** is marked by hypercellular marrow with small, round, mature lymphocytes with a thin rim of blue cytoplasm.
- **Myelofibrosis** is often the cause of a "dry tap." Bone marrow biopsy will reveal marrow infiltration with collagen and fibrous tissue.
- **Essential thrombocytosis:** Megakaryocyte hyperplasia is a common finding.
- **Polycythemia vera** is characterized by a hypercellular marrow.
- **Multiple myeloma:** The marrow is replaced by large numbers of abnormal, often immature plasma cells with eccentric nuclei containing a cartwheel pattern of nuclear chromatin. Flame cells contain pink, flamelike cytoplasm and are associated with an IgA paraprotein.
- **Megaloblastic anemia:** Findings include hypercellular marrow with abnormalities in myeloid and erythroid precursors. Megaloblasts are erythroid cells that are larger than normal, with more nuclear chromatin. There is loss of synchrony between nuclear and cytoplasmic maturation.
- **Storage diseases:** Patients with Gaucher disease may have macrophages with striated cytoplasm due to accumulation of cerebrosides. Individuals with Niemann–Pick disease may have macrophages with a foamy cytoplasm secondary to contained sphingomyelin.

White Blood Cell Disorders: Leukopenia and Leukocytosis

2

George Ansstas

LEUKOPENIA

General Principles

- The normal white blood cell (WBC) count varies with gender and ethnicity but, in general, ranges from 4×10^9 to 11×10^9 cells/L (Table 2-1) and is composed of those cells committed to the leukocyte lineage: granulocytes (neutrophils, eosinophils, and basophils), monocytes, and lymphocytes. Neutrophils make up about 60% of the peripheral blood nucleated cells. A person's gender and ethnic background should be taken into consideration when determining normal ranges.
- Leukopenia is **defined as a WBC count $<3.8 \times 10^9$ cells/L.** This lower limit of normal varies with age (infants have lower absolute neutrophil counts [ANCs] than adults) and race (lower ANCs in persons of African ancestry, West Indians, Arab Jordanian, and Yemenite Jews),[1] and 5% of the normal population may fall outside of the normal reference range. Leukopenias can be divided according to clinically relevant cell lineages: neutrophils and lymphocytes.

NEUTROPENIA

General Principles

Definition

The ANC is obtained by taking the percentage of neutrophils identified on a 100-cell differential or by the Coulter counter and multiplying by the total WBC count. Neutropenia is classified as **mild** (ANC, $<1.5 \times 10^9$ to 1×10^9/L), **moderate** (ANC, 1×10^9 to 0.5×10^9/L), or **severe** (ANC, $<0.5 \times 10^9$/L). **Agranulocytosis** is the total absence of granulocytes.

Epidemiology

Neutropenia is five times more prevalent in African Americans than Caucasians.

Etiology

Causes of neutropenia in adults are reported in Table 2-2. Severe neutropenia can be congenital or acquired. Congenital causes are usually suggested by family history. Most cases of neutropenia are acquired and related to decreased granulocyte production and, less often, increased destruction. Pseudo-neutropenia may be obtained by analyzing blood several hours old and in the presence of paraproteinemia and certain anticoagulants that can cause clumping. Lower ANCs occur in African Americans as a result of defective release of neutrophils from the marrow, a poor marrow reserve, or an increased marginated pool of neutrophils.[2]

TABLE 2-1 AVERAGE ADULT WBC COUNT

Cell	Percentage	Absolute Count ($\times 10^9$/L)
Leukocytes		3.8–9.8
Neutrophils	40–75	1.8–6.6
Monocytes	4–13	0.2–1.2
Eosinophils	0–6	<0.5
Basophils	0–3	<0.2
Lymphocytes	20–54	1.2–3.3

Adapted from Barnes-Jewish Hospital Laboratory References, Barnes-Jewish Hospital, St. Louis, MO.

TABLE 2-2 CAUSE OF NEUTROPENIA

Primary hematological disorders	Congenital/Inherited
	Severe congenital neutropenia (Kostmann syndrome)
	Cyclic neutropenia
	Familial benign neutropenia
	Diamond–Blackfan syndrome
	Schwachman–Diamond syndrome
	Chédiak–Higashi syndrome
	Glycogen storage disease type Ib
	Fanconi anemia
	Acquired
	Acute leukemia
	Myelodysplastic syndromes
	Chronic lymphocytic leukemia
	Hodgkin lymphoma
	Non-Hodgkin lymphoma
	Aplastic anemia and pure white cell aplasia
	Chronic idiopathic neutropenia
	Nutritional: copper, vitamin B_{12}, and folate
Secondary disorders	Immune neutropenias
	Isoimmune neutropenia of the neonate (transplacental IgG specific for paternal neutrophil antigens)
	Autoimmune neutropenia
	Neutropenia with autoimmune diseases
	Systemic lupus erythematosus
	Rheumatoid arthritis
	Felty syndrome
	Sjögren syndrome
	Neutropenia with clonal large granular lymphocytosis
	Marrow infiltrative process
	Drug induced (see Table 2-3)
	Neutropenia with infectious diseases
	Sepsis
	Viral: EBV, parvovirus, and HIV
	Hypersplenism

EBV, Epstein-Barr virus

Pathophysiology

Neutropenia results from decreased production, ineffective granulopoiesis, increased margination to peripheral pools, or increased peripheral destruction. Acquired neutropenias are usually a result of infection, toxins/drugs, or immune disorders. Viral, parasitic, or bacterial infections may cause neutropenia, and this is usually short lived. The underlying mechanism involves increased margination, sequestration, and increased destruction by circulating antibodies. Drug and toxin exposure usually follows a temporal course, with neutropenia developing after continued drug exposure of days to months. The mechanism of drug-induced neutropenia is either antibody-mediated or direct toxic effects on the marrow. Certain drugs at higher risk of causing neutropenia are highlighted in Table 2-3. Primary immune disorders mediate neutropenia through antibody-mediated neutrophil destruction.

Diagnosis

Clinical Presentation

- Neutropenia is often incidentally discovered on a complete blood count (CBC) but may present with fever or infection. **Signs of infection,** such as purulence, may be less evident, given the low neutrophil count. The risk of infection is directly related to the degree and duration of neutropenia. The risk of infection increases at an ANC $<1 \times 10^9$/L, but clinical symptoms usually do not become manifest until the ANC falls below 0.5×10^9/L.[3]
- The initial evaluation should include a complete history and physical exam. The **history** should focus on systemic symptoms of infection, recent exposures or new medications, history of neutropenia, and family history of neutropenia. The **physical exam** may suggest the cause of neutropenia, and attention should be paid to vital signs that would suggest sepsis or infection, oral cavity exam for gingivitis or tooth abscess, macroglossia to suggest vitamin deficiency, lymphadenopathy to suggest malignancy or infection, skin and joint changes suggesting a rheumatologic disorder, and splenomegaly (sequestration and Felty's syndrome).

Diagnostic Testing

Initial laboratory evaluation starts with the **CBC** with complete differential and review of the peripheral blood smear. Additional testing to consider includes nutritional studies of vitamin B_{12}, folate, and possibly copper. If a clonal process is suspected, lymphocyte immunophenotyping by flow cytometry and T-cell receptor gene rearrangement studies may be useful. Antinuclear antibody and antineutrophil antibody testing can be sent to evaluate for autoimmune neutropenia. HIV and EBV serologies start the initial infectious workup. If anemia or thrombocytopenia occurs in combination with neutropenia, direct examination of the bone marrow via bone marrow biopsy is usually warranted unless a cause is obvious. In cases of asymptomatic mild neutropenia, serial CBC examination to rule out cyclic neutropenia may be considered. In mild cases of neutropenia that do not improve in a couple of months with observation, a bone marrow biopsy should be considered.

Treatment

- Treatment is guided by the underlying etiology and severity of neutropenia. This can range from close observation in patients with benign neutropenia to growth factor support and antibiotics in patients with neutropenic fevers.

TABLE 2-3 DRUGS CAUSING NEUTROPENIA

Drug Class	Common Examples
Analgesics and anti-inflammatory agents	Indomethacin, para-aminophenol derivatives, e.g., acetaminophen Pyrazolon derivatives, e.g., phenylbutazone
Antibiotics	Cephalosporins Chloramphenicol Penicillins Sulfonamides Trimethoprim-sulfamethoxazole Vancomycin
Anticonvulsants	Phenytonin Carbamazepine
Antidepressants	Amitriptyline Imipramine
Antihistamines, H_2-blockers	Cimetidine Ranitidine
Antimalarials	Dapsone Quinine Chloroquine
Antithyroid drugs	Carbimazole Methimazole Propylthiouracil
Cardiovascular drugs	Captopril Hydralazine Propranolol
Diuretics	Hydrochlorothiazide Acetazolamide
Hypnotics and sedatives	Chlordiazepoxide Benzodiazepines
Atypical antipsychotics	Chlorpromazine Olanzapine Clozapine
Other drugs	Allopurinol Colchicine Penicillamine Ticlopidine

- **Growth factors** can be used to speed count recovery in drug-induced neutropenia. The major complication associated with neutropenia is infection.
- **Supportive care** with broad-spectrum antibiotics in the ill or febrile patient is an essential part of initial care while the workup for a cause of neutropenia is under way. Common sites of infection include mucous membranes, skin, perirectal and genital areas, bloodstream, and lungs. Most commonly, endogenous bacterial flora is the pathogen (*Staphylococcus* from skin or gram-negative

organisms from the gut). Antibiotics should be continued until the ANC is >500/L for 2 days and the fever subsides. If fever and neutropenia persist, empiric antifungal coverage should be considered.

- Cases caused by drug toxicity should improve, with removal of the drug within 1 to 3 weeks. Drug-related neutropenia can be confirmed by testing antineutrophil-associated drug antibodies. Infectious etiologies resolve with treatment of the infection or shortly after a viral infection has subsided. Autoimmune diseases can be treated by immunosuppression with corticosteroids and can be confirmed by testing antineutrophil antibodies. Congenital etiologies are often supported with growth factors such as granulocyte colony-stimulating factor (G-CSF). The involvement of other blood cell lineages (RBCs and platelets) suggests aplastic anemia, leukemia, myelodysplastic syndromes, or megaloblastic anemia.

LYMPHOPENIA

General Principles

Definition

Lymphopenia is defined as an **absolute lymphocyte count <1.2 × 10^9/L.** The absolute lymphocyte count is 80% T cells and 20% B cells. Sixty-six percent of the T-cell population is $CD4^+$ cells and the remaining is mainly $CD8^+$ cells.

Etiology

Lymphopenia is most often acquired, but congenital causes should also be considered. Etiologies of lymphopenia are listed in Table 2-4 and are mainly acquired. Patients who appear to have low or absent CD4 cells should be evaluated for OKT4 epitope deficiency. This condition is found in 8% of individuals of African descent. Individuals with OKT4 epitope deficiency usually have normal $CD4^+$ number and do not develop infections.[4]

Treatment

Most causes of lymphocytopenia are acquired, and the management focuses on treating the underlying illness. The most common infectious cause is acquired immunodeficiency syndrome (AIDS). Other viral and bacterial diseases also cause lymphocytopenia, which usually resolves a couple of weeks after antimicrobial therapy. Zinc deficiency responds to repletion of zinc and should be part of the initial screen, along with examination of the peripheral blood smear. Inherited causes predispose to recurrent and opportunistic infections, and detailed discussion of management is beyond the scope of this text. In general, prophylactic antibiotics can be used, as well as best supportive care.

LEUKOCYTOSIS

General Principles

An elevated WBC most commonly reflects a normal bone marrow response to inflammation or infection. Occasionally leukemia or myeloproliferative disorders are to blame. The maturation of WBCs is influenced by G-CSFs, interleukins (ILs), tumor necrosis factor, and complement components.

Definition

Leukocytosis is defined as a WBC count >10 × 10^9 cells/L.

TABLE 2-4 CAUSES OF LYMPHOPENIA

Congenital	Severe combined immunodeficiency Common variable immune deficiency Congenital thymic aplasia (DiGeorge syndrome) X-Linked agammaglobulinemia (Brutun agammaglobulinemia) Wiskott–Aldrich syndrome Purine nucleoside phosphorylase deficiency Ataxia-telangiectasia
Acquired	Aplastic anemia Viral infection: HIV/AIDS, severe acute respiratory syndrome (SARS), hepatitis, influenza, Herpes simplex virus Bacterial infection: tuberculosis, pneumonia, richettsiosis, ehrlichiosis, sepsis malaria—acute phase Immunosuppressive agents Antilymphocyte globulin, alemtuzumab, glucocorticoids Chemotherapy Radiation Renal or hematopeitic stem cell transplantation Hemodialysis
Systemic diseases	Autoimmune diseases: systemic lupus erythematosus, periarteritis Hodgkin lymphoma Carcinoma Sarcoidosis
Nutritional	Ethanol abuse Zinc deficiency

Classification

Leukocytosis should be divided into granulocytosis, monocytosis, and lymphocytosis to guide the workup and differential diagnosis.

Etiology

Most cases of leukocytosis are a result of the bone marrow reacting to inflammation or infection. A **leukemoid reaction** is an excessive WBC response (usually >50,000) associated with a cause outside of the bone marrow (growth factors, infection, or differentiating agents such as all-trans retinoic acid [ATRA]). Leukocytosis may also be caused by physical and emotional stress and usually resolves in hours once the stress is eliminated. In postsplenectomy patients, a transient leukocytosis can be seen, lasting for weeks to months secondary to the demargination of leukocytes typically stored in the spleen. Other etiologies include medications, but leukocytes should not rise above 20,000 to 30,000 in this case. The leukocytosis seen in hemolytic anemias (sickle cell and autoimmune types) is related to the nonspecific effects of increased erythropoiesis and inflammation. Nonhematopoietic malignancy can also cause a leukocytosis that is multifactorial in etiology. Finally, acute and chronic leukemias and myeloproliferative disorders usually present with a leukocytosis.

TABLE 2-5 CAUSES OF LEUKOCYTOSIS
Normally responding bone marrow
Infection
Inflammation
Tissue necrosis, infarction, burns, arthritis
Stress
Overexertion, seizures, anxiety, anesthesia
Drugs
Corticosteroids, lithium, beta-agonists
Trauma
Splenectomy
Hemolytic anemia
Malignancy
Leukocytosis of pregnancy
Abnormal bone marrow
Acute leukemias
Chronic leukemias
Myeloproliferative disorders

Pathophysiology

The pathophysiology of leukocytosis stems from the production, maturation, and survival of leukocytes. Stem cells give rise to erythroblasts, myeloblasts, and megakaryoblasts. Seventy-five percent of nucleated cells in the bone marrow are committed to production of leukocytes. At any given time, 90% of WBCs remain in storage in the bone marrow, with 7% to 8% in the tissue compartment and the remainder in circulation. This large storage pool allows for a rapid increase in WBCs (mostly neutrophils). In addition, a percentage of circulating WBCs is marginated along blood vessel walls and is mobilized by inflammatory stimuli. The two basic causes of leukocytosis are a normal bone marrow response to external stimuli or the effect of a primary bone marrow disorder.

Diagnosis

The differential diagnosis of leukocytosis is extensive, and common causes are listed in Table 2-5. Increases in the absolute numbers of lymphocytes, eosinophils, monocytes, or basophils are less common in leukocytosis than neutrophilia and help to direct the differential diagnosis.

NEUTROPHILIA

General Principles

Definition

Neutrophilia is defined as an **ANC >6.6 × 10^9/L.** The neutrophil count is influenced by shifts in neutrophils among four major compartments: the bone marrow, the circulation, the marginated pool, and the tissues. Only about 5% of neutrophils are in circulation at any given time, with a half-life of 6 to 10 hours. Most neutrophils and their precursors are contained in storage pools in the bone marrow at 10 to 20 times their circulating numbers. About 50% of peripheral blood neutrophils are circulating, and the other 50% marginated along vessel walls and in the spleen. This pool can be rapidly increased, within hours from the bone marrow stores or within minutes from demarginating neutrophils along blood vessel walls. Neutrophils move to sites of inflammation and infection and act as phagocytes. Their trafficking depends on chemotaxins and surface molecules such as selectins to mediate rolling and integrins to mediate adhesion and transmigration of blood vessels.

Pathophysiology

The pathophysiology of **primary neutrophilia** may be related to inherited deficiencies in adhesion molecules or, in the case of myeloproliferative disorders, constitutive expression and activation of a growth-promoting receptor tyrosine kinase such as *bcr/abl* or Jak2. **Secondary neutrophilia,** seen in infection and inflammation, is related to demargination from storage pools in the bone marrow and peripheral blood signaled by endotoxin and proinflammatory cytokines such as tumor necrosis factor-alpha, IL-6, IL-1B, IL-8, G-CSF, and granulocyte/macrophage colony-stimulating factor (GM-CSF).

Diagnosis

Differential Diagnosis

- Neutrophilia can be spurious, of primary hematologic origin, or related to secondary causes. Etiologies of neutrophilia are listed in Table 2-6. **Spurious leukocytosis** can be a result of the automated cell counter (Coulter counter) counting clumps of platelets as leukocytes and is usually associated with pseudo-thrombocytopenia. In addition, cryoglobulins can agglutinate and be counted as leukocytes at temperatures lower than body temperature.

TABLE 2-6 CAUSES OF NEUTROPHILIA

Spurious causes	Cryoglobulinemia Platelet clumping
Primary causes	Hereditary neutrophilia Chronic idiopathic neutrophilia Chronic myelogenous leukemia Myeloproliferative disorders (polycythemia vera and myelofibrosis) Leukocyte adhesion deficiency Down syndrome
Secondary causes	Infection Smoking Medications: glucocoticoids, beta-agonists, lithium, granulocyte colony-stimulating factor (G-CSF)/ granulocyte-macrophage CSF (GM-CSF), all-trans retinoic acid (ATRA) Nonhematologic malignancy: large cell lung cancer Stress Exercise Hemolytic anemia/sickle cell disease Leukoerythroblastic reaction: marrow invasion by tumor, fibrosis, and granulomatous reaction Asplenia

- **Primary causes** of neutrophilia may be hereditary (usually resulting in splenomegaly and leukocyte counts of 20×10^9 to 100×10^9/L) or associated with familial syndromes. Other primary causes include myeloproliferative disorders (e.g., chronic myeloid leukemia [CML]) and leukocyte adhesion deficiency.
- **Secondary causes** are by far the most common cause of neutrophilia. Common secondary causes include infection, smoking (25% increase), chronic inflammation (e.g., rheumatoid arthritis and inflammatory bowel disease), stress, medications, chronic marrow stimulation (hemolytic anemia and idiopathic thrombocytopenic purpura), asplenia, marrow invasion, and nonhematologic malignancy.

Diagnostic Testing

Initial laboratory evaluation starts with review of the **peripheral blood smear** to confirm automated counts and rule out spurious leukocytosis. The smear may suggest a secondary cause such as infection or inflammation with increased bands, vacuolization, Döhle bodies, and toxic granulations in neutrophils. A marrow-infiltrating process is suggested by a leukoerythroblastic reaction that shows a "left shift" (increased myelocytes and metamyelocytes in the marrow and bands in the peripheral blood) and nucleated RBCs. Acute leukemia is suggested by circulating blasts, which may be incorrectly counted as monocytes or neutrophils by the Coulter counter. If no secondary causes of neutrophilia can be identified, peripheral blood analysis for *bcr/abl* **by fluorescence in situ hybridization (FISH) or cytogenetics** may be helpful to exclude CML. A **leukocyte alkaline phosphatase (LAP) score** is of historical importance but is no longer commonly used because of intraoperator variability and the evolution of cytogenetic testing. A low LAP score can be seen in CML, and a high LAP score may suggest inflammation or infection.

Treatment

Treatment depends on the underlying etiology. Treatment of primary etiologies such as CML and myeloproliferative disorders are discussed elsewhere in this book. Treatment of neutrophilia related to a secondary cause revolves around treating the underlying cause.

EOSINOPHILIA

General Principles

Eosinophilia is defined as an **absolute eosinophil count >0.5 × 10^9/L.** Eosinophilia is most commonly due to secondary causes. Table 2-7 reviews causes of eosinophilia. Absolute eosinophil counts $>4 \times 10^9$/L suggest primary eosinophilia as a result of either clonal expansion (chronic leukemia variant or acute leukemia variant) or hypereosinophilic syndrome.[5]

Diagnosis

Initial evaluation of eosinophilia should include review of the **peripheral smear, stool examination** for ova and parasites, and **serum tryptase, cortisol, IgE, and IL-5 levels.** If no secondary source can be identified, T-cell immunophenotyping and T-cell receptor gene rearrangement analysis and bone marrow biopsy with cytogenetic analysis and FISH for the platelet-derived growth factor receptor-alpha (FIP1L1-PDGFRA) rearrangement and *bcr/abl* should be performed to evaluate for a clonal disorder.

TABLE 2-7 CAUSES OF EOSINOPHILIA

Allergic
Parasites
Dermatologic
Infections
Scarlet fever, chorea, leprosy, genitourinary infections, HIV and other retroviral infections
Immunologic disorders
Rheumatoid arthritis, periarteritis, lupus erythematosus, eosinophilia-myalgia syndrome
Pleural and pulmonary conditions
Loffler syndrome, pulmonary infiltrates, and eosinophilia
Malignancies
Non-Hodgkin lymphoma, Hodgkin lymphoma, acute eosinophilic leukemia (a variant of FABM4 phenotype of acute monocytic leukemia)
Myeloproliferative disorders
Chronic myelogenous leukemia, polycythemia vera, myelofibrosis
Adrenal insufficiency: Addison disease
Sarcoidosis

FAB, French-American-British classification

Treatment

Hypereosinophilic syndrome can cause end organ damage, including cardiac involvement causing conduction defects and cardiomyopathy, as well as pulmonary involvement. In patients with evidence of end organ damage, treatment with corticosteroids and hydroxyurea may be needed to decrease the eosinophil count rapidly. Leukopheresis may be used as well to lower the eosinophil count rapidly. Recent evidence suggests that patients with idiopathic hypereosinophilic syndrome and chronic eosinophilic leukemia with the FIP1L1-PDGFRA rearrangement may be effectively treated with the tyrosine kinase inhibitor imatinib.[6]

BASOPHILIA

General Principles

Definition

Basophilia is defined as an **absolute basophil count >0.2 × 10^9/L.** Basophils are inflammatory mediators, and their granules contain histamine, glycosaminoglycans, major basic protein, proteases, and other inflammatory and vasoactive substances. They primarily function to activate the type 1 hypersensitivity reaction mediated through surface receptors for IgE.

Etiology

Basophilia can be associated with hypersensitivity reactions to drugs and food. It may also be seen in chronic inflammatory states such as tuberculosis and ulcerative colitis. However, these reactions are rare, and the most common setting of basophilia is in myeloproliferative disorders such as CML.

Diagnosis

Review of the peripheral smear confirms basophilia and management focuses on the underlying etiology. Peripheral blood can be sent for **Jak2 and** ***bcr/abl*** to evaluate for a myeloproliferative disorder. If suspicion of a myeloproliferative disorder is high, a bone marrow biopsy is necessary.

MONOCYTOSIS

General Principles

Definition

Monocytosis is defined as an **absolute monocyte count >0.8 × 10^9/L.** Monocytes are cells in transit to the tissues and are capable of transformation to macrophages in the tissues. They play a role in acute and chronic inflammatory reactions.

Etiology

Monocytosis usually represents a myeloproliferative disorder such as CML or acute monocytic leukemia. Secondary causes include infection (bacterial or tuberculosis) and relative monocytosis as seen with initial count recovery after chemotherapy and drug-induced neutropenia.

Diagnosis

Review of the peripheral smear confirms monocytosis, and treatment is focused on the underlying etiology. Peripheral blood can be sent for **Jak2 and** ***bcr/abl*** to evaluate for a myeloproliferative disorder. If suspicion of a myeloproliferative disorder is high, a bone marrow biopsy is necessary.

LYMPHOCYTOSIS

General Principles

Lymphocytosis is defined as an **absolute lymphocyte count** >3.3 × 10^9/L. Lymphocytosis may be of primary or secondary origin. Table 2-8 reviews causes of lymphocytosis. Cell surface markers are important in determining primary from secondary lymphocytosis.

Diagnosis

The blood smear should be reviewed to look for evidence of reactive lymphocytes associated with infection, large granular lymphocytes associated with large granular lymphocytic leukemia, smudge cells associated with chronic lymphocytic leukemia (CLL), or blasts associated with acute leukemia. **Peripheral blood flow cytometry immunophenotyping** allows identification of clonal disorders. Immunoglobulin or T-cell receptor gene rearrangements support a clonal disorder.

Treatment

Management of hematological malignancies including CLL is discussed in Chapter 29. Resolution of infectious etiologies results in resolution of the lymphocytosis. Finally, removal of allergens such as drugs or venom results in resolution of the lymphocytosis associated with hypersensitivity reactions.

TABLE 2-8 CAUSES OF LYMPHOCYTOSIS

Primary lymphocytosis	Malignancy Acute lymphocytic leukemia Chronic lymphocytic leukemia Prolymphocytic leukemia Hairy cell leukemia Adult T-cell leukemia Large granular lymphocytic leukemia Essential monoclonal B cell lymphocytosis Persistent polyclonal B cell lymphocytosis
Secondary or reactive lymphocytosis	Mononucleosis syndromes EBV CMV Herpes simplex virus HIV Rubella Toxoplasma Adenovirus Hepatitis virus Varicella zoster Human herpesvirus (HHV)-6 and HHV-8 Bordetella pertussis Stress lymphocytosis Surgery, myocardial infarction, septic shock, sickle cell crisis Hypersensitivity reactions Insect bite and drugs Cancer: thymoma Smoking Hyposplenism Chronic infection

EBV, Epstein-Barr virus; CMV, cytomegalovirus

REFERENCES

1. Shoenfeld Y, Alkan ML, Asaly A, et al. Benign familial leukopenia and neutropenia in different ethnic groups. *Eur J Haematol.* 1988;41(3):273–277.
2. Andersohn F, Konzen C, Garbe E. Systematic review: agranulocytosis induced by nonchemotherapy drugs. *Ann Intern Med.* 2007;146(9):657–665.
3. Brown AE. Neutropenia, fever, and infection. *Am J Med.* 1984;76(3):421–428.
4. Bach MA, Phan-Dinh-Tuy F, Bach JF, et al. Unusual phenotypes of human inducer T cells as measured by OKT4 and related monoclonal antibodies. *J Immunol.* 1981;127(3):980–982.
5. Tefferi A, Patnaik MM, Pardanani A. Eosinophilia: secondary, clonal and idiopathic. *Br J Haematol.* 2006;133(5):468–492.
6. Jovanovic JV, Score J, Waghorn K, et al. Low-dose imatinib mesylate leads to rapid induction of major molecular responses and achievement of complete molecular remission in FIP1L1-PDGFRA-positive chronic eosinophilic leukemia. *Blood.* 2007;109(11):4635–4640.

Red Blood Cell Disorders

3

George Ansstas

ANEMIA

GENERAL PRINCIPLES

Definition

Anemia is defined as a decrease in circulating RBC mass, the usual criteria being an Hgb <12 g/dL or Hct <36% for women and an Hgb <14 g/dL or Hct <41% for men. Anemia is commonly encountered in inpatient medicine and thus a frequent reason for hematology consults. A systematic approach to anemia is best at narrowing down the diagnosis and guiding the subsequent diagnostic workup.

Etiology

While there can be some overlap, anemia can be divided into three broad categories: **blood loss (acute or chronic)**, **increased destruction of RBCs (hemolysis)**, and **decreased production of RBCs.** Blood loss can be evaluated by a careful evaluation of the patient, including volume status. The reticulocyte count will usually help differentiate between states with decreased production (reticulocyte index [RI] <2%; see below for description of RI) and those associated with increased destruction (implied when the RI is >2%).

DIAGNOSIS

Clinical Presentation

History

As with any other medical condition, the history and physical exam play key roles in approaching anemia. Based on symptomatology, one can discern the time line (acute, subacute, or chronic), the severity, and even the underlying etiology. Patients can be asymptomatic, but those patients with an Hgb <7 g/dL will usually have symptoms. Acute clinical manifestations include those typical of hypovolemia (pallor, visual impairment, syncope, hypotension, and tachycardia) and require immediate attention. Chronic symptoms will reflect tissue hypoxia (fatigue, headache, dyspnea, lightheadedness, and angina). In addition to the usual symptoms of anemia, iron deficiency is often associated with **pica** (consumption of nonfood substances such as corn starch or ice). A careful history of the clinical manifestations including initial presentation, time of onset, potential source of blood loss, family history, and medication history must be evaluated carefully.

Physical Exam

On exam, one can note pallor, alopecia, atrophic glossitis, angular cheilosis, congestive heart failure (with severe and chronic anemia), koilonychias (spoon nails), Plummer-Vinson or Patterson-Kelly syndrome (dysphagia, esophageal web, and atrophic glossitis with iron deficiency anemia), blue sclera, and brittle nails, as well as hypotension and tachycardia.

Diagnostic Testing

- The **complete blood count** (CBC) measures WBCs, Hgb, Hct, platelets, as well as measures of the *red cell indices.* The Hgb is a measurement of mass of Hgb in blood (grams per deciliter), whereas the Hct is the physical amount of space that the Hgb occupies as a percentage of the whole that the red cells occupy. Remember that the Hgb and Hct are unreliable indicators of red cell volume in the setting of rapid shifts of intravascular volume (i.e., acute bleeding).
- The most useful red cell indices include the **mean corpuscular volume** (MCV), **red cell distribution width** (RDW), and **mean cell Hgb concentration** (MCHC). MCV is the mean size of the red cells and the normal range is 80 to 100 fL. RBCs can be classified as microcytic when the MCV is <80 fL and macrocytic when it is >100 fL. RDW is a measure of variability in the size of the red cells and is calculated as: RDW = (standard deviation of red cell volume ÷ mean cell volume) × 100. An elevated RDW indicates increased variability in RBC size. The MCHC describes the concentration of Hgb in each cell.
- The **reticulocyte count** measures the immature red cells in the blood as a percentage of the whole and reflects the bone marrow's (BM's) response to anemia (i.e., a normal BM response is to increase the production of red cells in anemia so that the observed reticulocyte count goes up). A nascent RBC lives on average for 120 days, and the BM is constantly replenishing the bloodstream with new RBCs, with the normal reticulocyte count being ~1%. In the setting of anemia or blood loss, the BM should increase its production of RBC in proportion to loss of RBC, and thus a 1% reticulocyte count in the setting of anemia is inappropriate. The RI is calculated as percentage reticulocytes × (actual Hct/normal Hct) and is important in determining if a patient's BM is responding appropriately to the level of anemia. In normal individuals, an RI of 1.0 to 2.0 is acceptable; however, an RI of <2 with anemia indicates decreased production of RBCs. An RI of >2 with anemia may indicate hemolysis or loss of RBC leading to increased compensatory production of reticulocytes.
- The **peripheral smear** is a required part of the initial hematologic evaluation. Shapes, size, and orientation of cells in relation to each other are important factors to look for in a smear. RBCs can appear in many abnormal forms, such as acanthocytes, schistocytes, spherocytes, and teardrop cells, and abnormal orientations such as rouleaux formation.
- A **bone marrow biopsy** may be indicated in cases of normocytic anemias with a low RI without an identifiable cause or anemia associated with other cytopenias. The biopsy may confirm myelophthisic process (i.e., presence of teardrop or fragmented cells, normoblasts, or immature WBCs on peripheral blood smear) in the setting of pancytopenias.

ANEMIAS ASSOCIATED WITH DECREASED PRODUCTION

The approach to an anemia associated with decreased production of red cells is to divide them into categories based on red cell size with the MCV. Depending on the MCV, **microcytic** (<80 fL), **normocytic** (80 to 100 fL), and **macrocytic** (>100 fL) anemias have distinct differential diagnoses.

TABLE 3-1 CAUSES OF MICROCYTIC ANEMIAS BY MEAN CORPUSCULAR VOLUME (MCV)

MCV, 70–80	MCV, <70
Iron deficiency	Thalassemia
Anemia of chronic disease	Iron deficiency
Thalassemia	
Sideroblastic anemia	

MICROCYTIC ANEMIAS

Iron-deficiency anemia, sideroblastic anemia, and anemia of chronic disease make up the bulk of the microcytic anemias. The degree of microcytosis may give a clue to the possible underlying diagnoses. A very low MCV typically does not represent anemia of chronic disease or sideroblastic anemia (Table 3-1).

Iron-Deficiency Anemia

Etiology

- Iron-deficiency anemia can be caused by decreased intake/absorption of iron or loss of iron from chronic blood loss. **Dietary deficiency** is usually seen in infants who are milk-fed. In early childhood, it can be seen in meat-deficient diets. It can also occur in the setting of increased requirements, such as pregnancy and early childhood. **Malabsorption** of iron can occur in the setting of partial gastrectomy, as hypochlorhydria/achlorhydria impairs iron absorption. Iron is most actively absorbed in the duodenum. Decreased transit time through duodenum, as seen in chronic diarrhea, may result in iron deficiency. Gastrointestinal causes for iron deficiency (e.g., atrophic gastritis, *Helicobacter pylori* gastritis, celiac disease) should be considered in patients with otherwise unexplained iron deficiency, especially when there is refractoriness to oral iron therapy.[1]
- **Chronic blood loss** is the most common cause of iron deficiency in adults. It is usually lost via the GI tract by ulcerative disease, gastritis, cancer, hemorrhoids, or arteriovenous malformation, with ulcers and colon malignancies being the most common. Menorrhagia/menstruation, hematuria due to genitourinary cancer, frequent blood donation, and frequent phlebotomy in hospitalized patients are additional causes of chronic blood loss. **It should be noted that the diagnosis of iron deficiency in an adult mandates evaluation for GI malignancy.**

Diagnosis

Diagnosis involves serum testing of iron with an iron panel and ferritin level. The iron panel includes **serum iron level, total iron binding capacity** (TIBC), **unsaturated iron binding capacity** (UIBC), and **transferrin saturation** (Tsat).

- Serum iron levels reflect the level of iron immediately available for blood production. TIBC is an indirect method of determining the transferrin level in serum. Transferrin is an iron-transporting protein that is capable of associating reversibly with up to 1.254 g of iron per 1 g of protein. In one series, a transferrin saturation less than 15% was 80% sensitive as an indicator of iron deficiency, but only 50% to 65% specific.

- Serum **ferritin** (intracellular iron storage protein) should also be checked and, when low, almost always signifies iron deficiency. Virtually all patients with serum ferritin concentrations less than 10 to 15 ng/mL are iron deficient, with a sensitivity of 59% and a specificity of 99%.[2] However, it is an acute phase reactant and can be falsely elevated in inflammatory states. The effect of inflammation is to elevate serum ferritin approximately threefold. A useful rule of thumb in such patients is to divide the patient's serum ferritin concentration by 3; a resulting value of 20 or less suggests concomitant iron deficiency.
- Serum transferrin receptor (sTfR) provides a quantitative measure of total erythropoietic activity, since its concentration in serum is directly proportional to erythropoietic rate and inversely proportional to tissue iron availability. Typically, in iron-deficiency anemia, the iron level is low, the TIBC is in the normal to high range, sTfR is high, and ferritin is depleted. The Tsat, the percentage of transferrin that is bound to iron, can be a somewhat less reliable measure of iron. Low transferrin saturation is associated with iron-deficiency states, while high saturation is associated with excess iron. The gold standard for diagnosis of an iron-deficiency anemia is a BM biopsy with iron staining; however, this is rarely necessary.
- Of note, patients can have microcytic normochromic (concentration of Hgb in the erythrocytes is within the normal range of 32% to 36%) anemia that eventually progresses to microcytic hypochromic as the anemia progresses. With worsening iron-deficiency anemia, there is a gradual increase in anisocytosis and poikilocytosis (abnormally shaped cells).

Treatment

- In addition to diagnosing the patient with iron-deficiency anemia, it is important to discover and treat the underlying cause of the iron deficiency, if possible. **Iron replacement** may be given by oral iron salts, which should be given between meals because food or antacids may decrease absorption. Ascorbic acid given with iron sulfate may increase absorption. One replacement regimen is ferrous sulfate, 325 mg PO tid (equivalent of 65 mg elemental iron tid). Enteric-coated forms are not well absorbed and should not be used.
- **Parenteral iron** is given when the patient is intolerant of oral iron, when iron losses exceed the capacity to replete orally, or in the setting of malabsorption. There is ~1 in 300 risks of a serious reaction including anaphylaxis. The absolute risk for life-threatening adverse reactions for iron sucrose, ferric gluconate complex, low MW dextran, and high MW dextran is 0.6, 0.9, 3.3, and 11.3 per million doses, respectively.
- The amount of Fe needed can be calculated as the amount of Fe needed to replace the missing Hgb added to the amount necessary to replete the total body Fe stores (usually estimated as approximately 1000 mg) by the formula:

$$\textbf{Total dose (mg)} = \{[\textbf{normal Hgb(g/dL)} - \textbf{patient Hgb(g/dL)}] \times \textbf{body weight [kg]} \times \textbf{2.2)}\} + \textbf{1000 mg}$$

  However, in practice, iron is often infused at a dose of 1 to 1.2 g without formal calculation of iron repletion.
- One can expect an increase in the reticulocyte count within 7 to 10 days, and correction of anemia usually occurs within 6 to 8 weeks if ongoing blood loss is stopped. Treatment should continue for approximately 6 months (on PO iron) to fully restore tissue stores.

Sideroblastic Anemias

Sideroblastic anemias are characterized by ineffective erythropoiesis and the presence of ringed sideroblasts in the BM. The term *ringed* refers to the accumulation of iron in the mitochondria that surrounds the periphery of the nucleus. There are hereditary and idiopathic forms, as well as forms associated with drugs or toxins such as alcohol, lead, isoniazid (INH), zinc toxicity with resulting copper deficiency, and chloramphenicol. There is no cure for hereditary sideroblastic anemia, and treatment is aimed at preventing end-organ damage from iron overload (chelation therapy). Drug-induced sideroblastic anemias are commonly reversible when the offending agent is discontinued. For sideroblastic anemia caused by isoniazid treatment, high-dose pyridoxine supplementation (up to 200 mg/d PO) often reverses the anemia and allows for continuation of the drug.

Lead Poisoning

An additional diagnosis to consider in cases of microcytic, hypochromic anemias is lead poisoning. This is a rare but treatable form of microcytic anemia in adults and usually results from a work or an environmental exposure. The diagnosis is suggested by finding basophilic stippling on the peripheral smear.

Anemia of Chronic Disease

Anemia of chronic disease usually presents as a normocytic anemia; however, it can be microcytic (usually mild) in a minority of cases.

Thalassemias

Epidemiology

Beta-thalassemia is more common in Mediterranean, African, and Southeast Asian populations and is thought to offer resistance to falciparum malaria.

Pathophysiology

- The major hemoglobin in adults is hemoglobin A, a tetramer consisting of one pair of alpha-globin chains and one pair of beta-globin chains.[3] In normal subjects, globin chain synthesis is very tightly controlled, such that the ratio of production of alpha to non-alpha chains is 1.00 ± 0.05. Thalassemia refers to a spectrum of diseases characterized by reduced or absent production of one or more globin chains, thus disrupting this closely regulated ratio.
- **Beta-thalassemia major** results from a total lack of production of beta-globin chain. It causes lack of adequate Hgb A formation, leading to microcytic, hypochromic cells. Complications of severe beta-thalassemia include skeletal deformities resulting from erythropoietin-stimulated expansion of BM, hepatosplenomegaly from extramedullary hematopoiesis, and secondary hemochromatosis from repeat blood transfusions and increased dietary absorption of iron.
- **Beta-thalassemia minor** is loss of only one of the two alleles coding for the beta-globulin gene. It is usually an asymptomatic condition manifested by microcytosis and a normal red cell distribution width. It is accompanied by a mild anemia (if any). On electrophoresis in patients with beta-thalassemia minor, over 90% of the hemoglobin will be hemoglobin A along with an elevation in the hemoglobin A2 value, sometime as high as 7% or 8%, and an increase in hemoglobin F in about 50% of patients.

- □ **Alpha-thalassemia** results from decreased production of alpha-globin chains, of which there are four in total. The severity of anemia depends on the number of defective alpha genes. Hemoglobin H disease is due to the loss of three of the four alpha-globin loci. Adult patients have moderate degree of anemia, and their hemoglobin electrophoresis pattern shows 5% to 30% hemoglobin H (beta-4 tetramers). Hydrops fetalis with hemoglobin Barts (gamma-4 tetramers) is due to loss of all four alpha-globin loci. This condition is incompatible with extrauterine life. Diagnosis is by Hgb electrophoresis for beta-thalassemia and severe alpha-thalassemia. Mild alpha-thalassemia may be detected by alpha:beta ratio or by molecular testing, although neither is widely available.

Treatment

The treatment of thalassemias usually depends on the severity of the genetic defect and resultant clinical sequelae. The minor thalassemias are commonly asymptomatic and require no therapy. The major thalassemias may be treated by chronic transfusions, chelation therapy to avoid iron overload (due to transfusions), and splenectomy. For ferritin concentrations >1000 ng/mL, chelation therapy may reduce the long-term complications of iron overload. Options for chelation include the intramuscular or subcutaneous iron chelator deferoxamine and oral iron chelator deferasirox.

NORMOCYTIC ANEMIAS

Normocytic anemias can be associated with an elevated reticulocyte count, which represents hemolytic anemia (HA) or bleeding, whereas a decreased reticulocyte count typically represents a hypoproliferative disorder (Table 3-2). Normocytic anemia may be an early finding in BM failure. Aplastic anemia is actually a BM failure syndrome and is discussed in Chapter 8. Pure RBC aplasia involves a selective destruction of RBC precursors and can be congenital or acquired. It is often associated with viral infections (e.g., parvovirus). Symptoms are related to the anemia. Diagnosis is via BM biopsy showing absence of erythroid elements but with preservation of other cell lines. Treatment includes supportive measures with transfusions as needed.

TABLE 3-2 CAUSES OF NORMOCYTIC ANEMIA ASSOCIATED WITH A DECREASED RETICULOCYTE COUNT

Malignancies and other marrow infiltrative diseases
- Leukemia and lymphoma
- Metastatic cancer
- Plasma cell disorders
- Granulomatous disease

Stem cell disorders
- Myelofibrosis
- Aplastic anemia
- Pure red cell plasma
- Myelodysplasia

Due to other medical conditions
- Anemia of renal disease
- Anemia of chronic disease
- Endocrine disorders

Anemia of Chronic Disease (Anemia of Chronic Inflammation)

This condition is often associated with malignancy, infection, and inflammatory states. It may occur in patients with chronic infections (e.g., osteomyelitis), HIV, or inflammatory diseases (e.g., lupus or rheumatoid arthritis). These disorders have in common the inhibition of normal RBC synthesis due to the underlying disorder. They may act by inadequate release of or insensitivity to erythropoietin. Other etiologies include deficiency in mobilization of iron from the reticuloendothelial system. One acute phase protein that appears to be most directly involved in iron metabolism is hepcidin.[4,5]

The anemia is most often a normocytic, normochromic anemia with a decreased reticulocyte count but may also present as a mild microcytic anemia. The serum iron concentration and total iron-binding capacity are usually both low, often giving a normal transferrin saturation (although this may be low or low-normal range). Serum ferritin, however, is an acute phase reactant and is often elevated in inflammatory diseases and infections. BM exam, if done, typically shows present iron stores. Symptoms and physical exam of the anemia of chronic disease patient are dependent on the patient's underlying condition. The anemia is typically mild and does not require blood transfusion. The more appropriate treatment is to treat the underlying condition.

Myelophthisic Anemias

Myelophthisic anemias refer to those with evidence of hematopoiesis outside the BM or infiltration of the BM by nonhematologic cells. The most common cause is metastatic carcinoma to the BM (e.g., breast, lung, prostate, and kidney). Other causes include myeloproliferative disorders, multiple myeloma, leukemias, and lymphoma. These are often suspected by a typical appearance of the peripheral smear (nucleated RBC, teardrop-shaped RBCs, and immature WBCs) and a "dry tap" on BM aspiration. BM biopsy results are dependent on the underlying disease. Treatment is directed toward the underlying disorder.

Anemia of Chronic Renal Failure

Anemia of chronic renal failure is due to erythropoietin deficiency. The anemia **generally starts when CrCl <45 mL/min and worsens with declining renal function.** When possible, treatment involves first treating the underlying renal dysfunction. **Erythropoietin** can be given at 50 to 100 U/kg IV or SC 3×/wk, with readjustments based on response. In follow-up, expect an increase in Hct in 8 to 12 weeks.

Endocrine Disorders

Anemia due to endocrine disorders is seen in hypothyroidism, adrenal insufficiency, and gonadal dysfunction. Estrogens tend to inhibit red cell synthesis, and testosterone tends to stimulate it. Correction of the underlying endocrine disorder may improve the anemia.

MACROCYTIC ANEMIAS

Anemias that have an **MCV of more than ~100 fL** are macrocytic anemias. These may be separated into two categories based on features seen on peripheral smear: megaloblastic and nonmegaloblastic. ***Megaloblastic*** features include the presence of oval macrocytes and hypersegmentation of the PMNs. They are a consequence of abnormal maturation of these cells and nuclear/cellular asynchrony. Examples of megaloblastic anemia include vitamin B_{12} deficiency, folate deficiency, and drug-induced megaloblastic anemia. *Nonmegaloblastic* features include the presence of round macrocytes without hypersegmentation of the PMNs. Causes of nonmegaloblastic macrocytic anemia include liver disease, hypothyroidism, alcohol-induced reticulocytosis and reticulocytosis secondary to HA, and myelodysplastic syndrome (see Chap. 8 for further discussion).

Vitamin B_{12} Deficiency

The daily requirement of vitamin B_{12} is 2 μg/d, and a typical diet provides 5 to 15 μg/d, with the liver capable of storing ~2000 to 5000 μg. Thus, it takes up to 3 to 6 years for deficiency to develop once absorption completely ceases.

Etiology

Etiologies include pernicious anemia (the most common cause), gastrectomy or gastric bypass surgery, ileal disorders (sprue, inflammatory bowel disease, and lymphoma), bacterial overgrowth in the small intestine, fish tapeworms, and inadequate intake (this is very rare and only occurs in the strict vegetarian).

Clinical Presentation

Symptoms include burning sensation of the tongue, vague abdominal pain, diarrhea, numbness, paresthesia, and mental impairment. On exam, one can note glossitis, smooth tongue, dorsal column findings (decreased vibration and proprioception), and corticospinal tract findings (motor weakness, spasticity, positive Babinski sign). Of note, patients can present with neurologic signs without overt anemia.

Diagnostic Testing

In cases of borderline-low B_{12} values, one can measure **serum methylmalonic acid** and **homocysteine levels,** which are elevated in vitamin B_{12} deficiency. Once deficiency is established, an attempt should be made to identify the etiology. The presence of **anti-intrinsic factor antibodies** or **anti-parietal cell antibodies** lends support to the diagnosis of pernicious anemia. Surgical history can reveal postsurgical etiologies. Suspicion of ileal disorder can be evaluated by endoscopy. Stool ova and parasites should be performed if suspicious for parasitic infection. A therapeutic trial of antibiotics may be given if bacterial overgrowth is suspected. The Schilling test is rarely used today but may delineate the underlying pathology.

Treatment

Treatment usually includes vitamin B_{12}, 1 mg IM or SC daily for 7 days, then weekly for 1 month, followed by monthly doses thereafter. There are data suggesting that oral vitamin B_{12} at doses of 1 to 2 mg daily is just as effective as IM administration.[6] Failure to correct or identify the underlying mechanism of deficiency may result in lifelong therapy.

Monitoring/Follow-up

Reticulocytosis should occur in 5 to 7 days, with resolution of hematologic abnormalities in ~2 months. Resolution of neurologic abnormalities depends on their duration before treatment and may take up to 18 months but can also be permanent.

Folate Deficiency

The daily requirement of folate is 50 to 100 μg/d, with body stores of ~5 to 10 mg. Depletion can occur after ~2 to 4 months of persistent negative balance.

Etiologies include inadequate intake (e.g., alcoholics), decreased absorption (e.g., sprue, bacterial overgrowth, certain drugs such as phenytoin and oral contraceptives), or states of increased requirements (HA, pregnancy, chronic dialysis, exfoliative dermatitis). Folate deficiency can also be iatrogenic, such as treatment with folic acid antagonists (e.g., methotrexate, trimethoprim).

Symptoms and physical exam are similar to vitamin B_{12} deficiency except that **neurologic features are not present.** Both serum and RBC folate levels must be measured. Serum folate is more labile and subject to acute rise after a folate-rich meal; RBC folate is a better indicator of tissue stores.

It is important to **rule out vitamin B_{12} deficiency** before repletion with folate, because folate may improve the hematologic abnormalities in vitamin B_{12} deficiency but will not correct the neurologic manifestations.

Treatment is with oral folate (1 mg/d), with resolution of hematologic abnormalities in ~2 months.

Drug-Induced Disorders

Several drugs can cause a macrocytic anemia by affecting DNA synthesis. Offenders include purine analogs (e.g., 6-mercaptopurine, azathioprine), pyrimidine analogs (5-fluorouracil, cytarabine), hydroxyurea, and anticonvulsants (phenytoin, phenobarbital). Reverse transcriptase inhibitors (AZT, etc.) may cause macrocytosis without anemia. Therapy is cessation of the offending agent or toleration of a mild anemia if the drug is therapeutically needed.

Nonmegaloblastic Anemia

Nonmegaloblastic anemias typically have round macrocytes without hypersegmentation of PMNs on peripheral smear. MCV of nonmegaloblastic anemias is rarely >110 to 115. A value higher than this would tend to support a megaloblastic etiology. When the reticulocyte count is elevated, it suggests an etiology such as alcohol, hypothyroidism, or liver disease. HA can produce a macrocytosis via increased production of reticulocytes. Nonmegaloblastic anemias are usually treated by identifying and treating the underlying etiology, such as discontinuation of alcohol use and thyroid hormone replacement.

ANEMIAS ASSOCIATED WITH INCREASED DESTRUCTION

Table 3-3 lists causes of anemia associated with increased RBC destruction. Hemolytic anemias can be classified by the location of hemolysis or the mechanism of hemolysis.

Location of Hemolysis

Extravascular—Cell destruction occurs in the reticuloendothelial system, usually in the spleen.

Intravascular—RBC destruction takes place within the circulation.

Mechanism of Hemolysis

Intrinsic—Hemolysis is caused by a defect in the RBC membrane or contents.

Extrinsic—Factors outside the RBC, such as serum antibody, trauma within circulation, infection, etc., lead to RBC damage.

In general, most intrinsic causes are hereditary, and most extrinsic causes are acquired.

TABLE 3-3 CAUSES OF INCREASED RBC DESTRUCTION

Hereditary	Acquired
RBC membrane disorders	Immune related
Spherocytosis	Warm antibody
Elliptocytosis	Cold agglutinin
RBC enzyme disorders	Transfusion reaction
Pyruvate kinase deficiency	Nonimmune
Hexokinase deficiency	Microangiopathic hemolytic anemia
G-6-PD deficiency	Infection
Disordered Hgb synthesis	Hypersplenism
Hemoglobinopathy (i.e., sickle cell)	Paroxysmal nocturnal hemoglobinuria
Thalassemias	

Hemolytic Anemias

General Principles

Hemolytic anemias are disorders in which the **destruction of RBCs leads to a decrease in circulating RBC mass.** Acute hemolysis may be accompanied by a wide variety of signs and symptoms, many of which may point to the underlying etiology.

Diagnosis

Patients may present with fever, chills, jaundice, back and abdominal pain, splenomegaly, and brown or red urine. Peripheral blood smear remains a useful tool both to confirm the diagnosis of hemolysis and to aid in discerning the underlying etiology. Some signs commonly found on peripheral smears include spherocytes (autoimmune HA, hereditary spherocytosis), helmet cells or schistocytes (microangiopathic HA), sickle cells and Howell-Jolly bodies (sickle cell anemia), spur cells (in liver diseases), bite cells or Heinz bodies (glucose-6-phosphate dehydrogenase [G-6-PD] deficiency), and agglutination (cold agglutinin). Laboratory abnormalities suggestive of hemolysis, though not specific, include increased lactate dehydrogenase, decreased haptoglobin, and increased unconjugated bilirubin. In addition, signs of compensatory increased RBC production such as an increase in reticulocyte count are typically present. Other useful lab tests include the **direct Coombs test,** which is a direct antiglobulin test that detects antibodies (usually IgG) or complement (usually C3) bound to the surface of circulating RBCs by mixing *patient RBCs* with *anti-IgG.* Positive results occur when allo- or autoantibodies to RBC antigens are present, or when there is nonspecific adherence of other Ig or immune complexes to the RBC surface. The **indirect Coombs test,** which mixes the patient's serum with normal RBCs, is used to detect the presence of any anti-RBC antibody in the serum.

Sickle Cell Anemia

Sickle cell anemia is caused by a defect in the beta-globin chain, resulting in sickling of RBC under oxidative stress. See Chapter 11 for further details.

Glucose-6-Phosphate Dehydrogenase Deficiency

G-6-PD deficiency is an X-linked disorder that is fully expressed in males and homozygous females and variably expressed in heterozygous females. G-6-PD is the rate-limiting enzyme in the pentose phosphate pathway that helps maintain intracellular levels of glutathione, which serves to protect RBC against oxidative damage.

In patients with G-6-PD deficiency, the presence of oxidative stress results in an inability to maintain Hgb in a reduced state, which, in turn, leads to Hgb precipitation within RBCs (Heinz body formation) and intravascular hemolysis. Two main variants of G-6-PD lead to clinically significant hemolysis: *G-6-PD A^-* and *G-6-PD Mediterranean.* G-6-PD A^-, which occurs in 10% of black individuals, has normal enzyme activity in young RBCs but a marked deficiency of enzyme activity in older cells. Therefore, when oxidatively challenged, only the older cells lyse. This form is typically milder and self-limited. The G-6-PD Mediterranean variant occurs in people of Middle Eastern and Mediterranean descent, and is characterized by a nearly complete lack of G-6-PD. Hemolysis in this form tends to be more severe compared to the A^- variant.

The diagnosis of G-6-PD deficiency is suspected when hemolysis occurs after any form of oxidative stress, most commonly from starting on drugs known to precipitate hemolysis in a G-6-PD-deficient patient (Table 3-4). Other triggers of hemolytic crises include certain foods, most notably fava beans, illnesses such as severe infections, and diabetic ketoacidosis. Findings on the peripheral blood smear suggestive of the diagnosis include Heinz bodies and "bite" cells. Heinz bodies are Hgb precipitants in the RBC, while bite cells are deformed RBCs that result from attempts by macrophages in the spleen to remove the Heinz bodies.

Definitive diagnosis is made by measuring G-6-PD enzyme activity level. **In suspected G-6-PD A_2 variant, enzyme levels should not be measured during acute hemolysis.** In these patients, older RBCs containing the defective enzymes have mostly been lysed during acute hemolysis, and the normal enzyme activities in the remaining younger RBCs and reticulocytes will provide a false-negative result. It is, therefore, advisable to wait 3 to 4 weeks after the acute episode to get a true representation of the enzyme activity level. The same does not apply to the Mediterranean variant, as both younger and older red cells are affected.

Treatment is supportive, with transfusions as needed, and preventive, with avoidance of oxidative precipitant.

Hereditary Spherocytosis (Membrane Defect)

Hereditary spherocytosis is an autosomal dominant disorder most common in patients of Northern European descent. In these patients, a defect in a membrane cytoskeletal protein leads to loss of surface area on the RBCs, resulting in spherocyte formation. Hemolysis of the spherocytic RBCs occurs primarily in the spleen.

TABLE 3-4 PRECIPITANTS OF HEMOLYSIS IN GLUCOSE-6-PHOSPHATE DEHYDROGENASE DEFICIENCY

Infection: *E. coli,* salmonella, *S. pneumoniae,* viral hepatitis

Drug-induced
- Antimalarials: primaquine and chloroquine
- Antibiotics: sulfonamides, dapsone (dapsone USP, DDS), nitrofurantoin (Macrodantin)
- Phenazopyridine (Pyridium)
- Analgesics: in some cases, salicylates

Fava beans (in the Mediterranean variant only)
Naphthalene

Clinical presentation may vary from asymptomatic to profound anemia and jaundice, depending on the severity of spherocytosis. Some patients may present with cholelithiasis. **Splenomegaly** is detected in most patients due to extravascular hemolysis. Peripheral blood smears reveal spherocytes. The MCV is normal or slightly low and is of little diagnostic value. However, considering the degree of reticulocytosis, the MCV is actually low. In unsplenectomized children, for example, elevations in MCHC (>35 g/dL [normal 31.1–34 g/dL]) and RDW (>14 [normal mean 12.6]) have a sensitivity of 63% and specificity of 100% for the diagnosis of HS, making these combined indices a powerful screening tool.[7] The ***osmotic fragility test***, which measures the RBC resistance to hemolysis when incubated in hypotonic saline, will show increased hemolysis.

Treatment is largely supportive, with transfusions as needed and folate supplement to support increased erythropoiesis. Splenectomy, which corrects the anemia but not the underlying defect, can be curative and may be considered in patients with severe anemia.

Acquired Immune Hemolytic Anemia

Warm Antibody

Warm antibody is the most common form of autoimmune HA. The most common antibodies involved are IgG and they are most active at 37°C. Sixty percent of cases are *idiopathic* (or *primary*), whereas 40% are *secondary*. Secondary causes include chronic lymphocytic leukemia, non-Hodgkin lymphoma, Hodgkin lymphoma, autoimmune disorders (such as systemic lupus erythematosus), and drugs. **Drug-related antibodies** can occur by three main mechanisms:

Autoantibody—Antibody against Rhesus (e.g., methyldopa) is produced.

Hapten—Drug binds to the RBC membrane, acting as hapten, which serves as a target for antibodies. Hemolysis typically occurs 1 to 2 weeks after treatment (e.g., penicillin, cephalosporins).

Immune complex—Drug binds to plasma protein, evoking an antibody response. The drug-protein-antibody complex then nonspecifically coats RBCs, resulting in complement-mediated lysis (e.g., quinidine, INH, sulfonamides).

Warm antibodies usually cause extravascular hemolysis by the spleen, leading to splenomegaly. Almost all are panagglutinins (i.e., react with most donor RBCs), thus making crossmatching difficult. Treatment for drug-induced hemolysis is withdrawal of the offending agent, as hemolysis will stop with clearance of the drug. Steroids (prednisone) and immunoglobulins remain the most commonly used initial therapies. Prednisone up to 1 mg/kg/d may be used for severe hemolysis in idiopathic forms, until Hgb reaches normal levels over a few weeks, and then tapered. Intravenous immunoglobulins may be effective in controlling hemolysis, though its benefits tend to be short-lived. Splenectomy is an option for patients who fail or relapse after steroid taper. If steroids and splenectomy both fail, other immunosuppressives such as rituximab, cyclosporine, azathioprine, and cyclophosphamide should be considered. **Transfusions should be avoided**, if possible, as they may result in more hemolysis.

Cold Antibody

Most cold antibodies are IgM and active at <30°C. Acute onset is often associated with infectious causes such as mycoplasma pneumonia and infectious mononucleosis, whereas chronic forms occur with lymphoproliferative disorders or are idiopathic.

The two main manifestations are acrocyanosis (ears, nose, and distal extremities) and hemolysis (complement mediated). Symptoms mainly occur in distal body parts, where the temperature often drops below 30°C. In these cold temperatures, IgM will bind to the RBCs, leading to complement fixation and hemolysis. The antibody dissociates from the RBCs as the temperature rises above 30°C. Hemolysis is not usually seen unless cold agglutinin titers are above 1 in 1000. Treatment mainly involves avoidance of cold exposure and treatment of the underlying disorder. While certain immunosuppressive agents and plasmapheresis may be effective, splenectomy and steroids are of limited therapeutic value.

Acquired Nonimmune Hemolytic Anemia

Acquired causes of nonimmune HA are often secondary to physical damages from the environment, chemical changes, or infections. Microangiopathic and macroangiopathic HAs represent the most common causes of environmental damages. In these cases, changes in the vasculature result in the destruction of RBCs due to physical stress. Conditions associated with these forms of HAs include disseminated intravascular coagulation (DIC), thrombotic thrombocytopenic purpura (TTP), hemolytic-uremic syndrome (HUS), prosthetic heart valves, and severe aortic stenosis. DIC, TTP, and HUS are discussed in Chapter 4. Osmotic changes and certain snake and spider venom are examples of chemical damages to RBCs. HA is a characteristic feature of malarial infections. Table 3-5 lists the causes of acquired nonimmune HA.

TABLE 3-5 TYPES OF ACQUIRED NONIMMUNE HEMOLYTIC ANEMIAS

Microangiopathic hemolytic anemia
Thrombotic thrombocytopenic purpura
Disseminated intravascular coagulation
Hemolytic-uremic syndrome
Eclampsia
Malignant hypertension
Metastatic adenocarcinoma
Macroangiopathic hemolytic anemia
Prosthetic valve
Severe aortic stenosis
Physical and chemical
Snake and spider venom
Osmotic hemolysis from freshwater drowning
Damage to RBC membranes from third-degree burns
Infection
Malaria
Clostridium difficile
Babesiosis
Hypersplenism
Paroxysmal nocturnal hemoglobinuria

POLYCYTHEMIA

Secondary polycythemia refers to erythrocytosis, which is defined as increased RBC mass. Chronic generalized or local hypoxia causes the body to respond by producing RBC mass to compensate. Chronic hypoxia from congenital heart disease, lung diseases including chronic obstructive lung disease and smoking with increased carboxyhemoglobin levels, or even local hypoxia to kidneys may increase erythropoietin levels from the kidneys (appropriate or inappropriate), resulting in increased production of RBCs. On physical exam, a ruddy complexion can be seen in patients with secondary polycythemia. In patients who are suffering from chronic hypoxia at severe levels, clubbing or even cyanosis may be found. Usually, no therapy is indicated in patients with erythrocytosis, as it is a physiological response to hypoxia and is a compensatory mechanism.

Secondary polycythemia can be distinguished from primary polycythemia (polycythemia vera) by the erythropoietin level, which is elevated in secondary polycythemia and low or normal in polycythemia vera. Polycythemia vera is a stem cell disorder leading to increased RBC mass, which is discussed further in Chapter 9.

REFERENCES

1. Hershko C, Hoffbrand AV, Keret D, et al. Role of autoimmune gastritis, *Helicobacter pylori* and celiac disease in refractory or unexplained iron deficiency anemia. *Haematologica.* 2005;90:585–595.
2. Guyatt GH, Oxman AD, Ali M, et al. Laboratory diagnosis of iron-deficiency anemia: an overview. *J Gen Intern Med.* 1992;7:145–153.
3. Olivieri NF. The beta-thalassemias [published erratum appears in *N Engl J Med.* 1999;341(18):1407]. *N Engl J Med.* 1999;341:99–109.
4. Nemeth E, Valore EV, Territo M, et al. Hepcidin, a putative mediator of anemia of inflammation, is a type II acute-phase protein. *Blood.* 2003;101:2461–2463.
5. Ganz T. Hepcidin, a key regulator of iron metabolism and mediator of anemia of inflammation. *Blood.* 2003;102:783–788.
6. Kuzminski AM, Del Giacco EJ, Allen RH, et al. Effective treatment of cobalamin deficiency with oral cobalamin. *Blood.* 1998;92(4):1191–1198.
7. Michaels LA, Cohen AR, Zhao H, et al. Screening for hereditary spherocytosis by use of automated erythrocyte indexes. *J Pediatr.* 1997;130:957–960.

Platelets: Thrombocytopenia and Thrombocytosis

4

Gregory H. Miday and Paul Mehan

THROMBOCYTOPENIA

GENERAL PRINCIPLES

Definition

Platelets are essential for primary hemostasis—the process in which a platelet plug forms to initiate clotting. Normal platelet range is 150,000 to 450,000/μL. When the platelet number is decreased or the platelets are not functioning properly, bleeding may result.

Classification

Thrombocytopenia can generally be classified into one of the following processes: decreased platelet production or increased platelet destruction.

DIAGNOSIS

Clinical Presentation

Thrombocytopenia may present either asymptomatically on a routine CBC or with petechiae, purpura, or overt bleeding, especially of the mucosa. All patients with thrombocytopenia should undergo a thorough history and physical before choosing further diagnostic testing.

Differential Diagnosis

- **Decreased platelet production**
  - Infection: HIV, hepatitis C, parvovirus, varicella, rubella, mumps
  - Chemotherapy
  - Medications
  - Radiation
  - Congenital or acquired primary bone marrow failure: Fanconi anemia, megakaryocytic thrombocytopenia, paroxysmal nocturnal hemoglobinuria
  - Malignancy, particularly hematologic malignancies
  - Vitamin deficiencies: folate, B_{12}
  - Alcohol
- **Increased platelet destruction**
  - Medications: heparin, valproic acid, quinine
  - Autoimmune platelet destruction: immune thrombocytopenia (ITP), thrombotic thrombocytopenic purpura (TTP)/hemolytic-uremic syndrome (HUS)
  - HELLP (hemolysis, elevated liver enzymes, and low platelets) syndrome

- ○ Disseminated intravascular coagulation (DIC)
- ○ Pseudothrombocytopenia
- ○ Splenic sequestration
- ○ Platelet clumping

THROMBOTIC THROMBOCYTOPENIC PURPURA AND HEMOLYTIC-UREMIC SYNDROME

GENERAL PRINCIPLES

Definition

TTP and HUS are clinically similar disorders that are often grouped together as **TTP-HUS.** Although pathophysiology distinguishes the two disorders, both involve microvascular damage and platelet destruction. They are classically defined by thrombocytopenia and microangiopathic hemolytic anemia (MAHA) in the absence of another apparent cause. Neurologic and renal impairments are also characteristic. When neurologic impairment is present, the patient is more likely to be classified as TTP, whereas acute renal failure is considered to be a hallmark of HUS. In some cases, there is a significant overlap and patients can have both renal and neurological impairment.

Epidemiology

TTP has an incidence of ~4 cases/million persons. HUS is an uncommon disorder with two forms—a sporadic form more typical of adults and a childhood form that is often associated with verotoxin and *Escherichia coli* O157:H7. Both cause thrombocytopenia with MAHA but they are distinct entities. TTP-HUS once had a 90% mortality rate until the utility of plasma exchange was demonstrated. Six month mortality now is <30% with prompt initiation of appropriate treatment.[1]

Pathophysiology

- **Thrombotic thrombocytopenic purpura.** Endothelial cells produce ultralarge vWF (ULvWF) molecules that are cleaved by ADAMTS13 (a metalloprotease) into their typical-length multimers under normal circumstances (Fig. 4-1). In a significant number of TTP patients there is a marked decrease in ADAMTS13 activity(<5%). This protease deficiency may be inherited or due to acquired inhibitors such as IgG autoantibodies. When these ULvWF molecules persist, they induce abnormal platelet aggregation in the microcirculation in areas of high shear stress. This leads to platelet consumption and fragmenting and destruction of RBCs. It should be noted that some patients with clinical TTP do not have decreased ADAMTS13 activity, implicating other unidentified factors.[1]
- **Hemolytic-uremic syndrome.** Although HUS has long been thought to be related to TTP, ADAMTS13 inhibitors or deficiency does not appear to be the cause of HUS. HUS also differs from TTP in that it is associated with selective endothelial damage in the kidneys. Typical childhood HUS is associated with hemorrhagic diarrhea caused by shiga-toxin-producing bacteria such as *E. coli* 0157:H7. Atypical HUS occurs in children and adults without a preceding diarrheal prodrome and is thought to be related to complement regulatory abnormalities.[2] Atypical HUS is more likely to recur.

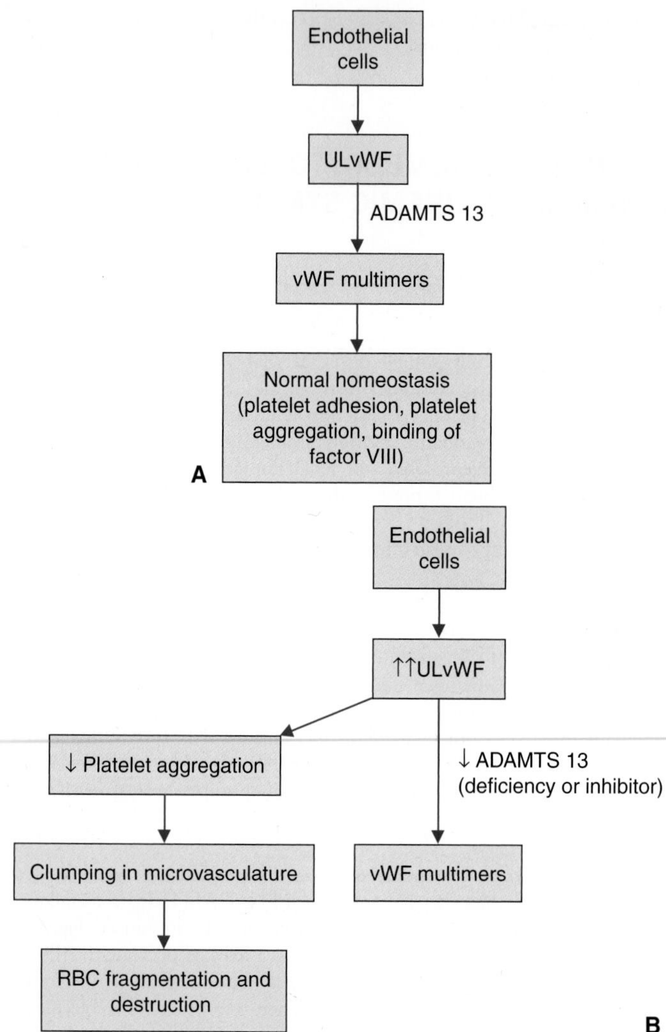

FIGURE 4-1. A: Role of ADAMTS13 in a normal subject. **B:** Role of ADAMTS13 deficiency in thrombotic thrombocytopenic purpura. ULvWF, ultralarge vWF; vWF, von Willebrand factor.

TABLE 4-1 ETIOLOGY OF TTP-HUS

Idiopathic (most common)
Estrogen use
Pregnancy
Infections (*E. coli* 0157:H7 in HUS, pneumococcal infection, HIV)
Stem cell transplantation
Autoimmune diseases (SLE, antiphospholipid syndrome)
Cardiac surgery
Drugs
- Quinine
- Ticlopidine
- Clopidogrel
- Cyclosporine
- Tacrolimus

Familial

SLE, systemic lupus erythematosus

Risk Factors and Associated Conditions

See Table 4-1.

DIAGNOSIS

Clinical Presentation

The classic findings of TTP-HUS include a pentad of physical examination and lab findings as reported in Table 4-2. The complete pentad does not have to be present for the diagnosis, and TTP-HUS often presents without fever or neurologic dysfunction. Renal failure may be oliguric or nonoliguric. TTP may be preceded by a few weeks of malaise, but neurologic symptoms (including headache, confusion, vision changes, tinnitus, seizures, and coma) are frequently the first symptoms that bring a patient to medical attention. These symptoms may wax and wane over the course of the illness. Bleeding, pancreatitis, and diarrhea can also be associated with TTP-HUS.

Diagnostic Criteria

Anemia and thrombocytopenia are universal. Elevated lactate dehydrogenase (LDH), elevated indirect bilirubin, and decreased haptoglobin will help identify the hemolysis associated with the disorder, but a **peripheral blood smear is mandatory** for diagnosis to identify schistocytes consistent with MAHA. The reticulocyte count is

TABLE 4-2 TTP/HUS: THE CLASSIC PENTAD OF FINDINGS

Thrombocytopenia
Microangiopathic hemolytic anemia
Neurologic changes
Renal dysfunction (predominates in HUS)
Fever

usually elevated. Coagulation studies (PT/INR, PTT) are usually within normal limits, and a DIC panel, including fibrinogen, fibrinogen degradation products (FDPs), and D-dimer, is useful to rule out DIC as an alternate diagnosis. ADAMTS13 activity levels may be undetectable; however, treatment should not be delayed while waiting for this test. Further classification of thrombotic microangiopathy as either TTP or HUS is usually based upon age, past medical history, clinical presentation, and the presence or absence of renal dysfunction or neurologic symptoms.

Differential Diagnosis

Differential diagnosis includes other etiologies of MAHA (DIC, prosthetic valve hemolysis, malignant hypertension, adenocarcinoma, and vasculitis). Although fever is part of the pentad, it should also prompt workup for sources of infection. Evans syndrome (immune thrombocytopenia and autoimmune hemolytic anemia) should be distinguished by the presence of microspherocytes and absence of schistocytes in the peripheral smear.

TREATMENT

- The primary treatment for TTP-HUS is **plasma exchange (plasmapheresis)**, with one estimated plasma volume exchanged daily. Plasma exchange can be done twice daily in severe cases or in cases that progress despite daily treatments. Because of the high mortality of untreated TTP-HUS, thrombocytopenia and MAHA are all that is required to initiate plasma exchange if no other certain cause can be identified. ADAMTS13 levels should not alter decision to perform plasma exchange. Plasma exchange has also shown benefits in other thrombotic microangiopathies so it should not be withheld in urgent cases. The goal of daily plasma exchange should be to reverse the thrombocytopenia and hemolysis. This can be monitored with LDH and CBC measurements; the platelet count is the most important factor. Plasma exchange can be tapered or stopped after the platelet count has been normal for 2 days. After remission, exacerbations due to discontinuing plasma exchange (<30 days) should lead to immediate resumption of plasma exchange.[2]
- Suspected ADAMTS13 deficiency can also be treated with systemic corticosteroid therapy in an effort to suppress inhibitors at a dose of 1 mg/kg of prednisone or potentially higher doses in critically ill patients.
- Platelet transfusions are relatively contraindicated, except in cases of life-threatening bleeding.
- In patients with refractory or relapsing TTP despite standard therapy, rituximab may be beneficial at achieving remission and decreasing the need for plasma exchange in patients with a demonstrated antibody to ADAMTS13.[3]

DISSEMINATED INTRAVASCULAR COAGULATION

GENERAL PRINCIPLES

Definition

DIC is an acquired and systemic disorder of hemostasis which produces both thrombosis and hemorrhage.

Epidemiology

DIC is associated with an underlying illness and is thus a condition most frequently diagnosed and treated in hospitalized patients. Around 1% of hospital admissions may be complicated by DIC, although rates approaching 35% may be seen in patients with severe sepsis syndrome.[4]

Pathophysiology and Etiology

In DIC, an underlying illness leads to systemic activation of the coagulation cascade, likely mediated by widespread endothelial damage and the release of inflammatory cytokines. This coagulation activation leads to increased fibrin formation and subsequent thrombosis, most notably in small and medium-sized vessels. The widespread thrombosis can lead to organ failure and MAHA. Widespread thrombosis can also deplete clotting factors and platelets leading to bleeding.[5]

Risk Factors/Associated Conditions

See Table 4-3.

TABLE 4-3 CONDITIONS ASSOCIATED WITH DISSEMINATED INTRAVASCULAR COAGULATION

- Systemic infection
  - Gram-negative sepsis related to endotoxin
  - Gram-positive organisms that may also cause sepsis
- Cancer
  - Solid tumors, including pancreatic, prostate, breast, and others
  - Hematologic malignancy, most notably acute promyelocytic leukemia (AML-M3)
- Trauma
  - Head injury, usually life threatening
  - Serious burns involving large parts of the body
  - Serious crushing injuries with substantial tissue damage
  - Serious fractures, most notably a femur fracture with fat embolism
- Obstetric complications
  - Amniotic fluid embolism
  - Placental abruption
- Vascular disorders
  - Aortic aneurysm
  - Hemangiomas, usually giant
- Immune-mediated reactions
  - Anaphylaxis, mediated by cytokine release
  - Transfusion reactions
  - Transplant rejection
- Toxins
  - Snake venom
- IV drugs, possibly related to a drug affect, but IV drug abuse–associated systemic infections should be considered.

DIAGNOSIS

Clinical Presentation

DIC can manifest with symptoms related to thrombosis or bleeding. Thrombosis can lead to digit gangrene, stroke, or organ failure. Bleeding may be in the form of petechiae, oozing from venipuncture or wound sites, or hemorrhage.

Diagnostic Criteria

- There are a number of useful laboratory tests to assist in the diagnosis of DIC. The **CBC** may reveal anemia or thrombocytopenia, often <100k, related to thrombotic microangiopathy. **Coagulation studies**, including PT/INR and PTT, may be prolonged due to consumption of coagulation factors. "DIC panels" often measure **fibrinogen, FDP, and D-dimer**. Fibrinogen levels are low as a result of consumption, while the FDP and D-dimers are markers of clot dissolution and are usually elevated. It should be noted that fibrinogen is an acute phase reactant and may be elevated due to underlying illness. In such situations, a declining fibrinogen level may provide a clue to the diagnosis of DIC. A peripheral smear often reveals schistocytes from the destruction of red cells.
- It is important to distinguish DIC from other conditions. Typical laboratory abnormalities with separate disease processes include: liver disease (low platelets and prolonged PT and PTT but normal fibrinogen—except in severe liver disease, which may show low fibrinogen), vitamin K deficiency (prolonged PT/PTT but normal platelets and fibrinogen), and TTP (MAHA and thrombocytopenia but normal PT, PTT, and fibrinogen).

TREATMENT

Management should be **focused predominantly on identifying and treating the underlying condition**. Symptomatic treatment of bleeding or thrombosis can be dictated by the clinical scenario. In patients with high bleeding risk or active bleeding, fresh-frozen plasma to replace clotting factors, cryoprecipitate to replace fibrinogen (target level >100 mg/dL), and platelet transfusions (target plt >50,000) are suggested. In patients, predominantly in the thrombotic phase of DIC, low dose heparin has been suggested, but this is controversial. Low-molecular-weight heparin (LMWH) may have less risk for bleeding, and some consider it an alternative. In cases in which the patient has low anti-thrombin III (ATIII) levels and severe DIC, some consider ATIII replacement (with FFP or ATIII concentrates) a reasonable option.

HEPARIN-INDUCED THROMBOCYTOPENIA (HIT)

GENERAL PRINCIPLES

Definition and Classification

Heparin-induced thrombocytopenia can be classified into two separate entities: HIT I and HIT II.

HIT I is non-immune mediated and characterized by a transient fall in platelet count. This form of HIT is not an indication for discontinuing heparin.

The remainder of this chapter focuses on HIT II, which will simply be referred to as HIT.

Epidemiology and Etiology

HIT is an acquired prothrombotic complication of heparin therapy. It is an immune-mediated disorder caused by **IgG Abs that bind to platelet factor 4 (PF4)–heparin complexes**. The frequency in one meta-analysis was 2.6% in patients treated with UFH and 0.2% in those treated with LMWH.[6]

Pathophysiology

- As a primary specific immune response, HIT syndrome generally has a delayed onset of 4 to 5 days after administration of heparin or LMWH.
- PF4 is a heparin-neutralizing chemokine protein found within the alpha-granules of platelets. This protein binds exogenous heparin (UFH > LWMH) and forms multimer complexes which can provoke an IgG antibody formation. Once formed, the HIT-IgG Ab (HIT Ab)–PF4–heparin complex can activate platelets and other cells, generate immunogenic multimolecular complexes, and promote tissue factor expression and thrombin generation, leading to significant risk for thrombotic events. Platelets targeted by HIT specific antibodies are cleared from the circulation, causing thrombocytopenia.[7]

Risk Factors

HIT is more common in adult medical and surgical patients than in obstetric or pediatric patients. UFH is ~10 times more likely than LMWH to produce HIT. Patients receiving IV heparin are more likely to develop HIT than those receiving SC heparin.[7]

DIAGNOSIS

Clinical Presentation

- Thrombocytopenia or a >50% fall in platelet count occur in ~95% of patients diagnosed with HIT. The average platelet count is 50,000 to 70,000.[7]
- There are three time courses of HIT: typical, rapid, and delayed-onset HIT.
  - In **typical-onset HIT**, thrombocytopenia develops ~5 to 10 days after initiation of heparin therapy, approximately the amount of time necessary to generate a humoral immune response.
  - A subset of patients experience **rapid-onset HIT**, where thrombocytopenia occurs within 24 hours, indicating a recent exposure to heparin during the preceding weeks.
  - **Delayed-onset HIT** occurs days after heparin has been stopped. This form of HIT is not well understood. These patients typically have high-titer platelet-activating HIT Ab. It is uncommon for HIT to occur if heparin has been discontinued for more than 2 weeks.
- HIT can present as **thrombosis**. The most common manifestation is venous thromboembolism (deep venous thrombosis and pulmonary embolism) in the postoperative setting. Though less common, arterial thrombosis can occur and is manifested as stroke, myocardial infarction, or limb ischemia.
- A clinical scoring system using the 4 Ts (Thombocytopenia, Timing of platelet fall, Thrombosis, and other causes) has been shown to help risk stratify patients with suspected HIT.[8]

Diagnostic Testing

Initial diagnosis should be made based on the clinical scenario and after other causes of thrombocytopenia have been ruled out. Presently, most medical centers employ an **immunoassay for the presence of PF4/heparin antibodies**. This test is rapid and sensitive (>99%) though it lacks specificity (40% to 70%).[7] Functional assays are more specific than HIT immunoassays but are not as widely available. Functional assays measure platelet activation at varying heparin concentrations. One such test, the **serotonin release assay**, utilizes radiolabeled serotonin to measure platelet activation. The test is considered positive when serotonin is released from donor platelets placed in patient serum when a low concentration of heparin is added. These tests are reported to have >95% sensitivity and specificity.[7]

TREATMENT

Medications

The first step in treating HIT is the **discontinuation of heparin**. Return of laboratory assay results often takes several days. Therefore, all heparin products, including heparin flushes and heparin-coated catheters, should be discontinued immediately if HIT is suspected. Because of cross-reactivity to the HIT Ab, LMWH should not be substituted. For patients who are strongly suspected of having HIT, **non-heparin anticoagulation** should be promptly instituted.

Agents which can treat HIT are classified as direct thrombin inhibitors (lepirudin, argatroban, and bivalirudin), indirect factor Xa inhibitors (danaparoid and fondaparinux), and vitamin K antagonists (warfarin).

- **Lepirudin** is a recombinant hirudin, a natural anticoagulant found in the salivary glands of medicinal leeches. This drug has been approved by the FDA for patients with HIT for the prevention and treatment of thrombosis. Lepirudin is renally cleared and should be dose-adjusted in patients with chronic kidney disease.
- **Argatroban** has also been approved by the FDA for the prevention and treatment of thrombosis associated with HIT. This drug is hepatically cleared and should be used with caution in patients with impaired hepatic function.
- **Bivalirudin** is a direct thrombin inhibitor specifically approved for patients undergoing percutaneous coronary intervention.
- Danaparoid is a heparinoid factor Xa inhibitor that is no longer marketed in the United States. It had previously been approved by the FDA for prophylaxis in HIT patients undergoing hip replacement surgery.
- **Fondaparinux** is a synthetic pentasaccharide Xa inhibitor which received a Grade 2C recommendation in the 2008 ACCP guidelines for treatment of HIT. It has not been FDA approved for this indication and controversy exists because several cases of HIT caused by Fondaparinux have been reported.
- **Warfarin** should not be used to treat a patient with HIT in the acute setting given the risk of venous limb gangrene and thrombosis with depletion of protein C. Warfarin can be started for long term anticoagulation when the patient has been anticoagulated with one of the above agents and the platelet count has reached a stable plateau >150,000. Warfarin should be started at a low dose (5 to 6 mg) and should overlap with one of the above agents for at least 5 days.[9]

IMMUNE THROMBOCYTOPENIA (ITP)

GENERAL PRINCIPLES

Definition

Immune thrombocytopenia (ITP) is an acquired disorder characterized by isolated thrombocytopenia. ITP is also known as immune thrombocytopenic purpura or idiopathic thrombocytopenic purpura, but changes in terminology have been proposed as more has become understood about ITP.[10]

Classification

- **Primary ITP** is an immune mediated disorder without clear cause.
- **Secondary ITP** is because of an underling disease, infection, or exposure.
- ITP can be further classified as **newly diagnosed** (<3 months), **persistent** (3 to 12 months), and **chronic** (>12 months).

DIAGNOSIS

Clinical Presentation

Patients often present with asymptomatic thrombocytopenia noted on routine CBC, but patients also frequently present with minor bleeding manifestations including petechiae, purpura, easy bruising, gingival bleeding, and menorrhagia. Less frequently, patients present with more severe bleeding including overt GI bleeding and intracranial hemorrhage.

History

Patient history should include a focus on bleeding symptoms and causes of secondary ITP or other hematologic disorders. Of particular importance are constitutional symptoms, prior thrombocytopenia, autoimmune diseases, hematologic diseases, liver disease, recent or chronic infections, recent transfusion, recent immunization, and medication exposures.

Physical Examination

Bleeding manifestations are frequently noted in ITP, but other abnormal exam findings should raise suspicion for secondary ITP or alternative causes of thrombocytopenia.

Diagnostic Testing

- ITP is a **diagnosis of exclusion** and no gold standard test exists.
- The CBC should reveal isolated thrombocytopenia unless bleeding is severe enough to produce concurrent anemia.
- Review of the **peripheral blood smear** is essential to rule out other causes of thrombocytopenia including pseudothrombocytopenia from platelet clumping and other diagnoses including TTP/HUS.
- A **bone marrow biopsy** can be considered in patients >60 years old or when the history and physical or other diagnostic data raise suspicion for a separate underlying hematologic disease.
- **HIV, HCV, and *Helicobacter pylori* testing** should be considered in at risk patients. Baseline thyroid function testing and quantitative serum immunoglobulin testing should also be considered.

TREATMENT

The primary goal of treatment in ITP is to prevent bleeding. When the platelet count is $>50 \times 10^9$/L treatment is not always necessary, but treatment should be considered if the patient is at increased risk for bleeding such as in known platelet dysfunction, trauma or predisposition to trauma, necessity for anticoagulation, or planned surgery. Multiple therapeutic modalities exist, and treatment should be tailored for each individual patient.[10]

First-Line Therapy

- **Corticosteroids:** Prednisone 1 mg/kg/d can be given until normalization of platelet count at which point steroids can be tapered to avoid side effects. Dexamethasone and methylprednisolone are other considerations.
- **IVIg:** IVIg can be given at dose of 1 g/kg/d $\times$ 2 days or 0.4 g/kg/d $\times$ 5 days with consideration of maintenance dosing.
- **IV anti-D:** 50 to 75 μg/kg/d of IV anti-D can be considered in Rh(D) positive patients who have not undergone splenectomy and who do not have history of autoimmune hemolytic anemia.

Second-Line Therapy

- **Splenectomy**
    - Eighty percent initial response rates are reported after splenectomy while sustained response is observed in around two-thirds of patients. Laparotomy has higher complication and mortality rates than laparoscopy. Prophylactic vaccinations should be administered after splenectomy to prevent subsequent infections.
- **Medical therapy**
    - Multiple drugs can be considered as second line agents including azathioprine, cyclosporine A, cyclophosphamide, danazol, dapsone, mycophenolate mofetil, rituximab, and vinca alkaloid regimens.
    - Thrombopoietin-receptor agonists including romiplostim and eltrombopag can be considered and may be particularly useful in those who cannot tolerate long-term immunomodulatory therapy.

Refractory ITP

For patients with severe refractory disease combination chemotherapy, alemtuzumab, and allogeneic stem cell transplantation can be considered.

Emergency Therapy

In emergent situations such as in life threatening bleeding or emergency surgery, combination therapies and platelet transfusions should be considered. Aminocaproic acid may be useful in preventing rebleeding in persistently thrombocytopenic patients.[11]

THROMBOSIS

GENERAL PRINCIPLES

A platelet count exceeding the reference range is called thrombocytosis. Thrombocytosis may be reactive or due to autonomous production of platelets by clonal megakaryocytes (essential thrombocythemia or other myeloproliferative disorders).

Reactive thrombocytosis is thrombocytosis in the absence of a chronic myeloproliferative disorder. It can be seen in the setting of infection, surgery, malignancy, blood loss, and iron deficiency or postsplenectomy. The platelet count is expected to normalize when the underlying process is corrected.

REFERENCES

1. Sadler JE. Von Willebrand factor, ADAMTS13, and thrombotic thrombocytopenic purpura. *Blood.* 2008;112:11–18.
2. George JN. How I treat patients with thrombotic thrombocytopenic purpura. *Blood.* 2010;116;4060–4069.
3. Scully M, Cohen H, Cavenagh J, et al. Remission in acute refractory and relapsing thrombotic thrombocytopenic purpura following rituximab is associated with a reduction in IgG antibodies to ADAMTS-13. *Br J Haematol.* 2007;136:451–461.
4. Levi M. Disseminated intravascular coagulation. *Crit Care Med.* 2007;35:2191–2195.
5. Franchini M, Lippi G, Manzato F. Recent acquisitions in the pathophysiology, diagnosis and treatment of disseminated intravascular coagulation. *Thromb J.* 2006;4:4.
6. Martel N, Lee J, Wells PS. Risk for heparin-induced thrombocytopenia with unfractionated and low-molecular-weight heparin thromboprophylaxis: a meta-analysis. *Blood.* 2005;106(8): 2710–2715.
7. Arepally GM, Ortel TL. Heparin-induced thrombocytopenia. *Annu Rev Med.* 2010;61:77–90.
8. Lo GK, Juhl D, Warkentin TE, et al. Evaluation of pretest clinical score (4 Ts) for the diagnosis of heparin-induced thrombocytopenia in two clinical settings. *J Thromb Haemost.* 2006;4:759–765.
9. Warkentin TE, Greinacher A, Koster A, Lincoff AM. American College of Chest Physicians. Treatment and prevention of heparin-induced thrombocytopenia: American College of Chest Physicians Evidence-Based Clinical Practice Guidelines. *Chest.* 2008;133(6 Suppl): 340–380.
10. Provan D, Stasi R, Newland AC, Blanchette VS. International consensus report on the investigation and management of primary immune thrombocytopenia. *Blood.* 2010;115: 168–186.
11. Rodeghiero F, Stasi R, Gernsheimer T, Michel M. Standardization of terminology, definitions and outcome criteria in immune thrombocytopenic purpura of adults and children: report from an international working group. *Blood.* 2009;113:2386–2393.

Introduction to Coagulation and Laboratory Evaluation of Coagulation

5

Tzu-Fei Wang

GENERAL PRINCIPLES

The hemostatic system is a complex, regulated, sequence of reactions involving interactions among platelets, endothelium, and coagulation factors (Table 5-1).

DIAGNOSIS

- **Workup of suspected hemostasis disorders** (Table 5-2; Fig. 5-1)
  - **Complete blood count (CBC)**
    - Reveals thrombocytopenia if present.
    - Assesses whether the patient has developed clinically significant anemia
    - Leukocytosis or leukopenia may implicate a hematologic malignancy as the cause of a patient's coagulopathy or thrombocytopenia.
    - Peripheral smear reveals the presence of microangiopathy, platelet clumping, and red and white blood cell morphology.
  - **Prothrombin time/international normalized ratio (PT/INR)**
    - Historically, PT values have varied from institution to institution due to differences in commercial thromboplastin. The INR system has markedly reduced interlaboratory variability. This ratio standardizes all PT assays and is calculated as

      $$\text{INR} = [(\text{PT patient})/(\text{PT laboratory mean})]^{\text{ISI}}$$

      (ISI—International Sensitivity Index for the thromboplastin reagent used)
  - **Activated partial thromboplastin time (aPTT)**
  - **Thrombin time (TT)**
- **Workup of elevated PT or aPTT**[1]
  - First, pre-analytical variables should be considered, such as
    - incomplete filling of blood collection tubes
    - heparin contamination
    - other confounding factors include a high hematocrit (>55%) and plasma turbidity (lipemic, hemolyzed, or icteric specimens)
  - Second, determine which pathway of the coagulation cascade is defective (see Table 5-2):
    - prolonged PT alone—extrinsic pathway
    - prolonged aPTT alone—intrinsic pathway
    - prolonged PTT and aPTT—both pathways
  - Third, perform a mixing study to determine whether the abnormality is due to an inhibitor present in the patient's plasma or a factor deficiency (Figs. 5-2 through 5-4).

TABLE 5-1 HEMOSTASIS

Process	Description	Abnormality	Symptoms of Dysfunction
Primary hemostasis	Platelet activation and aggregation	• Thrombocytopenia • Platelet dysfunction • von Willebrand factor (vWF) abnormalities	• Mucosal bleeding • Epistaxis • Gum bleeding, • Hematochezia • Melena • Petechiae
Secondary hemostasis	Activation of the coagulation cascade and formation of a stable fibrin complex	Coagulation factor deficiency or dysfunction	• Hemarthroses • Intramuscular hemorrhage • Bleeding into deeper structures
Fibrinolysis	Lysis of fibrin plug, limiting the extent of thrombosis		

- **Mixing studies** (Table 5-3)
  - Goal: to determine whether a prolonged PT or aPTT is due to factor deficiencies or inhibitors.
  - Method: patient's plasma is mixed with normal plasma at a 1:1 ratio and the PT or the aPTT is performed immediately and after incubation at 37°C for 1 hour.

- **Workup of lupus anticoagulants (LAs)**

LAs may occur in the presence or absence of systemic lupus erythematosus or other autoimmune diseases. They are associated with recurrent fetal loss and venous or arterial thromboembolic disease.

Routine aPTT and PT reagents are not sensitive enough to be used to screen for LA, so modifications have been made to develop LA-sensitive clotting tests with the following steps: (a) demonstration of prolonged phospholipid-dependent clotting time (such as modified aPTT, PT, or common pathway clotting test); (b) persistent prolongation of the clotting time after mixing with normal pooled plasma; (c) neutralization of the inhibitor by addition of excess phospholipid; (d) ruling out of a specific factor inhibitor (such as anti-factor VIII autoantibody). No LA test will detect 100% of LAs, therefore current guidelines require using at least two different sensitive clotting tests to screen for and confirm the presence of LA. If one or both tests are positive, testing should be repeated at least 12 weeks later. It is only clinically significant if positive LA is persistent and associated with an increased risk of future thrombotic complications.

TABLE 5-2 WORKUP OF HEMOSTASIS DISORDERS

Test	Measured Pathway	Components Added	Involved Factors	Conditions of Prolongation
PT	Extrinsic and common pathway (Fig. 5-1)	• Plasma • Thromboplastin (tissue factor and phospholipid) • Calcium	• Factor VII • Factors V • Factor X • Prothrombin • Fibrinogen	• Liver disease • Vitamin K deficiency • Coumadins • Rare congenital deficiency or inhibitor (factor VII)
aPTT	Intrinsic and common pathway (Fig. 5-1)	• Plasma • Phospholipid mixture and a surface activating agent (e.g., silica) • Calcium	• Factor XII • Factor XI • Factor VIII • Factor IX • Factor V • Factor X • Prothrombin • Fibrinogen	• Factor deficiencies (VIII, IX, XI, XII) • Factor inhibitors • Heparin type products • Lupus anticoagulant (LA) • vWD (if factor VIII is decreased)
TT	Common pathway (Fig. 5-1) Time of conversion of fibrinogen to fibrin	• Plasma • Thrombin (human or bovine)	• Fibrinogen	• Hypo- or dysfibrino-genemia • Increased fibrinogen degradation products • Monoclonal gammopathies • Heparin or heparin-like inhibitors • Direct thrombin inhibitors (lepirudin, argatroban, and bivalirudin) • Thrombin antibodies

vWF, von Willebrand factor.

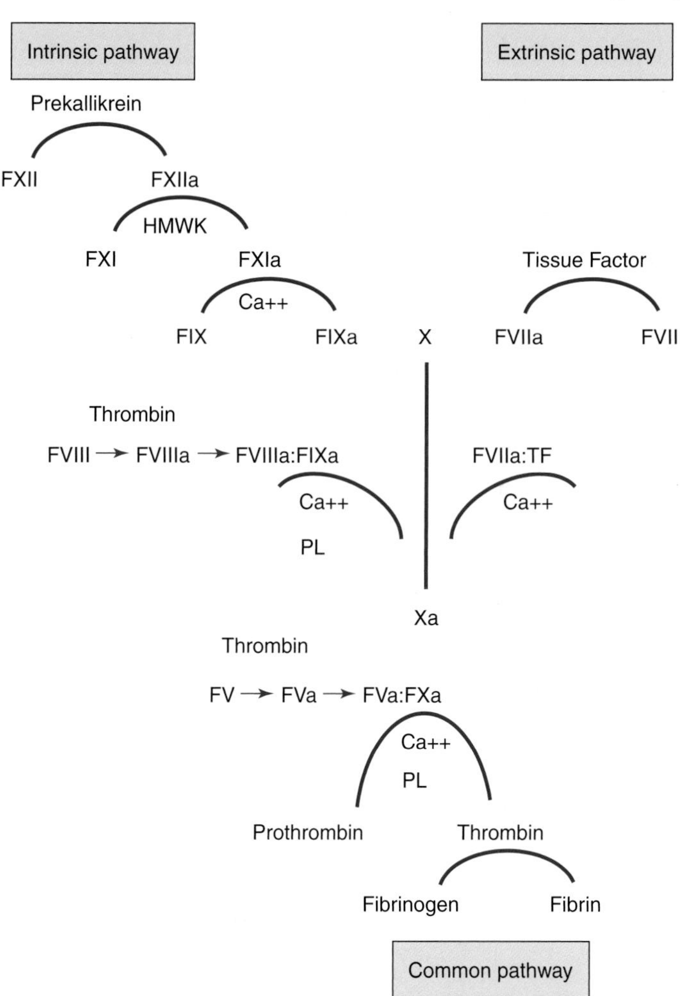

FIGURE 5-1. The normal coagulation cascade is split into the *intrinsic pathway* and the *extrinsic pathway,* either of which leads to activation of factor X to Xa. The factors after that point are referred to as the *common pathway.* Disorders of the intrinsic pathway are manifest as prolongation of the aPTT. Disorders of the extrinsic pathway are reflected by prolongation of the PT, whereas disorders of the common pathway will prolong both tests.

- **Coagulation factor assays**

  These are clot-based assays to determine the functional levels of the factors in the coagulation cascade. These tests are usually obtained when there is a suspicion of factor deficiency or inhibitors.

  - **Factor VIII assay**
    - Goal is to determine factor VIII level.

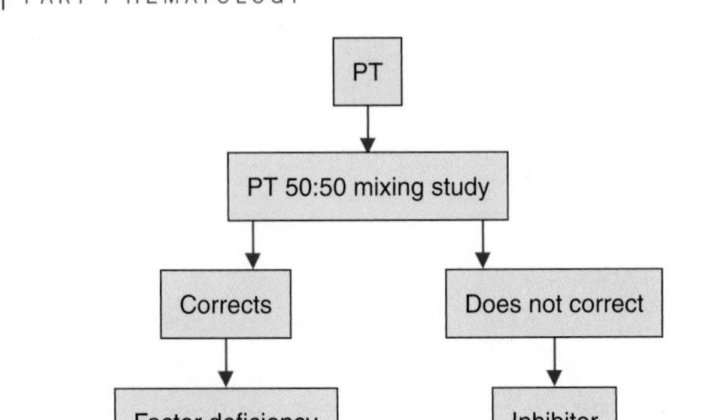

FIGURE 5-2. General workup of an elevated PT in the setting of a normal aPTT.

- Crucial test for diagnosing hemophilia A and von Willebrand disease (vWD) and for monitoring response to therapy in hemophilia.
- Method: Determine the level of factor VIII in the patient's plasma by mixing dilutions of the patient's plasma with factor VIII–deficient plasma and comparing the result to that of similar dilutions of normal pooled plasma mixed with factor VIII–deficient plasma.

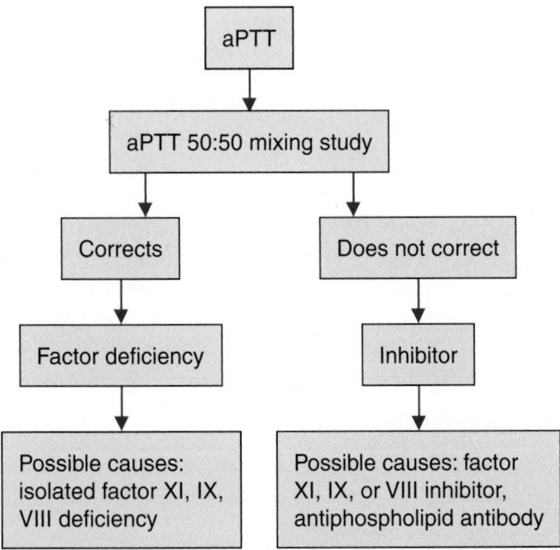

FIGURE 5-3. General workup of an elevated aPTT in the setting of a normal PT.

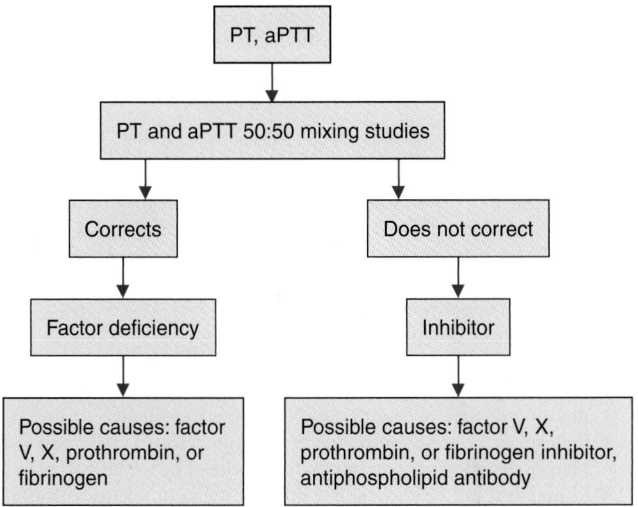

FIGURE 5-4. General workup of an elevation of both the PT and the aPTT.

- **Assessing deficiency of other factors**
  - The same procedure as described for the factor VIII assay is used to determine the activity of other intrinsic pathway coagulation factors, using the corresponding deficient plasma for dilutions.
  - The extrinsic and common pathway factor activities are determined by comparing PT results for patient and normal pooled plasma diluted in plasma depleted of factor VII, X, or V or prothrombin.
- **Factor VIII inhibitor quantification (Bethesda units)**
  - Indicated to test for factor VIII inhibitors. Factor VIII inhibitors are suspected when there is a normal PT; a prolonged aPTT that is partially corrected immediately after 1:1 mixing with normal plasma but prolonged again after 1 to 2 hours of incubation; and a very low factor VIII activity (usually <1%).

TABLE 5-3 MIXING STUDIES

Result of Mixing Studies	Interpretation
Correction immediately and after 1 h	Factor deficiency
Correction (or near to correction) immediately but no correction (PT or aPTT prolonged again) after 1 h	Factor inhibitors (specific inhibitory antibodies are time dependent, most typically factor VIII inhibitors)
No correction both immediately and after 1 h	Lupus anticoagulant

PT, prothrombin time; aPTT, activated partial thromboplastin time.

- Appropriate treatment requires determining the titer of the inhibitor, which is measured as arbitrary Bethesda units.
- Method: Serial dilutions of patient plasma are mixed with an equal volume of normal pooled plasma, and residual factor VIII activity is measured after 2 hours of incubation at 37°C.
- The Bethesda titer is the reciprocal of the plasma dilution that neutralizes 50% of the factor VIII activity of normal pooled plasma.
- A titer of BU <5 indicates a mild inhibitor that may be overwhelmed by larger infusions of factor VIII, whereas an inhibitor with a titer of BU >5 will likely require infusion of a bypass coagulation concentrate such as recombinant factor VIIa or activated prothrombin concentrate complex to achieve hemostasis.

- **Studies of platelet function**
  - **Bleeding time**
    - Method: Standardized incision is made in the patient's forearm, and the duration of time to cessation of bleeding is measured.
    - Indication: To detect primary hemostasis defects (vWD and qualitative platelet disorders) in patients with histories of recurrent mucosal bleeding.
    - Although it can be a useful test for identifying problems with primary hemostasis, many variables may artificially prolong the bleeding time, such as medications that interfere with platelet function, differences in operator procedure and interpretation, subcutaneous edema, or thinning of the skin.
    - It is not an accurate predictor of surgical bleeding risk in asymptomatic subjects; therefore, its use has markedly declined and replaced by PFA-100.
  - **Platelet function analyzer-100** (PFA-100)[2]
    - An in vitro screening test of primary hemostasis.
    - Method: Citrated whole blood is aspirated through a microscopic hole in a piece of nitrocellulose paper coated with collagen and epinephrine (COL/EPI) or collagen and ADP (COL/ADP). The flow conditions mimic the shear stress in a capillary bed. vWF adheres to the collagen, and platelets adhere to the vWF, followed by agonist-mediated activation, aggregation, and eventual closure of the hole. The time to occlusion is reported as the closure time. The COL/EPI cartridge is sensitive to qualitative platelet disorders, especially aspirin effect, and vWD. The COL/ADP cartridge is less sensitive to aspirin but remains sensitive to vWD. Neither cartridge is sensitive to ADP receptor inhibitors such as clopidogrel (Plavix).
    - Normal PFA-100 closure times do not rule out mild qualitative platelet disorders, and if clinical suspicion is high, platelet aggregation studies should be performed.
    - PFA-100 has not been validated for preoperative assessment of bleeding risk in asymptomatic patients.
    - A hematocrit of <30% or a platelet count of <100,000/μL can produce false-positive results.
  - **Platelet aggregation studies**
    - Indicated when an inherited qualitative defect in platelet function is suggested by the clinical and/or family history.
    - Method: Various aggregating agents (arachidonic acid, collagen, ADP, epinephrine, and ristocetin) are added to the initially turbid platelet-rich plasma specimen. The platelets clump, permitting more light to pass through the plasma. The results with each agent are displayed graphically and interpreted as normal or abnormal.

        - This qualitative test is very labor intensive and should only be performed in highly selected cases.
        - As many prescription or over-the-counter medications can affect in vitro measurements of platelet function, almost all inpatients should be excluded.
        - Outpatients must discontinue aspirin-containing medications and clopidogrel (Plavix) for at least 7 days and NSAIDs for at least 72 hours before testing to avoid false-positive results.

- **Laboratory evaluation of suspected von Willebrand disease** (see Table 5-4)[3] Important tests to evaluate vWD include vWF antigen (vWF:Ag), factor VIII activity, ristocetin cofactor activity assay, collagen-binding assay, vWF multimer assay, ristocetin-induced platelet aggregation (RIPA) analysis, and factor VIII binding ELISA. No single test is adequate to diagnose vWD by itself. When abnormal tests are found suggesting vWD, these tests should be repeated to confirm the diagnosis. If two sets of tests do not agree, testing symptomatic first-degree relatives for vWD may be appropriate. See Chapter 7 for detailed discussion of vWD.
    - **von Willebrand factor antigen concentration (vWF:Ag)**
        - vWF:Ag levels are measured against a normal reference sample and typically levels >50% of reference are considered normal.
        - Note that vWF:Ag reference intervals are blood type dependent. Healthy type O subjects may have vWF concentrations as low as 40% compared to normal pooled plasma, while the lower limit of the reference range for non-O controls will be ≥50%. Most laboratories do not provide blood type-specific reference intervals and are likely to have a lower limit ~50%. Therefore, some healthy individuals with blood type O and unimpressive personal and family histories of abnormal bleeding may have vWF:Ag, vWF activity, or factor VIII activity <50% due to their blood type but are incorrectly diagnosed with type 1 vWD.
        - The vWF:Ag concentration will be abnormally low in all type 3, most type 1, and some type 2 vWD.
    - **Ristocetin cofactor assay**
        - The ability of the patient's plasma (platelet poor plasma) to aggregate normal platelets in the presence of ristocetin is compared with that of a normal pooled plasma specimen.
        - Ristocetin is an antibiotic that that was off the market because it causes severe thrombocytopenia due to in vivo agglutination of platelets to vWF.
        - More than 50% is considered normal, but healthy blood type O patients may have lower activity (see discussion above).
        - This test is useful when used with the vWF:Ag test in the vWF ristocetin cofactor/vWF:Ag ratio. A ratio ≤0.7 suggests a qualitative defect of vWF, which indicates a diagnosis of vWD type 2A, 2B, or 2M and requires vWF multimer assay and RIPA analysis for final typing.
    - **Collagen-binding assay**
        - This ELISA is especially useful for identifying the presence of high molecular weight forms of vWF. Collagen is immobilized in the test well, and following incubation with plasma and washing, bound vWF is measured.
        - Patients with types 2A and 2B vWD are deficient in high molecular weight vWF, therefore this test is useful in their diagnosis. As described earlier, reference comparison with >50% levels are considered normal.
        - This test is used in comparison with the vWF:Ag test in the vWF collagen binding/vWF:Ag ratio (normal, >0.7).
        - This test is not popular and rarely used in the United States.

TABLE 5-4 LABORATORY EVALUATION OF VON WILLEBRAND DISEASE

	Factor VIII Activity	vWF Antigen	Ristocetin Cofactor Assay	RIPA	Multimer Pattern
Type 1: decrease in antigen and activity	Decreased/normal	Decreased	Decreased	Decreased or normal response	Normal
Type 3: absence of vWF	Markedly decreased	Very low or absent	Very low or absent	Absent	Absent
Type 2A: failure to make full length or increased cleavage	Decreased or normal	Usually low	Decreased	Decreased	Absent large + intermediate multimers
Type 2B: increased binding to platelets, enhanced clearance	Decreased or normal	Usually low	Decreased	Increased response	Absent large multimers
Type 2M: mutant vWF fails to bind platelets in the presence of shear stress or ristocetin	Decreased or normal	Usually low	Decreased	Decreased	Normal
Type 2N: mutant vWF fails to bind factor VIII	Decreased	Normal	Normal	Normal	Normal
Platelet Type: GP1b defect on platelets, spontaneous vWF binding	Decreased or normal	Decreased or normal	Decreased	Increased response	Absent large multimers

vWF, von Willebrand factor; RIPA, ristocetin-induced platelet aggregation.

TABLE 5-5 RIPA ANALYSIS RESULTS

Test Result	Type of vWD
Increased sensitivity to ristocetin; brisk platelet aggregative occurring at a low concentration of ristocetin (0.5 mg/mL)	2B
Decreased ristocetin sensitivity	2A (or 2M)

RIPA, ristocetin-induced platelet aggregation; vWF, von Willebrand factor.

- **von Willebrand factor multimer assay**
  - The multimer assay involves labor-intensive gel electrophoresis techniques to separate vWF into bands that normally range in size from 0.5 to 20 million daltons.
  - Loss of large and intermediate multimers is seen in type 2A and 2B vWD.
  - Normal distribution of vWF multimers is seen in type 2M cWD.
  - This should not be part of initial workup for vWD, only indicated for suspected type 2A/2B/2M, possibly type 3.
  - This test is not routinely performed at most institutions.
- **Ristocetin-induced platelet aggregation (RIPA) analysis** (Table 5-5)
  - The aggregation of the patient's platelets is tested in the presence of different concentrations of ristocetin.
  - Used for differentiating vWD type 2B from 2A or 2M.
  - RIPA is used only after the diagnosis of vWD is made and further clarification of subtype is necessary.
- **Factor VIII binding ELISA**
  - Indicated to assist in the diagnose type 2N vWD, which is characterized by impaired binding of vWF to factor VIII.
- **PFA-100 closure time**
  - Can be used to screen for vWD in patients with an appropriate bleeding history, and to monitor response to 1-desamino-8-D-arginine vasopressin (DDAVP; which stimulates release of vWF stored in endothelial cells) or infusion of vWF concentrate (Humate-P), since other vWF tests may not be available on a STAT basis.

REFERENCES

1. Kamal AH, Tefferi A, Pruthi RK. How to interpret and pursue an abnormal prothrombin time, activated partial thromboplastin time, and bleeding time in adults. *Mayo Clin Proc.* 2007;82:864–873.
2. Hayward CP, Harrison P, Cattaneo M, et al. Platelet function analyzer (PFA)-100 closure time in the evaluation of platelet disorders and platelet function. *J Thromb Haemost.* 2006; 4:312–319.
3. Sadler JE, Budde U, Eikenboom JC, et al. Update on the pathophysiology and classification of von Willebrand disease: a report of the Subcommittee on von Willebrand Factor. *J Thromb Haemost.* 2006;4:2103–2114.

Thrombotic Disease

6

Tzu-Fei Wang

GENERAL PRINCIPLES

Thrombotic disease refers to the inappropriate formation of a clot in the venous or arterial circulation. Arterial and venous thrombi form in the presence of **Virchow triad:** hypercoagulability, stasis, and endothelial damage. Embolism of these clots can occur, causing a pulmonary embolism (PE) when arising from the venous circulation or a systemic embolus when arising from the arterial circulation. Risk factors for venous thrombosis include immobility, surgery, increasing age, obesity, pregnancy, and an inherited or acquired hypercoagulable state (Table 6-1).[1] Thrombotic disease often results from an interaction of genetic predisposition and environmental factors. Evaluation of patients presenting with thrombosis includes identification of risk factors, recommendations on appropriate anticoagulant management and duration of therapy, and in carefully selected cases, workup for thrombophilia or hypercoagulable state.

DEEP VENOUS THROMBOSIS AND PULMONARY EMBOLUS

General Principles

Definition

The term venous thromboembolism (VTE) encompasses both deep venous thrombosis (DVT) and PE.

Epidemiology[1]

The annual incidence of DVT is approximately 100 per 100,000 persons per year. About 40% to 50% of people with a symptomatic DVT will have a silent PE, and 1% to 8% of patients with a PE will die of its complications.

Prevention

Primary prevention of VTE in the hospitalized patient with risk factors is essential. These risk factors include an acute infectious disease, congestive heart failure, malignancy, stroke, acute pulmonary disease, acute rheumatic disease, inflammatory bowel disease, and critical illness. Expert opinion recommends that all medical patients older than 40, who are expected to have at least 3 days of inpatient stay and have one risk factor, should be provided with DVT prophylaxis. Prophylaxis can be nonpharmacologic, with compression stockings or pneumatic compression devices. However, there are no large, blinded trials proving that these interventions prevent VTE in medical patients. For patients without a contraindication to low-dose anticoagulation who need prophylaxis, pharmacologic agents are recommended. Subcutaneous heparin three times a day, low-molecular-weight heparin (LMWH) once daily, and

TABLE 6-1 CAUSES OF HYPERCOAGULABILITY LEADING TO VENOUS THROMBOEMBOLISM

Acquired Cause	Inherited Cause
Surgery/trauma	Factor V Leiden mutation
Malignancy	Prothrombin G20210A mutation
Myeloproliferative disorders	Hyperhomocysteinemia[a]
Pregnancy	Protein C deficiency
Oral contraceptives	Protein S deficiency
Immobilization	Antithrombin deficiency
Congestive heart failure	Increased factor VIII activity
Nephrotic syndrome	
Obesity	
Antiphospholipid antibodies[a]	
Lupus anticoagulant	
Anticardiolipin antibodies	

[a]Hyperhomocysteinemia and antiphospholipid antibodies are considered risk factors for both venous and arterial thrombosis.

fondaparinux once daily have been shown to have equal efficacy in preventing VTE with minimal increased bleeding risk and have been wildly used as DVT prophylaxis in hospitalized patients.[2]

Diagnosis[3,4]

Clinical Presentation

History

Symptoms of acute DVT and PE can be variable; however, common symptoms include

- DVT—acute onset of pain, swelling, and pain at a unilateral extremity
- PE—dyspnea, pleuritic chest pain, cough, anxiety, and hemoptysis

Physical Examination

- DVT—unilateral extremity tenderness, erythema, and unequal circumference of extremities
- PE—tachypnea, tachycardia, and inspiratory crackles

Diagnostic Testing

Laboratories

D-dimer is a cheap and fast initial screening test, particularly in patients with low suspicion of VTE. D-dimer is the result of fibrin breakdown and is generated in many other circumstances, including infections, tumors, surgery, trauma, extensive burning, bruises, ischemic heart disease, stroke, peripheral artery disease, aneurysms, inflammatory disease, and pregnancy. The sensitivity of the D-dimer test in clinical trials ranges from 93% to 100%; however, the specificity ranges from 35% to 75%. Therefore, it is effective for ruling out the diagnosis if negative, but a positive D-dimer assay is not specific and requires additional workup. In cases of very high clinical suspicion, testing should be pursued despite a negative D-dimer.

Electrocardiography

The most common finding in PE is **sinus tachycardia.** The classic ECG changes associated with PE are S wave in lead I, Q wave in lead III, and inverted T wave in lead III (**SI, QIII, TIII**). However, these findings are neither sensitive nor specific for PE (present in 13.5% of patients with PE). **New right axis deviation** is another clue for right-sided heart strain from PE.

Imaging

- **Doppler ultrasonography** is the test of choice for diagnosing DVT.[3]
  - Sensitivity and specificity for DVT are >97%, with venography considered the gold standard.
  - A positive Doppler study should lead one to treat the patient.
  - A negative study largely rules out the diagnosis, and alternative diagnoses should be considered.
  - In cases of very high suspicion and negative Doppler study, venography or CT (or MR) venography can be considered.
- The most commonly used tests for the diagnosis of PE are **CT angiography** (CTA) of the lungs or **ventilation/perfusion scans** (V/Q scans), although the most useful algorithms and radiographic tests used to diagnose acute PE are still debatable and the subject of ongoing trials.[4,5]
  - Determining a clinical pretest probability of PE is necessary before performing any diagnostic tests. Objective criteria such as the **Wells Criteria** (Table 6-2) are commonly used to determine the pretest probability.
  - The **PIOPED trial** used V/Q scans in the diagnosis of acute PE (Table 6-3).[6]
  - The **PIOPED II trial** published in 2006 used CTA of the lungs and CT venography of the lower extremities to diagnose PE (Table 6-3).[7] As shown in Table 6-3, in patients with a high pretest probability and negative CTA, PE is still present in 40% of cases; therefore, these patients should undergo further testing such as venous compression ultrasonography of the lower extremities or CT venogram of lower extremities.
  - Based on the results of these trials, an algorithm for the diagnosis of PE has been recommended (Fig. 6-1).[8]

TABLE 6-2 SIMPLIFIED WELLS CRITERIA FOR PRETEST PROBABILITY OF PE

Variable	Points
Clinical signs and symptoms of DVT	3.0
Alternative diagnosis less likely than PE	3.0
Heart rate >100/min	1.5
Immobilization (>3 d) or surgery in previous 4 wk	1.5
Previous PE or DVT	1.5
Hemoptysis	1.0
Malignancy (receiving treatment, treated in the last 6 mo, or palliative)	1.0

Probability: ≤2 = low; 2–6 = intermediate; >6 = high.

DVT, deep venous thrombosis; PE, pulmonary embolus.

TABLE 6-3 PIOPED TRIALS

PIOPED, V/Q Scan for the Diagnosis of PE

	Clinical Probability of PE			
V/Q Scan Category	**80%–100%**	**20%–79%**	**0%–19%**	**All**
High probability	96%	88%	56%	87%
Intermediate probability	66%	28%	16%	30%
Low probability	40%	16%	4%	14%
Near normal/normal	0%	6%	2%	4%

PIOPED II, CT for the Diagnosis of PE

	PPV		NPV	
Clinical Probability	**CTA**	**CTA + CTV**	**CTA**	**CTA + CTV**
High probability	96%	96%	60%	82%
Intermediate probability	92%	90%	89%	92%
Low probability	58%	57%	96%	97%

PPV, positive predictive value; NPV, negative predictive value; CTA, CT angiography; CTV, CT lower extremity venogram.

In special cases such as patients with renal failure, patients with allergy to contrast dye, women of childbearing age, and pregnant women, the recommendations are guided by expert opinion. In these patients, the algorithm should begin with D-dimer testing followed by venous ultrasonography in the majority of cases. Patients with a positive D-dimer and a negative ultrasound will then need additional testing. Ventilation/perfusion scanning can then be used, with the realization that the testing may be nondiagnostic.

Treatment[9]

Treatment of VTE with unfractionated heparin or LMWH should begin promptly after the diagnosis is established or, in situations of high clinical suspicion, while awaiting confirmatory studies. Thrombolytics may be considered in selected patients with hemodynamically significant PE. Individuals who are actively bleeding or at high risk for bleeding should be considered for inferior vena cava (IVC) filter placement.

Medications

Most common medications used in the treatment of VTE are summarized in Table 6-4.

- **Low-molecular-weight heparin**
  - A recent meta-analysis concluded that LMWH is superior to unfractionated heparin for the treatment of DVT, with a lower overall mortality over the first 3 to 6 months and a reduced incidence of major bleeding during initial therapy.
  - In patients with cancer, LMWH for the duration of therapy is superior to oral coumarins in reducing the risk of recurrent thromboembolism without increasing the bleeding risk.[10]

TABLE 6-4 MOST COMMON MEDICATIONS USED IN THE TREATMENT OF VTE

Medication	Unfractionated Heparin	Low-Molecular-Weight Heparins	Warfarin (Coumadin)
Route	Intravenous continuous infusion ± initial bolus	Subcutaneous injection	Oral
Mechanism of action	Potentiate the action of antithrombin III, inhibiting thrombin (FIIa) and FXa	Inhibit FXa and thrombin (FIIa), stronger inhibitor for FXa than unfractionated heparin	Vitamin K antagonists
Advantage	Short half-life, commonly used in the hospital setting when future invasive procedures are planned	More predictable dose response, no need to monitor, longer half-lives	Oral
Disadvantage	Highly variable aPTT level, requiring frequent lab draws and may need extra time to achieve therapeutic level	Longer half-lives Renal excretion; caution or cannot be used in renal failure patients	Frequent monitoring needed Drug interactions Slow onset
Monitor	Target aPTT at 1.5–2.5 times the upper limit of normal value (heparin nomograms assist in rapid therapeutic heparin levels)	No monitoring necessary Antifactor Xa levels can be followed in patients with minor renal impairment or with extremes in weight (either morbidly obese or very thin) to assist with proper dosing	INR, target 2–3

FIIa, factor IIa; FXa, factor Xa.

- The **duration of anticoagulation** is variable and depends on a number of factors, including underlying thrombotic risk and risk of bleeding.[11]
  - Current recommendations suggest that 3 months of treatment is adequate for provoked DVT (i.e., an identifiable and reversible risk factor, such as trauma) and most suggest longer treatment, such as 6 months, for PE.

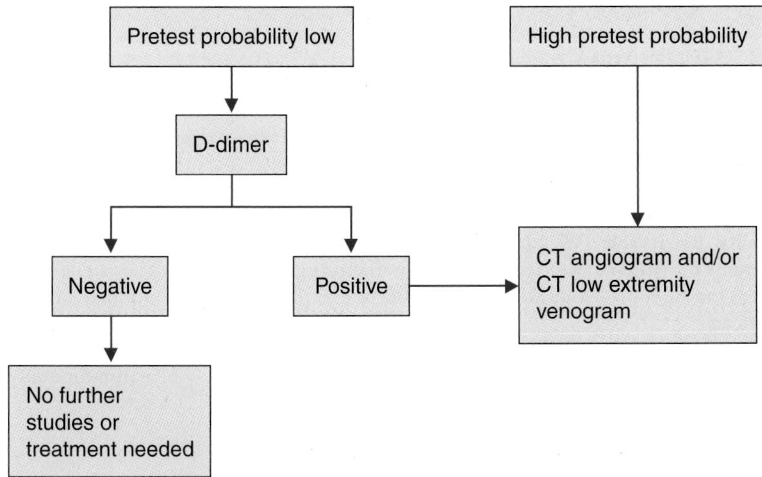

FIGURE 6-1. Algorithm for the diagnosis of PE. (Adapted from Writing Group for the Christopher Study Investigators. Effectiveness of managing suspected pulmonary embolism using an algorithm combining clinical probability, D-dimer testing, and computed tomography. *JAMA.* 2006;295:172–179.)

- Unprovoked VTE or a recurrent episode should be treated for an extended duration. The precise length of treatment is still debated. Many trials have treated patients for 3 months to 1 year after an initial unprovoked VTE. However, recurrent events occurred in similar numbers after treatment was stopped, regardless of the initial length of treatment. Therefore, most experts recommend treatment for 3 to 6 months for unprovoked VTE, with the realization that after completion of therapy there may be a recurrence.
- For patients with recurrent VTE, the recommendation is lifelong anticoagulation.

- **Thrombolytics**[12]
  - The role of thrombolytics in the management of VTE has not been fully elucidated. Thrombolytics dissolve clot faster than conventional anticoagulation; however, the risk of bleeding is significantly increased.
  - A recent meta-analysis suggested that thrombolytics should be reserved for patients with PE and circulatory shock, as there are data demonstrating a survival advantage in these patients.
  - Thrombolytics can be used for DVT to decrease symptoms and postthrombotic syndrome.
  - Prior to treatment with thrombolytics, clinicians must carefully evaluate the patient for any **contraindications to thrombolytic therapy,** including recent surgery, bleeding diathesis, recent stroke, active intracranial disease (including neoplasm, aneurysm), pregnancy, and uncontrolled hypertension. A careful risk/benefit analysis is warranted in every patient.

Other Nonpharmacologic Therapies

- **Inferior Vena Cava Filters**[13]

The use of IVC filters has increased significantly in the past 10 to 20 years, even as evidence supporting their use remains insufficient. Only one randomized controlled trial has compared the use of IVC filters with anticoagulation to the use of anticoagulation alone. At 2 years of follow-up, there was a mild increase in PEs (largely asymptomatic) in those without the filters and an increase in DVT and postthrombotic syndrome in those with the filters. There was no difference in mortality. **Retrievable IVC filters** have recently been studied with some encouraging results for patients with temporary contraindications to anticoagulation. These filters can be retrieved up to 2 months after initial placement with minimal adverse effects.

The only currently recommended indication for IVC filter placement is in patients with an absolute contraindication to anticoagulation. Potential indications that require additional study include the following:

- Patients who developed new VTE on therapeutic anticoagulation
- Patients undergoing pulmonary thromboembolectomy
- Prophylaxis in high-risk trauma patients
- Patients with extensive free-floating iliofemoral thrombus
- Patients undergoing thrombolysis of an iliocaval thrombus

Special Considerations

- **Acute Recurrent Thrombosis**

The diagnosis of recurrent venous thrombosis in the same vein can be difficult. Diagnostic tests currently available have difficulty differentiating between a venous occlusion caused by the initial venous thrombosis and a recurrence. The diagnosis of recurrent DVT commonly can only be made with certainty if there is a clot in an area that was documented to be free of thrombus on prior studies. The risk of new thrombosis in adequately anticoagulated patients is very low, but recurrence can occur, particularly in patients with cancer, heparin-induced thrombocytopenia, and the antiphospholipid antibody syndrome.

- **Venous Thrombosis During Pregnancy**

The risk of VTE is five times higher in pregnant women than nonpregnant women. As warfarin is teratogenic and can cause fetal hemorrhage, heparins have been the mainstay of therapy. Currently, the general recommendation is to use LMWH for the duration of pregnancy and then continue therapy with warfarin after delivery.

- **Thrombosis of Cerebral Veins and Sinuses**[14]

Although rare, the thrombosis of cerebral veins and sinuses is important to identify because, with appropriate treatment, patients often have a good neurologic outcome. Occlusion of cerebral veins leads to localized brain edema and venous infarction, whereas occlusion of the venous sinuses leads to intracranial hypertension. About 85% of patients have an identifiable risk factor, including a thrombophilia, oral contraceptive use, recent trauma (including lumbar puncture), and infection. The most common presenting symptom is unrelenting headache.

The diagnosis can be difficult to make, with an average delay of 7 days from initial presentation to diagnosis. **Venography** is the current recommended diagnostic modality.

Even with the theoretical risk of causing cerebral hemorrhage, the limited evidence suggests a benefit of rapid initiation of anticoagulation, with therapy continuing for at least 6 months. Endovascular thrombolysis has been attempted in some patients. In patients who develop intracranial hypertension, therapy including repeated lumbar punctures, acetazolamide, and possibly surgical creation of a lumboperitoneal shunt may be warranted. More than 80% of patients have a good neurologic outcome if appropriately treated.

A search for a thrombophilia should be pursued in these patients.

- **Budd–Chiari Syndrome**

Budd–Chiari syndrome encompasses various disease states that result in hepatic vein occlusion. Thrombosis of the hepatic veins leads to hepatomegaly, right-upper quadrant pain, and other sequelae of acute or chronic liver disease. The most common causes of Budd–Chiari syndrome in the Western world are the myeloproliferative disorders. All patients should undergo screening for thrombophilia and age-appropriate malignancy including myeloproliferative disorders. The decision to use anticoagulation should be based on the extent of liver disease and subsequent risk of bleeding. In certain cases, liver transplantation is the treatment of choice.

- **Mesenteric and Portal Venous Thrombosis**

Portal vein thrombosis often presents after the disease has caused splenomegaly and both esophageal and gastric varices. The main risk factors include local causes (pancreatitis, tumor, infection) as well as thrombophilic states such as myeloproliferative disorders. Treatment involves anticoagulation, assuming that the degree of thrombocytopenia related to splenomegaly and the extent of varices are minimal.

Mesenteric venous thrombosis presents acutely, with a mortality rate ranging from 20% to 50%. The usual presentation is severe abdominal pain and bloody diarrhea. Risk factors include intra-abdominal inflammation and thrombophilias. Myeloproliferative disorders are only rarely associated with thrombosis of the mesenteric veins. Treatment includes anticoagulation and surgery if the bowel becomes necrotic.

- **Renal Vein Thrombosis**

Renal vein thrombosis is frequently asymptomatic and incidentally discovered. These patients should be evaluated for nephrotic syndrome as well as other more common thrombophilias. Treatment involves anticoagulation, with thrombolysis reserved for patients with acute and marked deterioration in renal function due to the thrombosis.

- **Upper Extremity DVT**

DVTs occur in the upper extremity in 10% of cases. Risk factors specific to upper extremity DVT include indwelling central venous catheters and local trauma. Patients usually have unilateral upper extremity edema. Diagnosis is by ultrasonography or venography. Approximately one-third of upper extremity DVTs will cause PE, so treatment is essential. While there are limited studies guiding treatment, it is generally recommended to fully anticoagulate patients for at least 3 months. The use of thrombolytics is controversial.

- **Anticoagulation in Patients with Brain Metastases or Primary Brain Tumors**

The use of anticoagulation for patients with either primary brain malignancies or metastases to the brain has been controversial. In the past, it was thought that due to the risk of hemorrhage, anticoagulation should be absolutely contraindicated in these patients. However, the limited evidence currently available suggests that anticoagulation is preferable to IVC filters in the majority of cases. Highly vascular tumors such as melanoma, thyroid, and renal cell metastases are still felt to be contraindications to anticoagulation.

- **Cancer**

Patients with cancer have an increased risk of thrombotic events. In a recent cohort study, the incidence of VTE within the first 6 months of diagnosis was ~12%; the risk increased with chemotherapy and metastatic disease. Cancer of the ovary, pancreas, and lung, and hematologic cancers are associated with a high rate of VTE in the year prior to diagnosis. Thus, occult malignancy as a cause of VTE should always be a consideration in the appropriate clinical scenario.

Trousseau syndrome is a hypercoagulable state associated with malignancy and is characterized by DIC and recurrent arterial or venous thrombotic events. Multiple studies have shown that LMWH is superior to oral coumarins in the treatment of VTE in patients with cancer, with the main benefit in decreasing the recurrence of DVT, with similar overall mortality.[10]

Complications

- Chronic PEs can result in **pulmonary hypertension** leading to right-sided heart failure.
- **Postthrombotic syndrome** is one of the potential complications of DVT.[15]
  - Symptoms vary from venous stasis pigment changes and/or slight pain and swelling to more severe manifestations such as chronic pain, intractable edema, and leg ulcers. Symptoms can be similar to acute DVT; however, image studies showed no DVT. Symptoms can be profound and affect quality of life.
  - Treatment of the syndrome is largely supportive and often inadequate. Therefore, prevention by appropriately treating initial DVT is important.
  - Incidence of postthrombotic syndrome can be reduced with prompt anticoagulation and the use of compression stockings. Two trials have suggested that the use of compression stockings for 2 years after the diagnosis of DVT can decrease the incidence of postthrombotic syndrome by half.

THROMBOPHILIA

General Principles

The presence of inherited thrombotic disorders (thrombophilia) has been appreciated for only a few decades. Inherited causes of thrombophilia can be either gain-of-function disorders, in which mutations lead to prothrombotic activity (activated protein C resistance/factor V Leiden, prothrombin G20210A), or loss-of-function disorders, which result in deficiencies of endogenous anticoagulants (antithrombin, protein C, and protein S). Common mutations include factor V Leiden and prothrombin G20210A mutations, while other thrombophilias, such as antithrombin, protein C, and protein S deficiencies, are rare.

Etiology[16,17]

• **Activated Protein C Resistance/Factor V Leiden**

This is the most common hereditary thrombophilia in the Caucasian population (Table 6-5). More than 90% of patients with activated protein C resistance have the G1691A mutation in the factor V gene (factor V Leiden), which decreases the rate of proteolytic cleavage by activated protein C. Activated protein C resistance test should be used for screening before obtaining factor V Leiden mutation genotype. This test is performed by a clotting assay in which patient plasma is diluted in factor V-deficient plasma; in a positive test, the addition of activated protein C fails to cleave factor V, resulting in prolongation of PTT. Diagnosis is often confirmed by detection of the factor V Leiden mutation by a DNA-based assay. The risk for VTE in heterozygous patients who use oral contraceptives is increased 35-fold.

• **Prothrombin G20210A Mutation**

The prothrombin G20210A mutation is a substitution mutation that results in increased levels of plasma prothrombin, leading to increased generation of thrombin. Assays of prothrombin time or prothrombin antigen are neither specific nor sensitive enough for diagnosis; therefore, diagnosis is made by genotype analysis.

• **Antithrombin Deficiency**

Antithrombin is a plasma protease inhibitor that irreversibly binds and neutralizes thrombin and factors Xa, IXa, and XIa, resulting in reversal of coagulation cascade.

TABLE 6-5 THE PREVALENCE AND THE RISK OF THROMBOSIS OF DIFFERENT CAUSES OF THROMBOPHILIA

Causes of Thrombophilia	Prevalence	Prevalence in VTE Patients	Relative Risk of Thrombosis
Factor V Leiden	4% (in Caucasian, much less in other population)	20% (40% in patients with high risk of thrombophilia)	4–5 (heterozygous) 24–80 (homozygous)
Prothrombin G20210A mutation	2% (in Caucasian, much less in other population)	7%	2.8 (heterozygous)
Antithrombin deficiency	0.02%	2%	5
Protein C deficiency	0.2%–0.4%	3.7%	3.1
Protein S deficiency	0.16%–0.20%	2.3%	N/A
Elevated factor VIII levels	10%	25%	4.8

VTE, venous thromboembolism.

This reaction is accelerated by heparin. Therefore, antithrombin deficiency increases risk of thrombosis. Antithrombin deficiency is relatively rare but is considered one of the more severe thrombophilias.

Type I antithrombin deficiency is characterized by both decreased levels and decreased activity, whereas type II is characterized by decreased protease activity, with defects in either the active center or the heparin-binding site. Thus, resistance to the anticoagulant effects of heparin is seen in some patients. There is no difference in clinical severity between type I and type II.

Antithrombin activity assays and antigen levels are used to make the diagnosis. Acute thrombosis, heparin, liver disease, DIC, nephrotic syndrome, and preeclampsia can all decrease antithrombin levels; therefore, diagnosis should not be made on the basis of levels obtained under these conditions.

Prospective studies indicate that the incidence of VTE in these patients is 4% per year. Nearly 70% of patients present with the first thrombotic event before age 35 years.

- **Protein C and S Deficiency**

Proteins C and S are vitamin K-dependent endogenous anticoagulants. Homozygous protein C deficiency can cause neonatal purpura fulminans. Patients with either protein C or protein S deficiency can present with warfarin skin necrosis at the initiation of anticoagulation due to a transient hypercoagulable state.

Protein C deficiency is diagnosed by an assay to detect activity followed by immunoassays to differentiate type I (reduced antigen and activity) and type II (reduced activity) defects. Protein S binds to a plasma protein so that free protein S antigen and activity are used to screen for protein S deficiency and differentiate among type I (decreased antigen and activity), type II (decreased activity), and type III (low free protein S). DNA-based assays are not practical in both protein C and protein S deficiency, given that >150 mutations in the protein C gene have been described. Protein C and S levels are affected by liver disease, anticoagulation with warfarin, nephrotic syndrome, DIC, vitamin K deficiency, oral contraceptives, pregnancy, and hormone replacement therapy.

- **Elevated Factor VIII Levels**

Increased factor VIII levels have been associated with an increased risk of thrombosis (relative risk = 4.8). Elevated levels are found with increased age, obesity, pregnancy, surgery, inflammation, liver disease, hyperthyroidism, and diabetes. No gene alteration has been found, although familial clustering of increased factor VIII levels is noted. It is unclear how increased factor VIII levels lead to increased thrombotic risk and how elevated factor VIII levels may affect treatment of thromboembolism.

- **Hereditary Thrombotic Dysfibrinogenemia**

Dysfibrinogenemias are qualitative defects in the fibrin molecule. Multiple genetic defects have been described. These defects lead to VTE in 20% of patients and bleeding tendency in 25% of patients, but they are asymptomatic in 55%. Normal or low levels of fibrinogen and a prolonged thrombin time may be observed. This disorder is rare, and testing for it in patients with suspected thrombophilia is considered low priority.

Diagnosis

- Screening for thrombophilia should be done only in a carefully selected population rather than all patients with first onset of VTE. There are few clinical trial data available to guide the management of symptomatic or asymptomatic thrombophilic patients in different clinical scenarios. Consequently, there is debate about which patients should be screened. Screening symptomatic and asymptomatic individuals and their family members for the presence of thrombophilia has both benefits and drawbacks. Benefits include a focus on prophylaxis with anticoagulant therapy during high-risk situations, such as surgery, immobilization, and pregnancy to prevent a first-time event and an awareness of increased risk associated with oral contraceptive use, pregnancy, and hormone replacement therapy. Drawbacks may include difficulties in obtaining life insurance coverage and overanticoagulation, with exposure to unnecessary bleeding risk. Universal screening, even for women considering hormonal therapy, oral contraceptives, or pregnancy, is not currently recommended, as it is not cost-effective and may deny women birth control options.

- **Consideration of a hypercoagulable workup** is usually recommended in patients with
  - Recurrent VTE, especially unprovoked thrombosis
  - Thrombosis at a young age (<50 years)
  - Thrombosis at unusual sites (cerebral sinus, mesenteric vein, portal vein, hepatic vein)
  - Recurrent second or third trimester fetal loss, placental abruption, or severe preeclampsia
- The **optimal time for testing patients for hereditary defects** is not well defined, but performing the thrombophilic evaluation at the time of thrombosis is not advised because it often leads to misleading results. As discussed above, acute thrombosis can cause low levels of antithrombin, protein C, and protein S. Therapy with heparin reduces antithrombin levels, and warfarin reduces protein C and S levels. Therefore, it is usually recommended to test (if needed) at the time when patient is off anticoagulation for several weeks without recent thrombosis.

Treatment

There are few clinical trial data to provide evidence-based recommendations for the duration of anticoagulation in patients with hereditary thrombophilia.

- Many experts would recommend a **longer duration of anticoagulation in patients with**
  - Active cancer
  - Multiple allelic abnormalities
  - Antithrombin deficiency
  - Protein C or S deficiency
  - More than one thrombotic event
  - Antiphospholipid antibody syndrome
- Some experts recommend **lifelong anticoagulation for patients with**
  - Two or more unprovoked VTEs
  - Unprovoked VTE with antithrombin deficiency
  - Multiple genetic abnormalities
  - One life-threatening VTE
- In all patients with a history of a thromboembolic event, regardless of the presence or absence of hereditary thrombophilias, prophylaxis should be pursued

with unfractionated heparin or LMWH during high-risk situations, including surgery, trauma, and immobilization. Women should also be advised of the increased risk of recurrent thrombotic events with oral contraceptives, hormone replacement therapy, and pregnancy.

ARTERIAL THROMBOEMBOLISM

General Principles

Definition

Arterial thromboses are those that lodge in the arterial side of the circulatory system. There are two types:

- In situ thrombosis due to a damaged artery (e.g., by trauma, vasculitis, or foreign body)
- Embolization from a proximal source (e.g., from the atria in atrial fibrillation, a ventricular or arterial aneurysm, a proximal clot formed in an area of damaged artery, or a venous clot that passes into the arterial circulation through a heart defect)

Etiology

Possible hypercoagulable states leading to arterial thrombosis include hyperhomocysteinemia, antiphospholipid syndrome, HIT, myeloproliferative disorders, and paroxysmal nocturnal hemoglobinuria. Of note, these disorders may present with either venous or arterial thrombosis.

Risk Factors

- Smoking
- Hypertension
- Atherosclerosis
- Turbulent blood flow
- Diabetes
- Chronic inflammation
- Hyperlipidemia
- Hypercoagulable state

Diagnosis

Clinical Presentation

The symptoms are typically related to the acute ischemia of the organ in which the clot forms or lodges.

Treatment

The initial management of an arterial thrombus includes a search for either its source as an embolus from a distant site or its origin as a clot that formed in situ. The presence of a hypercoagulable state as the etiology of the arterial thrombus may be considered if there are no readily identifiable risk factors.

Special Considerations

- **Hyperhomocysteinemia**[18]
  - **General Principles**

Homocysteine is an intermediate formed in the metabolism of methionine. Elevated levels of homocysteine are associated with arterial and venous thrombosis. Hyperhomocysteinemia can be due to inheritance of enzyme defects involved in the homocysteine metabolic pathways or can be acquired. Severe hyperhomocysteinemia (plasma levels >100 μmol/L) is most commonly due to defects in cystathionine B-synthase, which results in homocystinuria, mental retardation, and thromboses at a young age. The most common genetic defect in mild homocysteinemia (plasma levels, 15 to 40 μmol/L) results in reduced activity of the enzyme methylenetetrahydrofolate reductase. Prospective studies show that the relative risk for VTE in patients with hyperhomocysteinemia is 3.4.

- **Acquired causes**
  - Vitamin B_{12}, vitamin B_6, and folate deficiencies
  - Chronic renal failure
  - Hypothyroidism
  - Cancer
  - Increasing age
  - Smoking
  - Inflammatory bowel disease
  - Psoriasis
  - Rheumatoid arthritis
  - Methotrexate, phenytoin, and theophylline
- The **diagnosis** is made by measuring fasting homocysteine plasma levels.
- **Treatment**

Patients deficient in folate, vitamin B_6, or vitamin B_{12} can be supplemented with these vitamins at sufficient doses to achieve normal levels. In the absence of specific deficiencies, plasma homocysteine levels can be reduced by up to 50% by administration of folate at doses of 1 to 2 mg/d, although it is uncertain whether this ultimately leads to a decreased frequency of adverse events. In patients with severe hyperhomocysteinemia due to cystathionine B-synthase deficiency, treatment with vitamin B supplements improves homocysteine levels and delays thrombotic events. In several recent studies, patients with first-time events, either arterial (stroke, myocardial infarction [MI]) or VTE, treated with vitamin supplementation had reductions in homocysteine levels but no protection from recurrent MI, recurrent venous thrombosis, or progression of peripheral vascular disease. Therefore, the role of homocysteine in thrombosis is still debated.

- **Antiphospholipid Syndrome**[19]
  - **General Principles**

Antiphospholipid syndrome is characterized by recurrent venous or arterial thrombosis and/or recurrent pregnancy morbidity/fetal loss and the presence of antiphospholipid antibodies (anticardiolipin antibodies, lupus anticoagulants, anti-B_2-glycoprotein 1). **Antiphospholipid antibodies** are autoantibodies that recognize phospholipids and/or phospholipid-binding proteins. Lupus anticoagulants are IgG or IgM antibodies that react with negatively charged phospholipids. In vitro they act as anticoagulants and interfere with membrane surfaces in clotting assays, resulting in false prolongation of the aPTT and, rarely, the PT. The pathogenesis of antiphospholipid antibodies is thought to involve the binding and subsequent activation of endothelial cells, platelets, and complement to promote thrombosis and the inhibition of the fibrinolytic pathway.

The syndrome is considered primary if there is no accompanying autoimmune disease and secondary if the patient has systemic lupus erythematosus (SLE).

- **Clinical Presentation**

Approximately 30% to 50% of patients develop DVT of the legs within 6 years of follow-up. Although venous thrombosis is more common, patients may present with arterial occlusions, the most frequent involving the brain, followed by coronary occlusions. Any vessel or vascular bed may be involved and diverse presentations, such as intestinal, pancreatic, or splenic infarction; ARDS; retinitis; and acute renal failure, may occur. Other features occasionally seen include thrombocytopenia, hemolytic anemia, and livedo reticularis. **Catastrophic antiphospholipid syndrome,** characterized by multiple simultaneous thromboses, occurs in <1% of patients and is associated with multiorgan failure and death.

- **Diagnosis** relies on meeting at least one of the clinical and one of the laboratory criteria as below.
  - **Clinical**
    - One or more episodes of venous, arterial, or small vessel thrombosis
    - Pregnancy morbidity—at least one unexplained death of a morphologically normal fetus beyond the 10th week of gestation; at least three unexplained spontaneous abortions before the 10th week of gestation; or one or more premature births secondary to eclampsia, preeclampsia, or placental insufficiency before the 34th week of gestation
  - **Laboratory**
    - **Lupus anticoagulant present on two or more occasions at least 12 weeks apart.** The presence of the lupus anticoagulant may be confirmed with the dilute Russell's viper venom assay or phospholipid neutralization assay.
    - **Anticardiolipin antibody** of IgG or IgM isotype presents at medium or high titer on two or more occasions at least 12 weeks apart.
    - **Anti-B_2-glycoprotein** 1 of IgG or IgM isotype presents on two or more occasions at least 12 weeks apart. Anticardiolipin and anti-B_2-glycoprotein 1 are detected by immunologic assays.

- **Treatment**

The treatment of antiphospholipid syndrome is lifelong anticoagulation, typically with warfarin, with the goal INR 2.0 to 3.0. Hydroxychloroquine and ASA may be used as adjunct therapy. Plasma exchange and rituximab have been used to treat patients with catastrophic antiphospholipid syndrome, although these approaches are based on case studies and not on clinical trials.

REFERENCES

1. Cushman M. Epidemiology and risk factors for venous thrombosis. *Semin Hematol.* 2007;44: 62–69.
2. Francis CW. Clinical practice. Prophylaxis for thromboembolism in hospitalized medical patients. *N Engl J Med.* 2007;356:1438–1444.
3. Palareti G, Cosmi B. Diagnosis of deep vein thrombosis. *Semin Thromb Hemost.* 2006;32: 659–672.
4. Bounameaux H, Perrier A. Diagnosis of pulmonary embolism: in transition. *Curr Opin Hematol.* 2006;13:344–350.
5. Stein PD, Fowler SE, Goodman LA, et al. Multidetector computed tomography for acute pulmonary embolism. *N Engl J Med.* 2006;354:2317–2327.

6. The PIOPED investigators. Value of the ventilation/perfusion scan in acute pulmonary embolism—results of the prospective investigation of pulmonary embolism diagnosis (PIOPED). *JAMA.* 1990;263:2753–2759.
7. Stein PD, Woodard PK, Weg JG, et al. Diagnostic pathways in acute pulmonary embolism: recommendations of the PIOPED II investigators. *Am J Med.* 2006;119:1048–1055.
8. Writing Group for the Christopher Study Investigators. Effectiveness of managing suspected pulmonary embolism using an algorithm combining clinical probability, D-dimer testing, and computed tomography. *JAMA.* 2006;295:172–179.
9. Segal JB, Streiff MB, Hofmann LV, et al. Management of venous thromboembolism: a systematic review for a practice guideline. *Ann Intern Med.* 2007;146:211–222.
10. Lee AY, Levine MN, Baker RI, et al. Low-molecular-weight heparin versus a coumarin for the prevention of recurrent venous thromboembolism in patients with cancer. *N Engl J Med.* 2003;349:146–153.
11. Streiff MB, Segal JB, Tamariz LJ, et al. Duration of vitamin K antagonist therapy for venous thromboembolism: a systematic review of the literature. *Am J Hematol.* 2006;81:684–691.
12. Arcasoy SM, Vachani A. Local and systemic thrombolytic therapy for acute venous thromboembolism. *Clin Chest Med.* 2003;24:73–91.
13. Hann CL, Streiff MB. The role of vena caval filters in the management of venous thromboembolism. *Blood Rev.* 2005;19:179–202.
14. Stam J. Current concepts: thrombosis of the cerebral veins and sinuses. *N Engl J Med.* 2005;352:1791–1798.
15. Pesavento R, Bernardi E, Concolato A, et al. Postthrombotic syndrome. *Semin Thromb Hemost.* 2006;32:744–751.
16. Bauer K. The thrombophilias: well-defined risk factors with uncertain therapeutic implications. *Ann Intern Med.* 2001;135:367–373.
17. Seligsohn U, Lubetsky A. Genetic susceptibility to venous thrombosis. *N Engl J Med.* 2001;334:1222–1229.
18. Gatt A, Makris M. Hyperhomocysteinemia and venous thrombosis. *Semin Hematol.* 2007;44: 70–76.
19. Levine S. The antiphospholipid syndrome. *N Engl J Med.* 2002;346:752–763.

Coagulopathy

7

Tzu-Fei Wang

GENERAL PRINCIPLES

Coagulopathy refers to disorders with excessive bleeding because of alterations of proteins involved in the coagulation pathway. It can be divided into two main categories: hereditary and acquired.

- Hereditary
  - von Willebrand disease (vWD)
  - Hemophilia A
  - Hemophilia B
- Acquired
  - Liver disease
  - Vitamin K deficiency
  - Disseminated intravascular coagulation
  - Acquired inhibitors of coagulation

HEREDITARY COAGULOPATHY

VON WILLEBRAND DISEASE (vWD)

GENERAL PRINCIPLES

vWD is caused by quantitative or qualitative abnormalities of von Willebrand factor (vWF), resulting in disorders of primary and secondary hemostasis. The usual inheritance pattern of vWD is autosomal dominant; incomplete penetrance may lead to phenotypic variability. The incidence is ~1 in 100 to 400.

Classification[1]

The subtypes of vWD are presented in Table 7-1.

Pathophysiology

vWF is a glycoprotein synthesized by endothelial cells and platelets. It is stored in the Weibel-Palade bodies of endothelial cells as well as platelet alpha granules. vWF plays a role in both primary and secondary hemostasis. It mediates the adhesion of platelets at sites of vascular injury, and it stabilizes and transports factor VIII (FVIII) in the circulation. vWF is synthesized as a 300-kD monomer, which then assembles into multimers of various sizes. The largest multimers mediate platelet adhesion.

TABLE 7-1 SUBTYPES OF vWD

Type	Description	Genetic Inheritance	DDAVP
1	Partial quantitative deficiency of vWF most common, ~70% of all vWD	Autosomal dominant	Effective
2	Qualitative abnormality of vWF	N/A	Not as effective, but a trial is reasonable, except for type 2B
2A	Abnormal assembly or reduced half life of high-molecular-weight vWF multimers (HMWM)	Autosomal dominant	Not as effective, but a trial is reasonable
2B	Increased binding of vWF to platelets, leading to deceased HMWM and platelets	Autosomal dominant	Contraindicated due to transient thrombocytopenia
2M	Decreased binding of vWF to platelets, normal multimer distribution	Autosomal dominant	Not as effective, but a trial is reasonable
2N	Decreased binding of vWF to FVIII, low FVIII level	Autosomal recessive	Not as effective, but a trial is reasonable
3	Complete quantitative deficiency of vWF	Autosomal recessive or compound heterozygous	Ineffective
Pseudo-vWD	Abnormal platelet GP Ib-Ix-V with increased affinity for large vWF multimers, phenotype indistinguishable from type 2B	N/A	N/A

vWD, von Willebrand disease.

DIAGNOSIS[2,3]

Clinical Presentation

- Recurrent mucocutaneous bleeding
- Prolonged bleeding after trauma or surgery
- Family history of a bleeding disorder is common.
- In contrast to hemophilia, musculoskeletal bleeding is rare.

- Although the majority of affected patients have mild vWD and minor bleeding, patients with the most severe form may suffer life-threatening hemorrhage.

Differential Diagnosis

- Hemophilia A

Diagnostic Testing

Laboratories (see Chap. 5 for details)

- CBC
- PT (usually normal), aPTT (can be slightly prolonged)
- Quantitative vWF antigen (vWF:Ag)
- Qualitative vWF assay: Ristocetin cofactor assay (vWF:RCof) and/or vWF collagen-binding assay (vWF:CBA)
- Factor VIII level
- vWF multimer assay
- Ristocetin-induced platelet aggregation (RIPA) analysis
- Factor VIII–binding ELISA
- vWF levels vary with physiological stress, estrogen levels, and other medical comorbidities, therefore levels should be repeated for confirmation.

TREATMENT[4]

- **DDAVP (Desmopressin)**[5]
  - Mechanism of action: Analog of antidiuretic hormone (vasopressin) that lacks vasoactive properties. It acts by releasing endothelial stores of vWF, thereby transiently increasing plasma levels of FVIII and vWF by a factor of 3 to 5 within 30 to 60 minutes of administration.
  - Dosage: 0.3 μg/kg IV or SC or 300 μg intranasally
  - Dosing frequency: 8 to 10 hours (guided by the half-life of FVIII after DDAVP administration)
  - DDAVP should not be used in patients with unstable coronary artery disease, due to concern for ultra large vWF multimer-mediated platelet aggregation in regions of high shear stress near atherosclerotic plaques.
  - At the time of vWD diagnosis or before elective treatment, a test dose of DDAVP should be administered to establish the individual pattern of response. FVIII levels and vWF:RCof should be measured at 1 and 4 hours after drug administration to determine peak factor levels and clearance rate.
- **FVIII and vWF concentrates**
  - The primary treatment for all vWD subtypes when significant bleeding or major surgery is involved
  - Virus-inactivated FVIII + vWF concentrates, such as *Humate-P* and *Alphanate,* are the products of choice, when available.
  - FVIII levels should be obtained every 12 hours on the day concentrates are administered and every 24 hours thereafter. Target FVIII levels are similar to those detailed for hemophilia A, below.
- **Cryoprecipitate,** which contains 5 to 10 times more FVIII and vWF than fresh-frozen plasma, can also be used, although techniques of virus inactivation are not routinely applied to this product.

- **Platelet transfusion** can be useful, especially when hemorrhage is not controlled despite adequate FVIII levels after FVIII and vWF concentrates.
- **Antifibrinolytic amino acids** (aminocaproic acid, tranexamic acid)

HEMOPHILIA A[6,7]

GENERAL PRINCIPLES

Hemophilia A is an inherited coagulation disorder caused by alterations of the gene encoding FVIII, leading to impaired intrinsic pathway function (see Figure 5-1 for intrinsic pathway). The inheritance pattern is X-linked recessive; the gene that encodes FVIII is located on the long arm of the X chromosome (Xq28). Thirty percent of cases are the result of spontaneous mutations. The incidence is approximately 1 in 5000 live male births among all ethnic groups.

DIAGNOSIS

Clinical Presentation

- Joint and muscle/soft tissue hemorrhages, easy bruising.
- Prolonged bleeding after trauma or surgery; however, usually no excessive bleeding after minor cuts or abrasions.
- Chronic disability can result from hemarthrosis-induced arthropathy and intramuscular bleeding.

Diagnostic Criteria

- Laboratory evaluations include
  - Platelet count—normal
  - PT—normal
  - PTT—prolonged
  - PTT mixing study—correct with normal plasma
  - FVIII level—decreased (confirmation of diagnosis)
  - von Willebrand factor (vWF) level—normal
  - Genetic analysis is used for carrier detection and prenatal diagnosis.
- Disease severity depends on FVIII level
  - Mild disease—level >5% of normal
  - Moderate disease—levels 1% to 5% of normal
  - Severe disease—≤1% of normal

Differential Diagnosis

- Hemophilia B
- von Willebrand disease (vWD) type 2N

TREATMENT[6]

- **Factor VIII replacement**
  - Used in severe hemophilia, for both major and minor bleeding.
  - Options consist of recombinant FVIII (agent of choice) or purified, virus-attenuated FVIII concentrates from pooled plasma.

- Dosage: Each unit/kg of FVIII replacement will raise the plasma FVIII level by 2%. Therefore, the bolus dose = target FVIII level (as below) × weight (kg) × 0.5.
- Target FVIII level:
  - minor bleeding: ≥30%
  - more severe bleeding (e.g., muscle and joint hemorrhages): ≥50%
  - surgical procedures or life-threatening bleeding: ≥80%
- The half life of FVIII is 8 to 12 hours, therefore, following a loading dose, repeat doses are administered every 8 to 12 hours, adjusted to measured factor VIII levels.
- FVIII replacement can also be provided by continuous infusion.
- Therapy should continue until hemostasis is achieved.
- Postoperative therapy is usually continued for 10 to 14 days. Measuring peak and trough FVIII levels after the first and selected subsequent doses permits dose adjustments to ensure cost-effective therapy.

- **Recombinant factor VIIa**[8]
  - Recombinant factor VIIa promotes hemostasis by activating the extrinsic pathway.
  - It is currently approved for use in hemophilia A and B patients who have developed inhibitors to FVIII or factor IX (FIX).
  - Dosage: 90 μg/kg every 2 to 3 hours until hemostasis is achieved.
- **DDAVP (Desmopressin)**
  - Used in patients with mild disease (FVIII level >5%) and minor bleeding episodes
  - Details as outlined above for vWD

COMPLICATIONS

- Infection from factor concentrates
- Antibody formation, primarily in patients with severe factor deficiency[9]
- Thrombosis
- Hemophilic arthropathy
  - Recurrent hemorrhage into one or more joints leading to chronic effusion, joint space narrowing, limited range of motion, atrophy of adjacent musculature, and end stage arthritis
  - Can be prevented by prophylactic factor infusions (three times a week for FVIII), intraarticular steroid injection, synovectomy, joint replacement.

HEMOPHILIA B (TABLE 7-2)

ACQUIRED COAGULOPATHIES

LIVER DISEASE[10]

All coagulation factors, with the exception of vWF and possibly FVIII, are produced in the liver. Liver dysfunction leads to a number of coagulation abnormalities secondary to decreased factor synthesis, decrease clearance of activated factors, dysregulation of fibrinolytic pathways, and production of abnormal fibrinogen. The coagulopathy of liver disease is usually stable unless the liver synthetic function is rapidly worsening, such as in fulminant hepatic failure. Patients with liver synthetic dysfunction frequently also have thrombocytopenia secondary to portal hypertension and splenic sequestration.

TABLE 7-2 HEMOPHILIAS

	Hemophilia A	Hemophilia B
Inherence pattern	X-linked recessive	X-linked recessive
Gene location	Xq28	Xq27
Incidence	1 in 5000 live male births	1 in 30,000 live male births
Presentations	Recurrent hemarthrosis, soft tissue hematomas	Recurrent hemarthrosis, soft tissue hematomas
Diagnosis	Decreased FVIII level	Decreased FIX level
Treatment	• FVIII concentrates • Each unit/kg of FVIII replacement raises plasma FVIII level by 2% • Bolus dose = target FVIII level (as above) × weight (kg) × 0.5 • Dosing frequency every 8–12 h • DDAVP can be used carefully in mild disease with minor bleeding	• FIX concentrates • Each unit/kg of FIX replacement raises plasma FIX level by 1% • Bolus dose = target FIX level (as above) × weight (kg) (multiply by 1.3 when recombinant is given) • Dosing frequency every 12–24 h • DDAVP is ineffective

Note: FIX is a small molecule with extensive extravascular distribution; therefore, multiplication by 1.3 is needed in dosage calculation.

VITAMIN K DEFICIENCY

- Vitamin K is a fat-soluble vitamin involved in the posttranslational modification of procoagulant factors II, VII, IX, and X, and anticoagulant proteins C and S. These reactions take place in the liver, where vitamin K serves as a cofactor for the conversion of glutamic acid residues to gamma-carboxyglutamic acid, which facilitates binding of coagulation factors to phospholipid, an essential step in coagulation. Vitamin K must then be recycled by vitamin K epoxide reductase (VKOR) for further gamma-carboxylation to occur. It follows that vitamin K deficiency would render these so-called vitamin K-dependent coagulation factors ineffective.
- Disorders of vitamin K most commonly results from the use of warfarin, a VKOR inhibitor. Other causes of Vitamin K deficiency are inadequate dietary intake, which may deplete vitamin K stores in as little as 7 days, malabsorption syndromes, or use of antibiotics, which can eliminate vitamin K–producing bowel flora.
- Vitamin K deficiency results in prolonged PT that corrects during mixing studies.
- Vitamin K repletion may be provided PO, SC, or IV. PO is the preferred route. IV vitamin K is effective but carries the risk of anaphylaxis. To minimize this risk, vitamin K may be diluted in a dextrose or saline solution and slowly administered via an infusion pump. If bleeding is significant or does not respond to vitamin K therapy, factor replacement in the form of fresh-frozen plasma should be administered.

DISSEMINATED INTRAVASCULAR COAGULATION[11]

DIC is a hemostatic derangement of multiple etiologies characterized by small- and medium-vessel thrombosis with consumption of platelets and coagulation factors. It leads to microangiopathic hemolytic anemia, thrombocytopenia, and coagulation abnormalities (see Chap. 4).

ACQUIRED INHIBITORS OF COAGULATION

Acquired inhibitors of coagulation are immunoglobulins, usually IgG, which exert their effects by inhibiting the activity or increasing the clearance of coagulation factors. They can be directed against any of the coagulation factors, with inhibitors of FVIII being most common. Inhibitors of coagulation can occur in the following settings:

- Extensive blood product exposure in patients with inherited factor deficiency, most commonly in hemophilia A
- Lymphoproliferative malignancies
- Autoimmune disorders such as rheumatoid arthritis or lupus
- Drug reactions
- Postpartum

Inhibitors cause prolongation of the PT, the aPTT, or both. If the abnormal coagulation studies do not correct with mixing, an inhibitor is likely, and the Bethesda assay can be run to quantify the inhibitor (see Chap. 5 for details). If antiphospholipid antibodies are suspected, a source of phospholipids (such as dilute Russell's viper venom) can be added to mixed plasma. Correction of the abnormal coagulation tests suggests the presence of antiphospholipid antibodies (see Chap. 6 for more information on antiphospholipid syndrome).

Patients may present with bleeding diathesis, which can be severe and life threatening.

Treatment varies depending on the type of inhibitor and severity of bleeding. Therapeutic options include recombinant factor VIIa, immunosuppression with corticosteroids and/or cyclophosphamide, plasma exchange, and intravenous immunoglobulin.

REFERENCES

1. Sadler JE, Budde U, Eikenboom JC, et al. Update on the pathophysiology and classification of von Willebrand disease: a report of the subcommittee on von Willebrand factor. *J Thromb Haemost.* 2006;4:2103–2114.
2. Budde U. Laboratory diagnosis of congenital von Willebrand disease. *Semin Thromb Hemost.* 2002;28:173–189.
3. Favaloro EJ. Laboratory assessment as a critical component of the appropriate diagnosis and sub-classification of von Willebrand's disease. *Blood Rev.* 1999;13:185–204.
4. Mannucci PM. Treatment of von Willebrand's disease. *N Engl J Med.* 2004;351:683–694.
5. Mannucci PM. Desmopressin (DDAVP) in the treatment of bleeding disorders: the first 20 years. *Blood.* 1997;90:2515–2521.
6. Hoyer L. Hemophilia A. *N Engl J Med.* 1994;330:38–47.
7. Bolton-Maggs PH, Perry DJ, Chalmers EA, et al. The rare coagulation disorders—review with guidelines for management from the United Kingdom Haemophilia Centre Doctors' Organization. *Haemophilia.* 2004;10:593–628.
8. Butenas S, Brummel KE, Branda RF, Paradis SG, Mann KG, et al. Mechanism of factor VIIa-dependent coagulation in hemophilia blood. *Blood.* 2002;99:923–930.
9. Sahud MA. Laboratory diagnosis of inhibitors. *Semin Thromb Hemost.* 2000;26:195–203.
10. Lechner K, Niessner H, Thaler E. Coagulation abnormalities in liver disease. *Semin Thromb Hemost.* 1977;4:40–56.
11. Levi M, Ten Cate H. Disseminated intravascular coagulation. *N Engl J Med.* 1999;341:586–592.

Myelodysplasia, Bone Marrow Failure Syndromes, and Other Causes of Pancytopenia

8

Yee Hong Chia

GENERAL PRINCIPLES

- **Pancytopenia is a reduction in all blood cell lines,** including red blood cells (RBCs), white blood cells (WBCs), and platelets. Patients can present in innumerable ways depending on the severity and type of cell lineages affected. Anemia can cause fatigue, shortness of breath, or lightheadedness. Patients with significant thrombocytopenia can present with bleeding and bruising. Neutropenia is associated with recurrent infections. Cytopenias may result from defects in bone marrow production or from peripheral causes.
- Bone marrow infiltration by disease processes such lymphoma, metastatic carcinoma, sarcoidosis, tuberculosis, myeloma, hairy cell leukemia, or in storage disorders (e.g., Gaucher, Niemann–Pick) can result in inadequate production. Vitamin B_{12} and/or folate deficiency leads to megaloblastic erythropoiesis and defective maturation of granulocytic and megakaryocytic lineages. Copper deficiency is a relatively uncommon cause of pancytopenia.
- Causes of increased destruction of blood cells in the periphery include hypersplenism, autoimmune diseases and overwhelming sepsis. Medications may also affect blood counts. For example, antipsychotics such as clozapine are known to cause agranulocytosis. Impaired production of blood cells is seen in bone marrow failure states, both inherited and acquired. **Bone marrow failure** is defined as the inability of the bone marrow to produce an adequate number of circulating blood cells. Inherited BM failure syndromes are as described in Table 8-1.[1] Acquired bone marrow failure states include myelodysplastic syndromes (MDS), acquired aplastic anemia (AA), and paroxysmal nocturnal hemoglobinuria (PNH).
- In most cases, initial laboratory evaluation should include a complete blood count, serum chemistries, peripheral smear and reticulocyte count. If clinically indicated, an evaluation of the patient's folate and B_{12} status, or an infectious workup (including HIV, hepatitis panel, other viral or fungal serologies) should be undertaken. If an etiology is not apparent, a bone marrow biopsy and aspirate should be obtained. In cases where a hematologic malignancy is suspected, flow cytometry and cytogenetics performed on the aspirate may be useful.
- Treatment and further laboratory or imaging evaluations will depend on the etiology of the cytopenia(s). In cases where a medication is the underlying cause, discontinuation of the offending drug may be curative. Cytopenias resulting from bone marrow infiltration or suppression by other conditions may improve with treatment of the underlying condition. Cytopenias resulting from nutritional deficiencies can be treated by addressing the underlying nutritional deficiencies. In cases where bone marrow failure is the etiology of the cytopenias, treatment will depend on the diagnosis. Features and management of selected bone marrow failure syndromes are described in the following sections.

TABLE 8-1 FEATURES OF INHERITED BONE MARROW FAILURE SYNDROMES

	Fanconi Anemia (FA)	Dyskeratosis Congenital (DC)	Shwachman–Diamond Syndrome	Congenital Amegakaryocytic Thrombocytopenia	Diamond–Blackfan Anemia (DBA)
Clinical effects	Microcephaly, thumb abnormalities, hypogonadism, skin changes	Triad of skin pigmentation, nail dystrophy, and mucosal leukoplakia	Exocrine pancreatic deficiency, skeletal abnormalities, skin changes	Cardiac and neurological abnormalities	Craniofacial, thumb, growth abnormalities
Associated malignancies	Leukemia, SCC, GI adenocarcinomas, liver, brain, Wilms tumor	Leukemia, lymphoma, SCC, GI adenocarcinomas, lung, skin, liver	Leukemia	Leukemia	Leukemia, osteosarcoma, soft tissue sarcoma
Inheritance	AR, rarely XLR	XLR, AD, AR	AR	AR	AD
Genetics	Multiple genes identified—FANCA, FANCC, FANCD1, FANCD2, FANCE, FANCF, FANCG, FANCI, FANCJ, FANCL, FANCM, FANCN, and FANCB. FA genes function coordinately to repair DNA damage. FA-B subtype is XLR	XLR form associated with mutations in dyskerin gene (DKC1); AD form associated with genes encoding RNA component of telomerase (TERC) and telomerase reverse transcriptase (TERT); AR form associated with NOP10/NOLA3 and NHP2/NOLA2	Up to 90% harbor biallelic mutations in the SBDS gene, which encodes a highly conserved protein thought to function in ribosome biogenesis	Mutations in c-MPL gene, which encodes the thrombopoietin receptor	Multiple genes identified—RPS19, RPS17, RPS24, RPL35A, and RPL11. DBA genes encode protein components of either the small 40S or large 60S ribosomal units

(*continued*)

Additional tests	Chromosome breakage	Telomere length	Serum trypsinogen, pancreatic isoamylase, fecal elastase, pancreatic imaging		Erythrocyte adenosine deaminase

SCC, squamous cell carcinomas; GI, gastrointestinal; AR, autosomal recessive; XLR, X-linked recessive; AD, autosomal dominant.

Modified from Shimamura A. Clinical approach to marrow failure. *Hematology Am Soc Hematol Educ Program.* 2009:329–337.

MYELODYSPLASTIC SYNDROMES

GENERAL PRINCIPLES

Myelodysplastic syndromes are neoplastic clonal stem cell disorders characterized by cytopenias and most commonly a hypercellular, dysplastic-appearing bone marrow. Peripheral blood features include monocytosis, Pelger Huet-like anomaly in neutrophils, circulating immature myeloid or erythroid cells, and macrocytosis. In MDS, the bone marrow is typically hypercellular with "megaloblastoid changes," atypical megakaryocytes, erythroid hyperplasia, and defective maturation in the myeloid series. Increased blasts or ringed sideroblasts can also be seen. Despite increased cell proliferation, there is also increased apoptosis, leading to the discrepancy between the cellular bone marrow and peripheral cytopenias.

Epidemiology

MDS is considered a disease of the elderly. Approximately 80% of patients are older than 60 years of age at diagnosis. The annual incidence rate of MDS in the United States is estimated to be 3.4/100,000. The median age at diagnosis is 76 years, with only 6% of cases diagnosed before age 50.[2] Risk factors include exposure to chemotherapy (especially alkylating agents and topoisomerase II inhibitors), chloramphenicol, radiation, benzene and other solvents, petroleum products, smoking, and immunosuppression. Inherited bone marrow failure syndromes are the primary risk factor for MDS in the pediatric age group.

Classification

The World Health Organization's (WHO's) International Agency for Research on Cancer (IARC) revised its classification of MDS in 2008. The revised classification is shown in Table 8-2.[3] **Therapy-related MDS** (tMDS) refers to MDS that arises after exposure to chemotherapy agents. tMDS occurs most frequently in patients diagnosed with tumors that are associated with a good prognosis, such as breast cancer, non-Hodgkin lymphoma, Hodgkin lymphoma, and testicular cancer. For instance, 1.7% of patients with breast cancer develop secondary bone marrow disease, with a mean time of 18 months. tMDS and acute myelogenous leukemia (AML) occur in about 5% to 10% of patients with Hodgkin's lymphoma and non-Hodgkin lymphoma. tMDS differs from sporadic MDS in that it tends to be associated with distinct chromosomal abnormalities. tMDS after exposure to alkylating agents is associated with deletions of chromosome 5 or 7 and occurs 3 to 5 years after therapy. Topoisomerase II inhibitors, such as daunorubicin, etoposide, and tenoposide, cause tMDS/AML with translocations involving the MLL gene at chromosome 11q23, usually manifesting 1 to 3 years after treatment.

Pathophysiology

Patients with MDS exhibit cytopenia(s) despite a cellular bone marrow. Chromosomal analysis suggests that MDS is a clonal disorder. The critical genetic lesions that initiate MDS are not well-characterized. The cytopenias seen in MDS are thought to arise from ineffective hematopoiesis arising from abnormal responses to cytokine growth factors, defects in the bone marrow microenvironment, and impaired cell survival.

TABLE 8-2 WHO CLASSIFICATION OF MYELODYSPLASTIC SYNDROMES

Category	Peripheral Blood	Bone Marrow
Refractory cytopenia with unilineage dysplasia: (refractory anemia [RA]; refractory neutropenia [RN]; refractory thrombocytopenia [RT])	Unicytopenia or bicytopenia No or rare blasts (<1%)	Unilineage dysplasia: ≥10% of cells in one myeloid lineage <5% blasts <15% of erythroid precursors are ringed sideroblasts
RA with ringed sideroblasts (RARS)	Anemia No blasts	<5% blasts ≥15% erythroid precursors are ringed sideroblasts Erythroid dysplasia only
Refractory cytopenia with multilineage dysplasia (RCMD)	Cytopenias No or rare blasts (<1%) Absence of Auer rods <1 × 10^9/L monocytes	Dysplasia in ≥10% of the cells in ≥2 myeloid lineages <5% blasts in marrow Absence of Auer rods ±15% ring sideroblasts
RA with excess blasts-1 (RAEB-1)	Cytopenia(s) <5% blasts Absence of Auer rods < 1 × 10^9/L monocytes	Unilineage or multilineage dysplasia 5%–9% blasts Absence of Auer rods
RA with excess blasts-2 (RAEB-2)	Cytopenia(s) 5%–19% blasts ±Auer rods <1 × 10^9/L monocytes	Unilineage or multilineage dysplasia 10%–19% blasts ±Auer rods
MDS, unclassified (MDS-U)	Cytopenias <1% blasts	Unequivocal dysplasia in <10% of cells in one or more myeloid lineages when accompanied by a cytogenetic abnormality considered as presumptive evidence for a diagnosis of MDS (see Table 8-3) <5% blasts
MDS with isolated del(5q)	Anemia No or rare blasts (<1%) Usually normal or increased platelet count	Normal to increased megakaryocytes with hypolobated nuclei <5% blasts No Auer rods Isolated del(5q) cytogenetic abnormality

Adapted from Vardiman JW, Thiele J, Arber DA, et al. The 2008 revision of the World Health Organization (WHO) classification of myeloid neoplasms and acute leukemia: rationale and important changes. *Blood*. 2009;114:937–951.

DIAGNOSIS

Clinical Presentation

MDS is clinically a heterogeneous disorder. Its clinical manifestations result from marrow failure and cytopenia(s). Sometimes, the diagnosis is made retrospectively after transformation to acute leukemia. Lymph node involvement and hepatosplenomegaly are rare.

Diagnostic Testing

In the absence of other causes, marrow failure (as evidenced by cytopenias) with bone marrow findings of normal or increased cellularity with dysplastic myeloid cells is a cornerstone in establishing the diagnosis of MDS. The CBC often reveals cytopenias, and an elevated mean corpuscular volume. Reticulocyte count is inappropriately low. Peripheral blood smear may show oval macrocytic red cells, hypogranular neutrophils, and giant platelets.

- **Bone marrow biopsy** is essential in the diagnostic evaluation. The cellularity is usually normal or increased, although it can be hypocellular. Dysplastic morphological changes may not be present in all patients with MDS, and the subjectivity of the findings may pose a significant diagnostic challenge. Morphological abnormalities include megaloblastic red cell precursors with multiple nuclei and asynchronous maturation of the nucleus or cytoplasm. Ringed sideroblasts (erythroid precursors with iron-laden mitochondria) are occasionally identified. There is often a predominance of immature myeloid cells, and granulocytic precursors may show asynchronous maturation of the nucleus and cytoplasm. Mature granulocytes are often hypogranular and hypolobulated. Megakaryocytes may be smaller and have fewer nuclear lobes.
- **Recurrent cytogenetic abnormalities** are present in 40% to 70% in de novo MDS and 95% of tMDS. In cases where the clinical and laboratory features are consistent with MDS but the morphological features are ambiguous, a presumptive diagnosis of MDS can be made if a specific clonal chromosomal abnormality (Table 8-3) is present.[4] Fluorescent in situ hybridization (**FISH**) is becoming an important diagnostic tool in the evaluation of MDS. Unlike cytogenetics, which can be performed only in mitotic cells, FISH can be performed in mitotic cells as well as cells in interphase. It also has the advantage of providing quick results and has a high sensitivity and specificity. It can detect clonal cryptic defects in about 3% to 15% of MDS patients with normal cytogenetics, and may detect chromosomal abnormalities earlier in the course of the disease. However, FISH will only detect what is being looked for and hence cannot replace cytogenetics.

TREATMENT

The Federal Drug Administration (FDA) has recently approved four drugs for the treatment of MDS patients: the hypomethylating agents 5-azacytidine (azaC) and decitabine; the immunomodulator lenalidomide for patients with del (5q) subtype; and deferasirox, an iron chelator for treating chronic iron overload resulting from multiple transfusions. Supportive treatment with transfusions and growth factors is also part of MDS management. Allogeneic hematopoietic stem cell transplant

TABLE 8-3 RECURRING CHROMOSOMAL ABNORMALITIES CONSIDERED AS PRESUMPTIVE EVIDENCE OF MDS IN THE SETTING OF PERSISTENT CYTOPENIA(S) OF UNDETERMINED ORIGIN

Unbalanced Abnormalities	WHO-Estimated Frequency in MDS (%)	Balanced Abnormalities	WHO-Estimated Frequency in MDS (%)
−7 or del(7q)	10; 50 in tMDS	t(11;16)(q23;p13.3)	3 in tMDS
−5 or del(5q)	10; 40 in tMDS	t(3;21)(q26.2;q22.1)	2 in tMDS
i(17q) or t(17p)	3–5	t(1;3)(p36.3;q21.1)	<1
−13 or del(13q)	3	t(2;11)(p21;q23)	<1
del(11q)	3	inv(3)(q21q26.2)	<1
del(12p) or t(12p)	3	t(6;9)(p23;q34)	<1
del(9q)	1–2		
idic(X)(q13)	1–2		

Adapted from Steensma DP. The changing classification of myelodysplastic syndromes: what's in a name? *Hematology Am Soc Hematol Educ Program.* 2009:645–655.

(HSCT) is the primary curative treatment for patients with MDS. Features to consider for HSCT include patient's age, IPSS (International Prognostic Scoring System) score, performance status, comorbidities, and availability of a suitable donor. Higher-risk patients ≤60 years of age should be offered a human leukocyte antigen (HLA) identical sibling transplant at diagnosis (if otherwise feasible), whereas delaying transplantation for several years and prior to disease progression would be appropriate for lower-risk patients. In patients who require reduction of their disease burden prior to HSCT, azaC, decitabine, or participation in clinical trials can be used as bridges to transplant.[5] The role of reduced-intensity regimens in patients of advanced age or with other comorbidities remains to be determined.

- **Lower-risk MDS**

For patients with lower-risk MDS, treatment is aimed at reducing transfusions, restoring effective blood cell production and maximizing quality of life. For lower-risk MDS patients with symptomatic anemia, treatment follows one of several pathways. In patients with MDS del(5q), lenalidomide, a derivative of thalidomide, is the treatment of choice. In this population, 70% experience transfusion independence or a decline in transfusion needs when treated with lenalidomide. Lenalidomide, like thalidomide, inhibits angiogenesis, alters cellular immune responses, modulates various cytokines, and has direct antileukemic, antiproliferative effects. In addition, lenalidomide also enhances erythropoietin (EPO) receptor signaling. It is more potent and has a favorable side-effect profile compared to thalidomide. Its dose-limiting side effects include neutropenia and thrombocytopenia.

- In other lower-risk MDS patients lacking del(5q), erythropoiesis stimulating agents (ESAs), which include epoetin and darbepoetin, may be appropriate. Patients with low transfusion needs, defined as <2 units of packed red blood cells (PRBCs) monthly, and a low baseline serum erythropoietin level (<500 IU) have a 74% chance of responding to ESAs. Consequently, ESAs, with or without granulocyte colony stimulating factor (GCSF), are appropriate initial treatment for these patients.
- On the other hand, patients with higher transfusion needs (≥2 units of PRBCs) and high serum erythropoietin level (≥500 IU) have only a 7% chance of responding to ESAs. Patients with age ≤60 years, hypocellular marrows, HLA-DR15 histocompatibility type, or PNH clone positivity, have a good probability of responding to immunosuppressive therapy (IST) with antithymocyte globulin (ATG) or cyclosporin A. Those who are deemed unlikely to respond to IST should be treated with hypomethylating agents. Lenalidomide can also be considered.

• **Higher-risk MDS**

For patients with higher-risk MDS, the goals of treatment are similar to patients with AML, and include attaining a partial or complete remission, prolonging survival and also maximizing quality of life if patients are candidates for high-intensity therapy, allogeneic HSCT is recommended if a suitable donor can be identified. Patients without a suitable donor should be treated with a hypomethylating agent such as azaC or decitabine, or high intensity chemotherapy. For higher-risk MDS patients who are not candidates for high-intensity therapy, treatment with hypomethylating agents is appropriate.

PROGNOSIS

Evolution to AML occurs in 10% to 50% of all cases of MDS; it varies with the MDS subtypes and correlates with the survival duration. The IPSS for MDS (Table 8-4) developed in 1997 continues to be one of the most widely used prognostic tools, despite its shortcomings.[6] It should be noted that the IPSS is only validated in previously untreated patients. Furthermore, in 2001, the WHO changed the acute leukemia-defining marrow blast threshold from 30% to 20%, making the IPSS appear dated. Much debate revolves around the classification of the patients with 20% to 30% blasts, who appear to represent a heterogeneous group with characteristics that differ from classic AML. The IPSS score does not take into account the severity of cytopenias, and has been criticized for overemphasizing the significance of marrow blast proportion while underemphasizing high-risk karyotypic findings. Lower-risk MDS patients (RA, RARS, RCUD, RCMD, MDS-U MDS del(5q), IPSS low or Int-1) have an estimated survival of 3 to 10 years. Higher-risk MDS patients (RAEB-1 or RAEB-2, IPSS Int-2 or high) have an estimated survival of <1.5 years, and a high rate of AML transformation.[7]

APLASTIC ANEMIAS

GENERAL PRINCIPLES

Aplastic anemias (AA) refer to conditions in which normal hematopoietic tissue is replaced by fat. They are characterized by pancytopenia and a hypocellular bone

TABLE 8-4 INTERNATIONAL PROGNOSTIC SCORING SYSTEM FOR MDS

Points	Bone Marrow Blasts (%)	Karyotype[a]	Cytopenias[b]
0	<5	Good	0 or 1
0.5	5–10	Intermediate	2 or 3
1.0	—	Poor	
1.5	11–20		
2.0	21–30		

Percentage marrow blasts, karyotype, and cytopenias are each assigned point values, which are then added together to derive the patient's risk score. Scores for risk groups are as follows: Low 0; INT-1 0.5–1.0; INT-2 1.5–2.0; and High >= 2.5.

[a]Good prognosis karyotypes = normal, –Y only, del(5q) only, del(20q) only; Intermediate = trisomy 8; Poor = complex defects, monosomy 7.

[b]Cytopenias defined as follows: hemoglobin <10 g/dL; absolute neutrophil count $<1.5 \times 10^9$; platelet count $<100 \times 10^9$/L.

Modified from Greenberg P, Cox C, LeBeau MM, et al. International scoring system for evaluating prognosis in myelodysplastic syndromes. *Blood.* 1997;89:2079–2088.

marrow in the absence of bone marrow infiltration and increased reticulin deposition. AA can be acquired or arise in the context of an inherited bone marrow failure syndrome. AA can coexist with other conditions such as PNH (discussed in the next section) and T-cell large granular lymphocyte (T-LGL) disease. Approximately 40% to 50% of patients with acquired AA have expanded populations of PNH cells.[8]

Epidemiology

Acquired AA is a rare disease. The incidence is estimated to be about two cases per million per year in Western countries, and about two- to threefold higher in Asia. Almost half of the cases occur during the first 3 decades of life.[8]

Classification

AA can be acquired or inherited. Table 8-1 outlines several forms of inherited AA.[1] In the presence of an empty marrow, pancytopenia, and transfusion dependence, the severity of the disease is based on the absolute neutrophil count (ANC). In nonsevere AA, the ANC is $>0.5 \times 10^9$/L. In severe AA, the ANC is between 0.2 and 0.5×10^9/L. In very severe AA, the ANC is $<0.2 \times 10^9$/L.[9]

Etiology

The genetic aberrations associated with inherited bone marrow failure are listed in Table 8-1. The rarity of acquired AA is accounted for by a combination of infrequent exposure events, diversity of predisposing genetic factors, and individual differences in immune response. Table 8-5 lists some of the factors thought to be associated with acquired AA.[10]

TABLE 8-5 FACTORS THOUGHT TO BE ASSOCIATED WITH DEVELOPMENT OF SEVERE APLASTIC ANEMIA

Idiopathic
Infections
Hepatitis A, B, C—nonserological
Epstein–Barr virus
Cytomegalovirus
Mycobacterial infections
Human immunodeficiency virus
Parvovirus B19
Drugs and chemicals
Gold salts
Chloramphenicol
Carbamazepine
Sulfonamides
Nonsteroidal anti-inflammatory drugs
Antiepileptic and psychotropic agents
Cardiovascular drugs
Penicillamine
Allopurinol
Benzene
Pesticides
PNH
Graft-versus-host disease (GVHD)
Pregnancy
Eosinophilic fasciitis

Modified from Valdez JM, Scheinberg P, Young NS, Walsh TJ. Infections in patients with aplastic anemia. *Semin Hematol.* 2009;46:269–76.

Pathophysiology

The pathophysiology of acquired AA is an immune-mediated attack on the hematopoietic stem cells in most cases, caused by activated cytotoxic T cells bearing the Th1 profile. These activated T cells produce cytokines such as interferon-gamma (IFN-γ) and tumor necrosis factor-alpha (TNF-α). Fas ligand expression is induced by IFN-γ and TNF-α. Binding of Fas ligand to the Fas receptor on hematopoietic stem cells could contribute to marrow aplasia by triggering apoptosis. The reason for T cell activation remains unclear. It is possible that an inciting event like an infection, toxin, or a drug exposure provokes the aberrant immune response. HLA-DR2 is overexpressed in patients with AA. Recent data also implicate intrinsic defects in hematopoietic stem cells. Mutations in the genes for telomerase, TERC and TERT, have been described in patients without overt clinical stigmata of dyskeratosis congenita. Telomere shortening is observed in one third to one half of patients with AA. Accelerated telomere shortening may result in premature death of rapidly proliferating cells.

DIAGNOSIS

Clinical Presentation

Patients with AA present with symptoms related to pancytopenia. The presence of weight loss, pain, loss of appetite, or fever suggests another diagnosis. Physical examination usually reveals pallor, mucosal bleeding, petechiae, and ecchymoses. The presence of lymphadenopathy, hepatomegaly, or splenomegaly strongly suggests another diagnosis such as lymphoma, leukemia, or bone marrow infiltration.

Diagnostic Testing

The diagnosis is established by **bone marrow aspiration and biopsy.** The findings include a profoundly hypocellular marrow with a decrease in all cellular elements, with marrow space being replaced by fat cells and stromal elements. The residual hematopoietic elements are morphologically normal. There is no increased reticulin formation or infiltrative elements. Evaluation for other etiologies of pancytopenia includes viral serologies for hepatitis, CMV, EBV, parvovirus, HIV, and herpes. Serum B_{12} and folate levels should be determined. As an underlying cause of AA is Fanconi anemia (FA), even in adults without other classic features of FA, diepoxybutane (DEB) or mitomyin C testing to exclude chromosome fragility should be considered. Evaluation for the presence of a PNH clone is also part of the workup. T-LGL, a rare condition characterized by an increase in the number of circulating T cells bearing the CD57 activation marker of effector/cytotoxic T cells, should be considered if increased large granular lymphocytes are noted on examination of the peripheral blood smear or if the patient has a history of rheumatoid arthritis.

TREATMENT

Management of AA includes supportive care as initial treatment to sustain an acutely ill, pancytopenic patient. Immunosuppression and allogeneic HSCT are the main therapeutic approaches.[8,9]

- **Supportive care.** Patients with symptomatic anemia will need transfusions. Patients with symptomatic thrombocytopenia or a platelet count of <10,000 should be given platelets. Blood products should be irradiated to prevent transfusion-associated GVHD. In patients who are considered for stem cell transplantation, only CMV-negative products should be administered to CMV IgG-negative patients, and blood products from family members should be avoided to prevent alloimmunization. EPO and myeloid factors are not used as a mainstay of treatment. No significant survival in survival has been seen in patients receiving G-CSF as compared to those who did not receive G-CSF.
- **Immunosuppression.** ATG with cyclosporine is indicated as first-line therapy for nonsevere AA patients who are transfusion dependent, severe AA patients >40 years of age, and severe AA patients <40 years of age who lack an HLA-identical sibling donor. Response to ATG occurs in around 50% of patients by 3 months, and 70% to 75% by 6 months. Relapses occur in up to 30% to 35% of patients when cyclosporine is withdrawn at 6 months.

- **HSCT.** Patients with severe AA <40 years of age with an HLA-matched sibling donor should be offered HSCT as first-line treatment. The 5-year survival is 77%. In children and minimally transfused patients, survival of 80% to 90% can be routinely achieved. Acute GVHD occurs in about 20% to 30% of patients. Chronic GVHD is a major cause of morbidity and mortality in patients who survived more than 2 years post transplantation, and life-long immunosuppression is often needed. Chronic GVHD occurs in about 30% to 40% of patients. As a matched sibling donor is available in only about 20% to 30% of cases, alternative sources of hematopoietic stem cells have been sought. HSCT from unrelated donor carries higher morbidity and mortality than HSCT from a matched sibling donor, and are therefore reserved for patients who lack a matched sibling donor and who failed to respond to one or more rounds of immunosuppression.

PROGNOSIS

Without treatment, patients with severe or very severe AA will eventually succumb to infections or hemorrhagic complications. Spontaneous remission can be seen with drug-induced AA and usually occurs within 2 months of presentation. Overall survival after immunosuppression for AA is approximately 75% at 5 years. This equates with survival after HSCT. For patients treated with immunosuppression, long-term follow-up data indicated an actuarial probability of developing hemolytic PNH at 11 years of 10%, MDS or AML 8%, and a solid tumor 11%.

PAROXYSMAL NOCTURNAL HEMOGLOBINURIA

GENERAL PRINCIPLES

PNH is an acquired disease characterized by nonmalignant clonal expansion of one or more hematopoietic stem cells that have undergone somatic mutation of the PIG-A gene. PNH can present with bone marrow failure, hemolytic anemia, smooth muscle dystonias, and thrombosis. PNH can arise de novo or in the setting of AA.[11]

Pathophysiology

The protein encoded by the PIG-A gene is essential for the synthesis of glycosyl phosphatidylinositol (GPI), and therefore GPI-linked proteins are lacking in the PIG-A mutant clone. PNH RBCs lack two GPI-anchored complement regulatory proteins, CD55 and CD59. Hemolysis in PNH results from increased susceptibility of PNH RBCs to complement-mediated destruction. Intravascular hemolysis releases free hemoglobin into circulation. Free plasma hemoglobin scavenges nitric oxide (NO) and the depletion of NO at the tissue level is postulated to account for multiple PNH manifestations, including esophageal spasm, male erectile dysfunction, renal insufficiency and thrombosis. The PNH clone is present in a considerable proportion of the general population without symptoms. In patients with PNH, the clone is expanded significantly. It is postulated that PNH patients have some degree of marrow failure and the PNH clone is selectively protected from bone marrow injury as result of the lack of GPI-linked proteins.

DIAGNOSIS

Clinical Presentation

The clinical manifestations of PNH are **intravascular hemolytic anemia, marrow failure,** and **thrombosis.** Bone marrow failure can be transient, mild, or severe. Thrombosis usually involves the venous system and occurs in about 40% of PNH patients. Thrombosis can occur in unusual sites such as intra-abdominal veins. The clinical course is unpredictable and patients can have spontaneous remissions. PNH can present with or without evidence of another disorder such as AA or MDS. Subclinical PNH (without clinical or laboratory evidence of hemolysis) can occur in association with other bone marrow failure syndromes.

Diagnostic Testing

Flow cytometry using monoclonal antibodies against specific GPI-linked proteins is the most sensitive and specific test to identify the PNH clone. Fluorescein-labeled proaerolysin variant (FLAER) is increasingly used as a flow cytometric assay to diagnose PNH. The hemolysis is intravascular (high reticulocyte count, increased lactate dehydrogenase and unconjugated bilirubin, and decreased haptoglobulin) and is Coombs negative. Iron studies are needed to evaluate for iron-deficiency anemia, which can result from renal loss of hemoglobin. Bone marrow biopsy is helpful in assessing for marrow failure.

TREATMENT

There are no clear evidence-based indications for treatment of PNH. For asymptomatic patients or those with mild symptoms, watchful waiting is an appropriate approach. For patients with underlying AA, treatment is directed toward the underlying bone marrow failure. **Indications for treatment** in classic PNH include disabling fatigue, thromboses, transfusion dependence, frequent pain paroxysms, renal insufficiency, or other end-organ complications. Corticosteroids can improve hemoglobin levels and reduce hemolysis in some PNH patients, but its long-term use is limited because of toxicity. Complement inhibition and HSCT are established effective therapies for PNH.

- **Complement inhibition. Eculizumab,** a humanized monoclonal antibody against complement C5, inhibits terminal complement activation.[12] It has been approved by the FDA for use in PNH. Eculizumab is effective in decreasing intravascular hemolysis, need for blood transfusions, and risk of thrombosis. Eculizumab is administered intravenously at a dose of 600 mg weekly for the first 4 weeks, then 900 mg biweekly starting on week 5. It is well tolerated, but must be continued indefinitely as it does not treat the underlying cause. Its serious adverse effects include risk of infection by encapsulated organisms. Patients receiving eculizumab should be vaccinated against *Neisseria meningitides* prior to starting therapy.
- **HSCT.** Allogeneic HSCT remain the only curative therapy for PNH, but it is associated with significant morbidity and mortality. Currently there is no definite indication for transplantation. Patients with life-threatening thrombosis and underlying severe BM failure should be considered for transplantation.

- **Treatment of thrombosis.** Thrombosis is a life-threatening complication of PNH and should be treated promptly with anticoagulation. However, anticoagulation is only partially effective in preventing clots, and treatment with eculizumab should be strongly considered in patients with thrombosis. The duration of anticoagulation after initiation of eculizumab is controversial in these patients. Likewise, the role of prophylactic anticoagulation in PNH is also controversial.

PROGNOSIS

The natural history of PNH is highly variable. Median survival is 10 to 15 years. Thrombosis is the leading cause of death. Patients with PNH may also develop life-threatening bone marrow failure, MDS, or leukemia. Patients with AA and a PNH clone typically do not exhibit signs or symptoms of PNH early in the natural history of their disease, but many will experience further expansion of the PIG-A mutant clone and progress to classic PNH.

REFERENCES

1. Shimamura A. Clinical approach to marrow failure. *Hematology Am Soc Hematol Educ Program.* 2009:329–337.
2. Strom SS, Velez-Bravo V, Estey EH. Epidemiology of myelodysplastic syndromes. *Semin Hematol.* 2008;45:8–13.
3. Vardiman JW, Thiele J, Arber DA, et al. The 2008 revision of the World Health Organization (WHO) classification of myeloid neoplasms and acute leukemia: rationale and important changes. *Blood.* 2009;114:937–951.
4. Steensma DP. The changing classification of myelodysplastic syndromes: what's in a name? *Hematology Am Soc Hematol Educ Program.* 2009:645–655.
5. Greenberg PL. Current therapeutic approaches for patients with myelodysplastic syndromes. *Br J Haematol.* 150:131–143.
6. Greenberg P, Cox C, LeBeau MM, et al. International scoring system for evaluating prognosis in myelodysplastic syndromes. *Blood.* 1997;89:2079–2088.
7. Sekeres MA. Treatment of MDS: something old, something new, something borrowed. *Hematology Am Soc Hematol Educ Program.* 2009:656–663.
8. Young NS, Scheinberg P, Calado RT. Aplastic anemia. *Curr Opin Hematol.* 2008;15:162–168.
9. Bacigalupo A. Aplastic anemia: pathogenesis and treatment. *Hematology Am Soc Hematol Educ Program.* 2007:23–28.
10. Vawldez JM, Scheinberg P, Young NS, Walsh TJ. Infections in patients with aplastic anemia. *Semin Hematol.* 2009;46:269–276.
11. Brodsky RA. How I treat paroxysmal nocturnal hemoglobinuria. *Blood.* 2009;113:6522–6527.
12. Brodsky RA, Young NS, Antonioli E, et al. Multicenter phase 3 study of the complement inhibitor eculizumab for the treatment of patients with paroxysmal nocturnal hemoglobinuria. *Blood.* 2008;111:1840–1847.

Myeloproliferative Disorders

9

George Ansstas

GENERAL PRINCIPLES

The myeloproliferative disorders (MPDs) are a group of clonal diseases characterized by overproduction of mature, largely functional cells arising from the transformation of a clonal hematopoietic stem cell. The World Health Organization (WHO) has designated seven conditions as MPDs (Table 9-1). Philadelphia chromosome-positive chronic myeloid leukemia (CML) is discussed in the chapter on leukemias (Chap. 29). Collectively, these disorders are uncommon. They share the signs and symptoms of hepatosplenomegaly, hypercatabolism, clonal marrow hyperplasia without dysplasia, and increased numbers of one or more cell lines. They are typically indolent and chronic in nature but may evolve into acute leukemia. Recent description of the activating Janus kinase 2 (JAK2) mutation V617F in many of these disorders links them with a common pathophysiology. Although of clear clinical importance, this mutation is still being incorporated into diagnostic, prognostic, and treatment algorithms.

POLYCYTHEMIA VERA

GENERAL PRINCIPLES

Definition

Polycythemia vera (PV) is a monoclonal stem cell disease characterized by proliferation of a multipotent stem cell with trilineage hyperplasia resulting primarily in expansion of the RBC line. Recently, the **activating JAK2 V617F mutation has been noted in nearly all patients.** JAK2 is an essential kinase in the erythropoietin (EPO) receptor signal transduction pathway. Constitutive JAK2 kinase activity results in EPO-independent proliferation of erythrocyte precursors. JAK2 is also involved in the JAK2-STAT5 pathways of the thrombopoietin (TPO) receptor (Mpl) and the granulocyte colony-stimulating factor receptor (GCSF-R). The V617F mutation can thus lead to proliferation of multiple cell lines, and patients with PV often have elevated platelets and leukocytes as well.[1]

Epidemiology

PV is the most common of the MPDs, with an incidence of ~2 in 100,000 people. The average age of PV patients is 60 years, but it occurs across all age groups, with a male predominance. Although familial clustering does exist, it is uncommon, and the JAK2 mutation is acquired somatically, suggesting a separate predisposition pathway.

TABLE 9-1 MUTATIONAL AND WHO CLASSIFICATION OF MYELOPROLIFERATIVE DISORDERS

BCR-ABL Positive	BCR-ABL Negative	JAK2V617F
Chronic myeloid leukemia	Polycythemia vera	~95%
	Essential thrombocythemia	50%–60%
	Chronic idiopathic myelofibrosis	35%–55%
		1%–5%
	Chronic neutrophilic leukemia	
	Chronic eosinophilic leukemia/hypereosinophilic syndrome	
	Myeloproliferative disease, unclassifiable	

Etiology

Etiology is not clear but the following observations have been made:

- Clonal cytogenetic abnormalities are associated with the disorder in ~30% of patients, mainly deletion of long arm of chromosome 20, trisomy of chromosome 8 or 9, or loss of heterozygosity on short arm of chromosome 9. The *JAK2* gene is located on the short arm of chromosome 9.
- Up to 97% of patients have an activating mutation in *JAK2* (V617F), which is also seen in other MPDs.
- There is impaired post-translational processing of the TPO receptor, Mpl, leading to decreased expression on platelets and megakaryocytes. Thus, proliferation of platelet in PV may be independent of TPO.
- BCL-X_L, an apoptosis-inhibiting oncoprotein, is overexpressed in erythroid cells.
- Bone marrow shows erythroid progenitor cell proliferation in the absence of EPO stimulation.

Risk Factors

None known.

Clinical Course

- PV is a chronic disorder and may be characterized as having phases during its course. The **preerythrocytic phase** is generally asymptomatic, with an isolated increase in platelets or RBCs. Patients may experience trivial pruritus and may have mild splenomegaly. This progresses to the **erythrocytic phase,** characterized by erythrocytosis requiring regular phlebotomy as well as increased granulocytes and platelet counts. Splenomegaly, pruritus, thrombosis, and hemorrhage may be present. This may last for a number of years. The **spent phase** is characterized by a reduced need for phlebotomy. Thrombocytosis and leukocytosis persist, and splenomegaly is progressive.
- Up to 50% of patients may progress to a clinical picture difficult to differentiate from that of idiopathic myelofibrosis. Anemia develops, and the peripheral

smear shows a leukoerythroblastic picture with teardrop poikilocytes, nucleated red cells, and anisocytosis. Immature granulocytes are seen, with a slight increase in basophils, and platelets are often abnormal in morphology. Splenomegaly worsens, and there are increased systemic symptoms. Acute myeloid leukemia (AML) may occur in up to 20% of patients, and the risk is increased in patients treated with alkylating agents. The incidence of progression to AML is higher in patients with myelofibrosis.

- Thrombotic risk is present throughout the course of PV and may be linked to elevated, dysfunctional leukocytes or platelets. Reduction of thrombotic risk is a mainstay of therapy, and recurrent thrombosis can be common.

DIAGNOSIS

Clinical Presentation

Patients are often asymptomatic at presentation; however, they may present with symptoms related to increased RBC mass and hyperviscosity. Symptoms may include headache, weakness, peptic ulcer disease, hyperhydrosis, vision changes, tinnitus, and vertigo. In addition, many patients experience pruritus, especially with exposure to hot water. Erythromelalgia, due to microarteriolar occlusion, is characterized by a burning sensation in the digits and may be severe. Patients are also predisposed to thrombosis and, less often, hemorrhage. Many of these symptoms have been attributed to hyperviscosity, but dysfunction of leukocytes and platelets may also play an important role. Physical exam findings include splenomegaly, hepatomegaly, hypertension, and plethora.

Diagnostic Criteria

The Polycythemia Vera Study Group established diagnostic criteria >30 years ago. These are currently in flux, as they include neither EPO levels nor the JAK2 mutation. At Washington University, we have adopted the Campbell-proposed criteria based on JAK2 status, with modifications of the Polycythemia Vera Study Group criteria (Table 9-2).[2] Patients with JAK2-positive PV have a hematocrit >52% in men or >48% in women or an increased red cell mass (>25% above predicted) and a documented mutation. Ninety-five percent to 97% of patients with PV test positive either in exon 14 or in exon 12. Patients with suspected PV and negative exon 14 V617F JAK2 mutation should be tested for JAK2 exon 12 mutations.[3] JAK2-negative PV is much less common and should prompt a careful examination for secondary causes of polycythemia.

Differential Diagnosis

Patients with secondary polycythemia typically have elevated EPO levels caused by chronic hypoxemia, heavy smoking, renal disease, or malignancies such as renal cell cancer, hepatocellular cancer, and hemangioblastoma. Rare conditions such as congenital polycythemia with augmented hypoxia sensing and high–oxygen affinity hemoglobin mutants should be considered. Relative polycythemia, or pseudopolycythemia, is associated with a normal red cell mass and decreased plasma volume secondary to causes such as dehydration, diuretics, and burns. In cases of JAK2-negative polycythemia with low-normal EPO levels, *BCR-ABL* rearrangements should be evaluated, as CML may present with many of the same features.

TABLE 9-2 DIAGNOSTIC CRITERIA FOR POLYCYTHEMIA VERA AND ESSENTIAL THROMBOCYTHEMIA

Polycythemia Vera	Essential Thrombocytosis
JAK2 positive	
Hct >52%, males Hct >48%, females	Platelets >450 × 10⁶/mL No other malignancy
JAK2 negative	
4 major or 3 major + 2 minor: *Major:* • Hct >60% (males) or >56% (females) • No secondary erythrocytosis • Palpable splenomegaly • Acquired genetic abnormalities (excluding JAK2 and BCR-ABL) *Minor:* • Platelets >450 × 10⁶/mL • Neutrophils >10 × 10⁶/mL • Radiographic splenomegaly • Low serum erythropoietin	All of the following: • Platelets >600 × 10⁶/mL on 2 occasions 1 month apart • No cause for reactive thrombocytosis • Ferritin >20 μg/L • No other myeloproliferative disease or myelodysplasia

—
Adapted from Campbell PJ, Green AR. The myeloproliferative disorders. *N Engl J Med.* 2006;355:2452–2466.

Diagnostic Testing

- The diagnosis is suspected when blood counts reveal an elevated hematocrit (Hct). The **EPO level is low** (<20 mU/mL) and often undetectable. The **JAK2 V617F mutation** is seen in nearly all patients. Leukocyte alkaline phosphatase scores, vitamin B_{12}, and uric acid levels may be elevated but are nonspecific findings. These patients also have an elevated RBC mass as demonstrated by ^{51}Cr labeling of RBCs and isotope dilution, although this is rarely tested now. In addition, ~60% of patients have elevated granulocyte counts, and 50% have thrombocytosis.
- The **peripheral smear** may show microcytic, hypochromic RBCs with anisocytosis and poikilocytosis, reflecting exhaustion of iron stores due to increased hemoglobin (Hgb) synthesis. WBCs generally have normal morphology, but there are often increased basophils, eosinophils, and immature forms. Platelets occasionally have an abnormal morphology, with megathrombocytes seen on the smear.
- **Bone marrow biopsy** findings are not diagnostic of PV, but biopsy is frequently performed to evaluate fibrosis and cytogenetics even when the diagnosis is not in question. Findings include hypercellular marrow with trilineage hyperplasia and clustered megakaryocytes with hypolobulated nuclei. Approximately 30% of PV patients will have an abnormal karyotype. Common karyotype changes include trisomy 9 (amplification of JAK2), trisomy 8 (also found in other MPDs, myelodysplastic syndrome, AML), trisomy 1q (unclear significance), del 5q and del 7q (more often seen after cytotoxic therapy), and del 13q (also associated with idiopathic myelofibrosis and chronic lymphocytic leukemia).

TREATMENT

The goals of treatment are to reduce the blood volume to normal and to prevent thrombotic and hemorrhagic complications. **Thrombotic risk** has been associated with an age >60 years, prior thrombosis, and a platelet count $>1000 \times 10^9$/L. Thrombocytosis clearly increases thrombotic risk, and this risk appears to be a continuum, with increased risk starting at 400×10^9/L and peaking at 900×10^9/L. Hemorrhagic risk increases with platelet counts $>1500 \times 10^9$/L. Emerging risk factors include leukocyte counts $>15 \times 10^9$/L and cardiovascular factors such as smoking, obesity, hypertension, hypercholesterolemia, diabetes, and coronary artery disease (Table 9-3).

- **Low-risk patients** are <60 years old and have no history of thrombosis, no cardiovascular risk factors, and platelet counts $<1500 \times 10^9$/L. These patients are managed with phlebotomy to an Hct of <45% and low-dose aspirin. Iron deficiency via phlebotomy is a goal of treatment.
- **High-risk patients** are ≥60 years old or have a history of a thrombotic event, or cardiovascular risk factors, or platelet counts $>1500 \times 10^9$/L. These patients typically require cytoreductive agents in addition to phlebotomy, and aspirin is usually held off until platelet counts are $<1500 \times 10^9$/L.
- Treatment for **intermediate-risk patients** must be individualized, as data are insufficient to clearly support either a conservative (low-risk) or an aggressive (high-risk) treatment plan. Typically, these patients are treated with phlebotomy, aspirin, and management of cardiovascular risk factors to limit thrombotic risk. Patients with elevated platelets ($>400 \times 10^9$ to 600×10^9/L) or elevated leukocytes ($>15 \times 10^9$/L) may need to be treated more like high-risk patients.

Medications

Hydroxyurea, interferon-alpha, and anagrelide are the most commonly used cytoreductive agents.

- **Hydroxyurea** acts to decrease all three blood lines. It has been particularly useful in patients with extensive pruritus. Long-term use of hydroxyurea has been

TABLE 9-3 THROMBOTIC RISK FACTORS IN POLYCYTHEMIA VERA AND ESSENTIAL THROMBOCYTHEMIA

Thrombotic risk factors typically requiring cytoreduction
Age >60
Prior thrombosis
Platelets $>400 \times 10^9$–600×10^9/L
Emerging thrombotic risk factors: treatment is individualized
Cardiovascular risk factors: smoking, obesity, hypertension, hypercholesterolemia, diabetes, coronary artery disease
Leukocytes $>15 \times 10^9$/L: polycythemia vera
Leukocytes $>8.7 \times 10^9$/L: essential thrombocythemia

suggested to increase the risk of leukemogenesis (mean time to transformation ~15 years). This has been difficult to assess in MPD patients, who already have an underlying propensity toward leukemic evolution. However, in other diseases, such as sickle cell anemia, leukemogenic risk has not been seen. Long follow-up of prospective trials will be required to definitively answer this question, and some authors currently prefer its use in the elderly more than in those younger than 60 years. Hydroxyurea is generally well tolerated but may cause erythema, hyperpigmentation, and distal leg ulcers. Gastrointestinal symptoms of nausea, vomiting, constipation, and diarrhea are very common with doses >60 mg/kg.

- **Interferon-alpha** decreases both the red cell number and the frequency of thrombohemorrhagic events. As in CML, it affects the stem cell compartment, and reversal of JAK2 mutational status can be seen. It must be administered subcutaneously and can cause fever, arthralgias, myalgias, alopecia, anorexia, peripheral neuropathies, and depression. ACE inhibitors should be avoided with interferon-alpha, as this may lead to granulocytopenia and thrombocytopenia.
- **Anagrelide** primarily effects platelet production and is more commonly used in PV for thrombocytosis. Side effects include palpitations, tachycardia, nausea, diarrhea, and fluid retention.
- Agents such as **radioactive phosphorus** and **alkylating agents** also are cytoreductive but are associated with increased transformation to AML and are rarely used today. Radioactive ^{32}P may have a role in noncompliant patients with life expectancy <10 years.
- Additional agents can be useful in symptom management. **Hyperuricemia** may be treated with allopurinol. **Erythromelalgia** may be treated with aspirin or other non-steroidal anti-inflammatory drugs. **Hemorrhage** should be managed with platelet transfusion, since platelets have abnormal function in PV. **Pruritus** is often poorly responsive to antihistamines but may respond to cimetidine or cyproheptadine. If these agents fail, cytoreductive agents may be needed.

SPECIAL CONSIDERATIONS

- **Surgery.** Elective surgery should be avoided in patients with poorly controlled polycythemia, as 75% will have hemorrhagic or thrombotic complications, and mortality is high. Platelet counts and Hct should be controlled for at least 2 months before surgery, if possible. Thromboembolic prophylaxis should be used as well. Splenectomy is rarely recommended in PV patients because of the high risk of surgical complications.
- **Polycythemia vera and pregnancy.** There is an increased incidence of premature births, preeclampsia, and hemorrhage in PV patients. Management should include phlebotomy and low-dose aspirin. Aspirin should be discontinued ~5 days prior to delivery to limit hemorrhagic risk. If cytotoxic treatment is needed, interferon-alpha is the agent of choice, as it has not been shown to be teratogenic or leukemogenic.

OUTCOME/PROGNOSIS

Patients with PV who are treated have a mortality rate similar to that of age-matched controls. Death is secondary to thrombosis in 30% to 40% of patients. Myelofibrosis is the cause of death in ~5% of patients, and hemorrhage is the cause in 2% to 10% of patients.

ESSENTIAL THROMBOCYTHEMIA OR ESSENTIAL THROMBOCYTOSIS

GENERAL PRINCIPLES

Definition

Essential thrombocythemia or essential thrombocytosis (ET) is a stem cell disorder whose distinguishing characteristic is a markedly elevated platelet count caused by excessive megakaryocyte proliferation. The activating JAK2 V617F mutation is seen in nearly half of patients with ET, and patients also may have other clinical features of PV. Studies of X chromosome inactivation suggest that ET is a heterogeneous disease and both monoclonal and polyclonal evolution has been noted.

Epidemiology

ET occurs at an incidence of between 1.5 and 2.5 cases per 100,000. Most patients are >50 years old, and there is a female predominance.

Pathophysiology

Neither TPO nor its receptor (c-Mpl) has been implicated in the pathogenesis of ET. Mutations involving the *c-Mpl* gene are only rarely identified in ET,[4] and endogenous megakaryocyte colony growth does not appear to be dependent on an autocrine stimulation involving TPO. This is in contrast to autosomal dominant familial ET where activating mutations in the genes for TPO or c-Mpl, or mutations in the genes for other proteins, are responsible for TPO-mediated thrombocytosis.

Serum TPO levels in ET have been reported to be inappropriately normal or elevated. This unexpected finding may be a result of increased bone marrow stromal production of TPO or decreased ligand clearance associated with reduced platelet c-Mpl expression in patients with ET.

DIAGNOSIS

Clinical Presentation

Symptoms generally are related to hemorrhage and vaso-occlusion, although most patients are asymptomatic at diagnosis. Bleeding is commonly from mucous membranes, skin, and GI tract and is rarely life threatening. Vaso-occlusion may cause erythromelalgia (burning pain, increased skin warmth, and erythema of the feet and hands), transient ischemic attacks, visual disturbances, headache, seizures, and dizziness. Large vessel involvement has also been reported with myocardial infarction and cerebrovascular accidents. A small percentage of patients may experience pruritus. Physical exam findings are generally limited to splenomegaly and easy bruising.

Diagnostic Testing

Patients have an **elevated platelet count,** with large platelets visible on **peripheral smear.** Granulocytes may be increased, with mild basophilia and rare early forms. Serum B_{12} and leukocyte alkaline phosphatase scores are generally normal. Iron deficiency must be ruled out. **Bone marrow findings** are commonly nondiagnostic and include hypercellularity with granulocyte hyperplasia and increased megakaryocytes. The megakaryocytes are large, are often clustered, and may exhibit mild atypia. JAK2 V619F is seen in nearly half of ET patients.

At Washington University, we have begun incorporating **JAK2 status** into the diagnostic criteria (Table 9-2). **Other causes of reactive (secondary) thrombocytosis should be carefully investigated** and include splenectomy, trauma, cancer, acute and chronic inflammation, infection, and iron deficiency. C-reactive protein and sedimentation rate can be useful in this evaluation. If iron stores are absent, iron replacement is initiated, which may uncover PV in some patients. Philadelphia chromosome also should be evaluated to rule out CML. Ultimately, bone marrow biopsy may be required to differentiate ET from myelodysplastic syndromes.

TREATMENT

The goals of treatment focus on maintaining platelet counts of $<600 \times 10^9$/L ($<400 \times 10^9$/L if possible) and limiting thrombo-hemorrhagic risk. **Thrombotic risk** has been linked to age (>60 years old), prior thrombosis, and platelet count $>400 \times 10^9$ to 600×10^9/L. Other risk factors that are still emerging and being validated include elevated leukocytes ($>8.7 \times 10^9$/L), positive JAK2 V617F mutation, and cardiovascular risk factors such as diabetes, obesity, smoking, hypertension, hyperlipidemia, and hypercholesterolemia (Table 9-3).

- **Low-risk patients** are <60 years old, with no prior thrombotic event and a platelet count $<400 \times 10^9$ to 600×10^9/L. These patients are managed with low-dose aspirin and observation.
- **High-risk patients** are >60 years old or have a history of thrombosis. These patients require cytoreductive agents such as hydroxyurea, interferon-alpha, and anagrelide, with aggressive treatment of reversible risk factors.
- **Intermediate-risk patients** require individualized therapy.
- **Aspirin** is commonly used to prevent thrombosis but should be withheld once platelet counts are $>1500 \times 10^9$/L due to bleeding risk. Extreme thrombocytosis may promote the abnormal adsorption of large von Willebrand factor (vWF) multimers and result in a hemostatic defect. Accordingly, such patients should be screened for the presence of acquired von Willebrand disease (vWD). Low-dose aspirin therapy (e.g., <100 mg/d) is acceptable if the ristocetin cofactor level is at least 30%; if <30%, all aspirin should be avoided. As discussed in the PV section above, **hydroxyurea** has been suggested to increase the risk of leukemic transformation in MPD patients (mean time to transformation ~15 years). In young patients, it is not unreasonable to start with **anagrelide,** which has not been linked to leukemogenesis. However, the combination of anagrelide and aspirin has been shown to increase the risk of bleeding compared to hydroxyurea and aspirin. In patients who require aspirin, especially those >60 years, hydroxyurea is still typically the first-line agent. In younger patients, alternatives include anagrelide monotherapy and interferon-alpha.

- **Management of thrombosis** typically requires either lifelong aspirin, for arterial thrombosis, or coumadin, for venous thrombosis. In addition, other risk factors should be aggressively managed, including platelet count, leukocyte count, and cardiovascular risk factors.
- Rarely, symptomatic, extreme thrombocytosis may be managed with **thrombopheresis**, although the results are short lived and must be combined with other modalities of therapy.
- Symptoms of **gout** may be managed with allopurinol. **Vaso-occlusive symptoms** may respond to aspirin alone. Like PV, **pruritus** may respond to cimetidine or cyproheptadine.

SPECIAL CONSIDERATIONS

- **Surgery.** Splenectomy poses a high risk for patients with ET and an increased platelet count and is contraindicated.
- **Essential thrombocythemia and pregnancy.** Pregnant patients are at higher risk of early miscarriage complications and are often treated with aspirin. As the pregnancy progresses, the platelet count usually decreases toward the normal range but may rebound quickly after delivery. Aspirin should be discontinued ~5 days prior to delivery to limit hemorrhagic risk.

OUTCOME/PROGNOSIS

Patients generally have an excellent prognosis and appear to have median survivals similar to those of age-matched controls. Morbidity and mortality are related to thrombotic and hemorrhagic events. Transformation to AML is relatively rare, but risk is increased in patients treated with multiple cytotoxic drugs.

CHRONIC IDIOPATHIC MYELOFIBROSIS (AGNOGENIC MYELOID METAPLASIA)

GENERAL PRINCIPLES

Definition

Chronic idiopathic myelofibrosis (CIMF) is a clonal disorder thought to arise from a primitive lymphohematopoietic precursor. Patients have clonal circulating red cells, granulocytes, and platelets, and their marrow is fibrotic due to a reactive, polyclonal proliferation of fibroblasts and other mesenchymal cells induced by the neoplastic cells. The neoplastic cells also emigrate from the marrow and establish sites of **extramedullary hematopoiesis** (myeloid metaplasia) in various sites throughout the body. One-third of cases of CIMF harbor cytogenetic abnormalities at diagnosis and often transform to AML. **Common genetic abnormalities** found in CIMF are mutations in JAK2 (35% to 55%), the retinoblastoma susceptibility gene, and the *p53* gene, as well as abnormalities of the RAS family of proto-oncogenes. Neoangiogenesis is particularly active in CIMF compared with the other myeloproliferative syndromes.

Epidemiology

CIMF is the least common of the MPDs, with an annual incidence of 0.2 to 1.5 cases per 100,000. The typical case is a male older than age 50 years. The median age at presentation is 67 years, and 70% of cases are diagnosed after age 60 years. No common etiologic factor has been identified, although there are sporadic reports of an association with radiation and benzene exposure.

DIAGNOSIS

Clinical Presentation

Two-thirds of patients are symptomatic at diagnosis from the effects of hypercatabolism, cytopenias, or extramedullary hematopoiesis (Table 9-4). Bone pain may also be a prominent feature. Splenomegaly is very common, with 85% to 100% of patients having it at diagnosis, and it is frequently progressive, with up to 35% of patients developing massive splenomegaly (extending into the pelvis). Two-thirds of patients will have hepatomegaly, and 10% will have peripheral lymphadenopathy. A minority of patients will develop portal hypertension, with the associated signs and symptoms.

Diagnostic Criteria

CIMF is diagnosed when the following are present:

- Presence of megakaryocyte proliferation and atypia, usually accompanied by reticulin and/or collagen
- WHO criteria for PV, CML, MDS, or other myeloid neoplasm not met
- Demonstration of a clonal marker (e.g., JAK2 or MPL)
- Leukoerythroblastosis
- Palpable splenomegaly
- Anemia
- Increased serum lactate dehydrogenase level

Other causes of bone marrow fibrosis should be excluded, including cancers metastatic to the marrow, CML, myelodysplasia with fibrosis, other MPDs, infection, autoimmune disorders, secondary hyperparathyroidism associated with vitamin D deficiency, and lymphoma. In addition, the marrow may not be fibrotic early in the course of the disease, further complicating the diagnosis. Careful morphologic exam of the bone marrow, as well as cytogenetic studies, may help to differentiate among disorders. The diagnosis of **osteosclerosis** is made when sclerotic lesions by x-ray are present along with the criteria for CIMF. These lesions occur in up to 50% of patients and may cause severe pain.

TABLE 9-4 CLINICAL MANIFESTATION OF CIMF

Hypercatabolic State	Extramedullary Hematopoiesis	Cytopenias
Fatigue	Splenomegaly	Anemia
Weight loss	Portal hypertension	Thrombocytopenia
Nocturnal sweating	Tumor mass effects	
Pruritus	Pulmonary hypertension	
Hyperuricemia		

Diagnostic Testing

- The **complete blood count** is usually abnormal in CIMF. Fifty percent to 70% of patients will be anemic at presentation, some severely, with 25% having an Hgb <8 g/dL. Other abnormalities are variably present: leukocytosis (50%), leucopenia (7%), thrombocytosis (28%), and thrombocytopenia (37%). The **peripheral smear** shows a leukoerythroblastic picture with teardrop poikilocytes, nucleated red cells, and anisocytosis. **Abnormalities in immunologic studies** are found in 50% of patients and include autoantibodies, polyclonal hyperglobulinemia, a positive Coombs test, and monoclonal antibodies.
- During **bone marrow biopsy,** marrow may not be attainable by aspiration secondary to fibrosis, resulting in a "dry tap." Findings on marrow exam include increased cellularity, granulocyte hyperplasia, and megakaryocyte dysplasia. Reticulin staining is increased, and variable degrees of fibrosis are present. The diagnosis is usually made by the constellation of increased marrow reticulin or collagen fibrosis, typical leukoerythroblastic peripheral blood findings, and splenomegaly in the absence of other known disorders such as ET, PV, CML, and AML-M7.

TREATMENT

Conventional therapy, including **supportive care,** does not alter the natural history of CIMF. Low-risk patients with only mild splenomegaly should initially be observed. Those with progressive organomegaly and/or leukocytosis or thrombocytosis should be initially managed with hydroxyurea. Those with painful or massive splenomegaly and those with portal hypertension should be considered for either splenic irradiation or splenectomy. Those who develop anemia in the setting of cytopenias should be treated with androgens, transfusion, and exogenous EPO. Those who develop anemia and increased WBC and/or platelet counts should be managed with corticosteroids and transfusions.

- **Splenectomy** may alleviate mass-related symptoms, portal hypertension, refractory anemia, and thrombocytopenia. Prolonged benefit has been seen; however, serious perioperative complications, including bleeding, thrombosis, and infection, occur in nearly 30% of persons. Therefore, it should be reserved for patients who have not responded to more conservative management for these symptoms. The median survival for patients undergoing splenectomy is 2 years. There is an increased risk for leukemic transformation in those individuals who undergo splenectomy.
- **Splenic irradiation** usually controls pain and other symptoms related to splenomegaly (94% of the time for a median of 6 months), but the associated toxicity is not trivial. Severe cytopenias may develop in up to 43% of irradiated patients, of which 13% may be fatal due to infections and hemorrhage. Toxicity is not related to radiation dose, so blood counts must be monitored closely with treatment. In addition, radiation therapy does not improve the anemia and, therefore, is generally used for patients who are not surgical candidates.
- **Thalidomide,** with or without a tapering course of steroids, has shown some promise in ameliorating both splenomegaly and cytopenias. Unfortunately it is poorly tolerated, with up to two-thirds of persons stopping the medication within 6 months. **Lenalidomide** may have similar benefits, with better tolerability. These

and other targeted therapies have been associated with a hyperproliferative syndrome requiring rescue hydroxyurea for leukocytosis and/or thrombocytosis.

- **Etanercept** (Enbrel, 25 mg SQ twice weekly) has been associated with improvement of constitutional symptoms (e.g., weight loss, night sweats, fatigue, fever).
- **JAK2 inhibitors** are being investigated in patients with myelofibrosis. Reductions in splenic size and relief of symptoms (e.g., pruritus, fatigue) have been reported.
- **Allogeneic stem cell transplantation** is the only therapy that offers the chance to eliminate marrow fibrosis and potentially cure patients. With standard myeloablative conditioning regimens, there is significant morbidity and mortality. Reduced-intensity conditioning regimens may abrogate some of these complications. Transplantation should be considered in young patients with a poor prognosis and a histocompatible donor.

OUTCOME/PROGNOSIS

- The course of CIMF is highly variable, and most of the morbidity and mortality is due to progressive marrow failure, thrombosis, hypersplenism, advanced age, and evolution into AML. The rate of progression to acute leukemia is ~20% over 10 years. Approximately 7% of patients will develop portal hypertension related to increased portal flow from massive splenomegaly as well as intrahepatic obstruction related to thrombosis in small portal veins. Associated ascites and variceal bleeding may occur. Progressive splenomegaly may lead to **splenic infarction,** which presents acutely with fever, nausea, and left upper quadrant pain. Patients may develop neutrophilic dermatoses, which appear as tender plaques. Extramedullary hematopoiesis may develop in many sites, including the spleen, liver, lymph nodes, serosal surfaces, paraspinal or epidural spaces, and urogenital system.
- CIMF carries the worst prognosis of all the MPDs, with a median survival of ~3.5 to 5.5 years. However, survival is variable and ranges from <3 to >10 years. The International Working Group for Myelofibrosis Research and Treatment has devised a prognostic scoring system (IPSS-PMF) from an evaluation of presenting signs and symptoms in 1054 consecutively studied patients diagnosed with CIMF at seven different centers. The following **five adverse prognostic features** were noted on multivariate analysis:[6]
  - Presence of constitutional symptoms (i.e., weight loss >10%, night sweats, or fever)
  - Age >65 years
  - Hemoglobin <10 g/dL
  - Leukocyte count >25,000/μL
  - Circulating blast cells ≥1%
- Subjects with 0 (low risk), 1 (intermediate risk-1), 2 (intermediate risk-2), or ≥3 (high risk) of these variables at presentation had nonoverlapping median survivals of 135, 95, 48, and 27 months, respectively.
- The degree of fibrosis does not appear to be related to prognosis. In addition, cytogenetic findings predict either good (sole abnormalities of del(20q), del(13q), trisomy 9) or poor (complex abnormalities, trisomy 8) prognosis. The prognostic value of other cytogenetic findings is unclear because of the small number of patients evaluated. Two studies have shown that a low burden of the

JAK 2V617F allele in PMF might indicate the presence of an overriding V617F-negative clone that confers a more aggressive disease phenotype with shortened overall survival, although the biologic mechanisms underlying this correlation remain to be established.

HYPEREOSINOPHILIC SYNDROMES

GENERAL PRINCIPLES

Definition

Two syndromes compose this category: **chronic eosinophilic leukemia** (CEL) and **idiopathic hypereosinophilic syndrome** (HES). They should be suspected when the peripheral eosinophil count is persistently >1500/µL. The diagnosis of these disorders requires ruling out other causes of eosinophilia, such as underlying infection, allergy, autoimmune disease, pulmonary disease, clonal lymphoid disorder, and other MPDs. Also, the peripheral eosinophilia should be accompanied by an elevated eosinophil count in bone marrow and characteristic end-organ damage.

Epidemiology

HES is rare and the prevalence is unknown. Most patients are diagnosed between the ages of 20 and 50 years, although HES can develop in children. PDGFRalpha (PDGFRA)-associated HES occurs almost exclusively in males, whereas lymphocytic variant HES and HES of unknown etiology appear to be equally distributed between the sexes.

Pathophysiology

Eosinophils are derived from myeloid progenitors in the bone marrow, through the action of three hematopoietic cytokines: granulocyte-macrophage colony-stimulating factor (GM-CSF), interleukin (IL)-3, and IL-5. Of these three, only IL-5 is specific for eosinophil differentiation.

Several mechanisms have been proposed to account for the dysregulated overproduction of eosinophils in patients with HES:[7]

- Clonal eosinophilic proliferation as a result of a primary molecular defect involving hematopoietic stem cells and/or defects in signal transduction from the receptors that mediate eosinophilopoiesis
- Overproduction of eosinophilopoietic cytokines, such as IL-5
- Functional abnormalities of the eosinophilopoietic cytokines, related to enhanced or prolonged biologic activity
- Defects in the normal suppressive regulation of eosinophilopoiesis or of eosinophil survival and activation

DIAGNOSIS

Clinical Presentation

Ninety percent of patients will have symptoms at diagnosis. Characteristically, patients will complain of various **nonspecific constitutional symptoms** such as fever,

TABLE 9-5 CLINICAL MANIFESTATION OF CHRONIC EOSINOPHILIC LEUKEMIA/HYPEREOSINOPHILIC SYNDROME (CEL/HES)

Cardiac	Skin
Constrictive pericarditis	Angioedema
Fibroblastic endocarditis	Urticaria
Myocarditis	Papulonodular lesions
Intramural thrombosis	Erythematous plaques
Central nervous system	Gastrointestinal
Mononeuritis multiplex	Ascites
Peripheral neuropathy	Diarrhea
Paraparesis	Gastritis
Cerebellar dysfunction	Colitis
Epilepsy	Pancreatitis
Dementia	Cholangitis
Cerebral vascular accident	Hepatitis
Eosinophilic meningitis	Musculoskeletal
Pulmonary	Arthritis
Infiltrates	Arthralgias
Fibrosis	Myalgias
Pleural effusions	Raynaud phenomenon
Pulmonary emboli	

fatigue, cough, pruritus, diarrhea, angioedema, and muscle pains. Infiltrating eosinophils will produce end-organ damage in the majority of patients within 3 years of diagnosis. Cardiac disease is the major cause of death, but virtually every organ system may be involved, leading to protean clinical manifestations (Table 9-5).

Diagnostic Criteria

Diagnosis relies on the exclusion of all possible causes of reactive eosinophilia. Also, patients must be evaluated and ruled out for T-cell lymphomas, Hodgkin lymphoma, mastocytosis, ALL, AML, CML, PV, ET, CIMF, and the myelodysplastic syndromes. If all of these exclusions are met, a diagnosis of HES can be made. If there is a clonal chromosomal abnormality or if there are >2% blasts in the peripheral blood or >5% but <19% blasts on bone marrow aspirate, then the diagnosis is CEL. If there are >20% blasts on bone marrow aspirate, then the diagnosis is AML.

Diagnostic Testing

The diagnosis is usually suspected based on **peripheral eosinophilia** and some constellation of the symptoms reviewed in Table 9-4. CEL is due to an autonomous proliferation of clonal cells. HES is diagnosed when the diagnostic criteria for CEL are satisfied, but without evidence of clonality or myeloid cell proliferation. A molecular defect has been identified in about half of CEL/HES cases. It is a specific interstitial deletion on chromosome 4 that results in the expression of a **FIP1L1-PDGFRA fusion tyrosine kinase.** This fusion kinase is sensitive to inhibition by imatinib.

TREATMENT

- Treatment is aimed at those with end-organ damage. **Corticosteroids** reduce peripheral eosinophil numbers and the toxicity of the eosinophilic granules. Steroid-resistant patients are treated with various single-agent or combination therapies, including hydroxyurea, interferon, vincristine, and etoposide.
- Several recent studies have shown the efficacy of **imatinib** in the treatment of both CEL and HES. Notably, responses are seen both in patients with recognized mutations of the FIP1L1-PDGFRA kinase, the assumed target of imatinib in this disease, and in those without it. These dramatic responses argue that imatinib should be the first-line therapy for symptomatic CEL and HES. For HES patients (with or without the FIP1L1/PDGFRA fusion) who fail pharmacologic management, **allogeneic hematopoietic cell transplant** offers a chance of long-term remission.

OUTCOMES/PROGNOSIS

The clinical course of both HES and CEL is markedly variable. Features that portend a better prognosis include the following:

- Prolonged eosinopenia in response to prednisone challenge
- The absence of findings associated with MPDs, including elevated serum vitamin B_{12}, abnormal leukocyte alkaline phosphatase scores, splenomegaly, cytogenetic abnormalities, myelofibrosis, and myeloid dysplasia
- The presence of angioedema, although this observation may have been due to the inclusion of patients with the entity of episodic angioedema with eosinophilia (Gleich's syndrome)

Blast transformation may come early or very late in the clinical course. Features that predict a poor prognosis are marked splenomegaly, cytogenetic abnormalities, dysplastic myeloid features, and increased peripheral or marrow blast counts. Long-term survival is possible. In one case series up to 42% of persons were still alive 15 years after diagnosis.

REFERENCES

1. Spivak JL. Narrative review: Thrombocytosis, polycythemia vera, and JAK2 mutations: The phenotypic mimicry of chronic myeloproliferation. *Ann Intern Med.* 2010;152(5):300–306.
2. Campbell PJ, Green AR. The myeloproliferative disorders. *N Engl J Med.* 2006;355:2452–2466.
3. Scott LM, Tong W, Levine RL, et al. JAK2 exon 12 mutations in polycythemia vera and idiopathic erythrocytosis. *N Engl J Med.* 2007;356(5):459–468.
4. Pardanani AD, Levine RL, Lasho T, et al. MPL515 mutations in myeloproliferative and other myeloid disorders: a study of 1182 patients. *Blood.* 2006;108(10):3472–3476.
5. Barbui T, Finazzi G. When and how to treat essential thrombocythemia. *N Engl J Med.* 2005;353(1):85–86.
6. Cervantes F, Dupriez B, Pereira A, et al. New prognostic scoring system for primary myelofibrosis based on a study of the International Working Group for Myelofibrosis Research and Treatment. *Blood.* 2009;113(13):2895–2901.
7. Ackerman SJ, Bochner BS. Mechanisms of eosinophilia in the pathogenesis of hypereosinophilic disorders. *Immunol Allergy Clin North Am.* 2007;27(3):357–375.

Transfusion Medicine

10

Ronald Jackups and Tzu-Fei Wang

GENERAL PRINCIPLES

Transfusion of donated blood products is used to treat many disorders, including anemia and impaired hemostasis. This treatment may be life saving, but all blood products carry the risk of transfusion complications, some of which may be life threatening. The functions of blood centers and hospital blood banks include consultation in appropriate blood product use and the delivery of blood products that have undergone adequate precautions for safety.

PRETRANSFUSION SCREENING AND TESTING

Donor Screening

Donors undergo extensive screening and testing to ensure the safety of both the donors and the eventual recipients of their donated products. At the time of donation, donors must meet requirements for age, weight, vital signs, and hematologic indices, and they are asked a battery of questions to assess their risk of transfusion-transmitted diseases and other conditions that may affect donation and transfusion safety. Their blood is screened for infectious diseases (Table 10-1). Transfusion-transmitted infections are extremely rare due to effective screening, but they cannot be completely eliminated because screening cannot identify new infections during the initial, undetectable "window period."

Compatibility Testing

Blood collection centers and blood banks provide routine laboratory testing of both donors and recipients to prevent hemolytic transfusion reactions due to ABO antibodies and other clinically relevant antibodies to RBC antigens, as well as to prevent the formation of alloantibodies against the Rh D antigen in Rh-negative recipients. This testing is performed by serology. RBCs from a patient or donor are incubated with plasma from a patient or donor or a reagent known to contain specific antibodies. If IgM antibodies (such as ABO antibodies) are present against an antigen on the RBCs, antibody binding will cause the formation of a visible cell clump due to agglutination after the sample is centrifuged. This technique is called **immediate spin,** and is primarily used to quickly identify ABO type, ABO antibodies, and Rh D type. IgG antibodies do not routinely cause visible agglutination, and therefore a reagent anti-human globulin (Coomb's reagent) is added, and the sample is incubated for 30 to 60 minutes at 37°C to strengthen the

TABLE 10-1	INFECTIOUS DISEASES TESTED BY DONOR SCREENING
Bacteremia	
Syphilis	
Hepatitis B (HBV)	
Hepatitis C (HCV)	
HIV	
Human T-cell leukemia virus (HTLV)	
West Nile virus (WNV)	
Cytomegalovirus (CMV)	
Chagas disease (*Trypanosoma cruzi*)	

reaction due to antibody crosslinking. This technique is called **Coomb's test,** and is primarily used to identify common clinically relevant antibodies responsible for non-ABO hemolytic transfusion reactions, such as Rh (D, C, and E), Kell, Duffy, and Kidd. The common compatibility tests performed in the blood bank are summarized in Table 10-2.

Emergency Release

In certain critical situations, the immediate need for transfusion supersedes the need for standard and potentially time-consuming compatibility testing. In these situations, it is appropriate for clinicians to request an emergency release of blood products before compatibility testing is completed. In these cases, **type O RBCs (which lack ABO antigens) and type AB plasma (which lacks ABO antibodies) are transfused until testing is complete, in order to avoid an acute hemolytic reaction due to ABO antibodies.**

BLOOD PRODUCTS

Most blood products are produced from whole blood, which is separated into components by centrifugation and manual separation. Packed RBCs, platelets, and plasma may also be collected separately by apheresis. Coagulation factor concentrates are produced by fractionation of multiple units of donated plasma or by synthesis of recombinant proteins. The most common blood products available are described in Table 10-3.

PRODUCT MODIFICATIONS

Depending on the clinical situation, modifications and specifications may be requested for blood products. The most common are described in Table 10-4.

TABLE 10-2 COMPATIBILITY TESTS

Test	Purpose	Indication	Technique
ABO/Rh type	To identify ABO and Rh D antigens on a patient's RBCs	All recipients, within 3 days of transfusion	Immediate spin on patient's RBCs
Antibody screen	To detect clinically relevant non-ABO antibodies in a patient's plasma	All recipients, within 3 days of transfusion	(Indirect) Coomb's test on 2–3 donor RBC lines with known antigen types
Antibody panel	To identify the specificity of antibodies detected by screen	Whenever antibody screen is positive	(Indirect) Coomb's test on more donor RBC lines
Direct antiglobulin test	To detect antibodies directly attached to a patient's RBCs	When autoimmune or alloimmune hemolysis is suspected	(Direct) Coomb's test on patient's RBCs
Full crossmatch	To confirm that a patient does not have any antibodies directed against a product's RBCs	When the recipient's antibody screen is positive, or the recipient has a history of previous antibodies	(Indirect) Coomb's test on RBCs from product
Immediate spin crossmatch	To confirm that a patient does not have ABO antibodies directed against a product's RBCs	When the recipient has no history of antibodies and has a negative antibody screen	Immediate spin on RBCs from product
Computer crossmatch[a]	To confirm that a patient does not have ABO antibodies directed against a product's RBCs	When the recipient has no history of antibodies and has a negative antibody screen	Computer comparison of records of recipient and product ABO type

[a]May be used in place of immediate spin crossmatch if eligibility criteria are met.

TABLE 10-3 BLOOD PRODUCTS

Type	Description	Indication	Dosing
Packed RBCs (pRBCs)	• 200 mL of red cells suspended in plasma and additives to a final volume of ~300 mL	• To augment O_2 delivery to tissues	• Each unit is expected to increase Hgb by 1 g/dL or Hct by 3%
Platelets	• Pooled platelets: concentrates separated from multiple units of whole blood	• To reduce the risk of spontaneous hemorrhage in individuals with thrombocytopenia	• Each unit is expected to increase platelet count by ~30,000–50,000/μL
	• Single-donor platelets: obtained from a single donor by apheresis • Shelf life: 5 d	• To facilitate hemostasis in patients with acute bleeding	• Transfusion thresholds: ○ Intracranial bleeding: <100,000 ○ Other bleeding or pre-procedure: <50,000 ○ All others: <10,000
Fresh frozen plasma (FFP)	• Fluid portion of blood that is separated and stored at less than −18°C • 1 mL of undiluted plasma contains ~1 IU of each coagulation factor	• To provide coagulation factors for patients with coagulopathy who are actively bleeding	• Recommendations vary, usually starting with 2–4 units depending on the severity of bleeding and coagulopathy • See Chapter 7 for details
Cryoprecipitate	• Produced by thawing FFP at 1–6°C and recovering the cold-insoluble precipitate • A rich source of factor VIII, fibrinogen, von Willebrand factor, and factor XIII	• Bleeding associated with fibrinogen deficiency and factor XIII deficiency	• One unit increases fibrinogen by ~7–8 mg/dL in a 70-kg patient • 10 units are usually given at one time • Goal fibrinogen concentration is >100 mg/dL

(*continued*)

TABLE 10-3 BLOOD PRODUCTS (*Continued*)

Type	Description	Indication	Dosing
Factor VIII and IX concentrates	• Recombinant products are the most widely used given no risk of viral infection • Viral-inactivated plasma purified products are also available	• For treatment of active bleeding or to prevent perioperative bleeding in hemophilia A (FVIII) and B (FIX) patients	• See Chapter 7 for dosing
Factor VIIa concentrate[1,2]	• Recombinant product • Activated factor that can immediately stimulate coagulation	• For treatment of bleeding in patients with factor VIII inhibitors or factor VII deficiency • To rapidly reverse life-threatening bleeding such as intracranial bleeding (off-label use)	• Hemophilia A or B with inhibitors or acquired hemophilia: 70–90 μg/kg • Intractable, life-threatening bleeding: dose suggestions vary, 20–120 μg/kg • Dose is usually given every 2 h until hemostasis is achieved
vWF-containing factor VIII concentrate	• Viral-inactivated product • Humate-P is the only product that is licensed by the FDA for use in vWD	• Indicated in type 2B, 2N, and type 3 vWD • May be used in type 1 or 2A vWD, unresponsive to desmopressin	• Dosing depends on clinical situation and coagulation studies
Granulocytes[3]	• Collected by apheresis • γ-irradiated to prevent graft-versus-host disease	• Patients with severe neutropenia (ANC <500/μL) and infection who do not respond to growth factors and antibiotic treatment	• Must be infused within 24 h, preferably within 4–6 h of collection due to rapid loss of function • One product per day until ANC >500/μL or clinical improvement

TABLE 10-4 MODIFICATIONS OF BLOOD PRODUCTS

Modification	Purpose	Indication	Products	Process
Leukoreduced	To prevent several transfusion complications due to the presence of donor WBCs[a]	All patients (recommended)	pRBCs, platelets	Leukoreduction filter before storage or at time of transfusion
Irradiated	To prevent transfusion-associated graft-versus-host disease (TA-GVHD) due to donor lymphocytes	Certain neonatal and immunosuppressed patients[b]	pRBCs, platelets, granulocytes	γ-irradiation of product (25–50 Gy)
CMV-seronegative	To prevent transmission of CMV[c]	CMV-negative patients receiving CMV-negative transplants, neonates, and pregnant women	pRBCs, platelets, granulocytes	Donor testing (CMV serology) at time of donation
Sickledex-negative	To prevent transfusion of Hgb S to recipients with sickle-cell disease	Patients with sickle-cell disease	pRBCs	Hb S solubility (Sickledex) testing of product
Plasma-reduced	To prevent transfusion of potentially allergy-causing plasma proteins	Patients with history of repeated, severe allergic reactions	pRBCs, platelets	Centrifugation, removal of plasma, and replacement with saline
IgA-deficient	To prevent anaphylaxis in IgA-deficient recipients	IgA-deficient patients	All plasma-containing products	Identification of IgA-deficient donors
HLA-matched	To prevent platelet refractoriness due to HLA antibodies	Patients with platelet refractoriness and positive HLA antibody screen	Platelets	Platelet crossmatching or matching of donor HLA antigens against recipient antibodies

[a]Leukoreduction is used to reduce the risk of viral infections (e.g., CMV), febrile transfusion reactions, and other forms of transfusion-related immunomodulation.

[b]Generally accepted indications for irradiation include intrauterine transfusions, premature neonates, hematologic malignancies and solid tumors, and bone marrow transplant recipients.

[c]It is generally accepted that leukoreduction and CMV-seronegativity are equally efficacious at preventing CMV transmission.

vWF, von Willebrand factor; vWD, von Willebrand disease; ANC, absolute neutrophil count; HLA, human leukocyte antigen.

TABLE 10-5 CAUSES OF PLATELET REFRACTORINESS

Immunologic	Non-immunologic
ABO antibodies	Acute bleeding
HLA antibodies	DIC
Platelet antibodies	Sepsis
	Medications

DIC, disseminated intravascular coagulation.

PLATELET REFRACTORINESS

In some patients, response to platelet transfusions may be lower than expected. This condition is known as platelet refractoriness and may have multiple causes (Table 10-5). Platelet refractoriness is typically suspected if a patient's platelet count rises by <30,000/μL 10 to 60 minutes following transfusion.

Because platelets do express some ABO and human leukocyte antigen (HLA) activity, platelet-refractory patients may respond better to ABO-matched and/or HLA-matched platelet transfusions. ABO matching is performed by serologic compatibility testing as with RBCs. It is advisable to begin with ABO matching, as the serologic techniques are easy and inexpensive to perform. If ABO matching is not successful, HLA matching is indicated; this is particularly common in patients who have received bone marrow transplants and/or multiple transfusions. HLA matching may be done by crossmatching selected units, or by obtaining an HLA antibody screen of the recipient, and selecting donors whose HLA type is compatible with the recipient's screen.

TRANSFUSION COMPLICATIONS

Every blood product carries with it the risk of transfusion complications, some of which may be severe and life-threatening. It is important to recognize the signs and symptoms of a transfusion complication and treat it appropriately. Recommendations for diagnosis and treatment are shown in Table 10-6. In all cases, **if a suspected transfusion reaction occurs during transfusion, it should be stopped immediately,** and appropriate measures taken.

TABLE 10-6 MANAGEMENT OF TRANSFUSION COMPLICATIONS

Reaction	Mechanism	Signs/Symptoms	Diagnosis	Treatment/Prevention
Acute hemolytic transfusion reaction	Pre-formed (usually ABO) antibody against incompatible transfusion	• Fever • Hypotension • Flank pain • Shock • Renal failure	• Clerical check • Hemoglobinuria • Hemoglobinemia • Repeat ABO type	• Hydration • Pressors
Delayed hemolytic transfusion reaction	Delayed (~2–10 d) RBC antibody response	• Usually asymptomatic	• Unexplained decrease in Hgb • Direct antiglobulin test	• Monitor Hgb
Febrile non-hemolytic transfusion reaction	Cytokines or antibodies against donor WBCs	• Fever • Chills	• Exclude hemolytic reaction or bacterial contamination	• Premedicate with acetaminophen • Transfuse leukoreduced products
Bacterial contamination	Transmission of bacteria during donation	• Fever • Shock • DIC	• Culture of product • Culture of patient	• Broad-spectrum antibiotics
Allergic reaction	Allergy to donor plasma proteins	• Urticaria • Pruritis • Hypotension	• Exclude hemolytic reaction	• Antihistamines • Corticosteroids if severe

(*continued*)

TABLE 10-6 MANAGEMENT OF TRANSFUSION COMPLICATIONS (*Continued*)

Reaction	Mechanism	Signs/Symptoms	Diagnosis	Treatment/Prevention
Anaphylactic reaction	Allergy to donor plasma proteins or antibody to IgA in IgA-deficient recipients	• Wheezing • Hypotension • Shock	• Exclude hemolytic reaction • Evaluate for IgA deficiency	• Hydration • Pressors • Oxygen • Intubation if necessary
Transfusion-associated circulatory overload (TACO)	Volume overload, especially in patients with a history of CHF	• Hypertension • Dyspnea • Hypoxia	• Pulmonary edema	• Diuretics • Transfuse slowly
Transfusion-related acute lung injury (TRALI)	Presumed to be due to donor anti-HLA or other antibodies directed against recipient neutrophils, causing lung damage	• Acute respiratory distress within 6 h of transfusion	• Pulmonary edema • Exclude TACO • HLA antibody screen on donor	• Supportive care • Self-limited
Transfusion-associated graft-versus-host disease (TA-GVHD)	Donor lymphocytes cause GVHD in immunosuppressed (BMT) recipients ~2 wk following transfusion	• Fever • Rash • Diarrhea • Pancytopenia	• Diagnosis usually made on clinical grounds	• Supportive care • Mortality ~100% • Prevent with γ–irradiation of blood products

CHF, congestive heart failure; BMT, bone marrow transplant.

REFERENCES

1. Rodriguez-Merchan EC, Rocino A, Ewenstein B, et al. Consensus perspectives on surgery in haemophilia patients with inhibitors: summary statement. *Haemophilia.* 2004;10(Suppl 2): 50.
2. Freeman WD, Brott TG, Barrett KM, et al. Recombinant factor VIIa for rapid reversal of warfarin anticoagulation in acute intracranial hemorrhage. *Mayo Clin Proc.* 2004;79(12): 1495–1500.
3. Vamvakas EC, Pineda AA. Meta-analysis of clinical studies of the efficacy of granulocyte transfusions in the treatment of bacterial sepsis. *J Clin Apher.* 1996;11(1):1–9.

Sickle Cell Disease

11

Kim French

GENERAL PRINCIPLES

Sickle cell disease (SCD) is a term for a group of genetic disorders characterized by the presence of at least one sickle gene and the predominance of hemoglobin (Hgb) S. Examples of SCD include sickle cell anemia (homozygous Hgb SS), sickle beta-thalassemia syndromes (Hgb S-beta$^+$ or S-beta^0), and Hgb SC disease.[1] There is tremendous variability in clinical severity among disease groups and among individual patients with the same Hgb abnormalities. In the United States, these disorders are most commonly observed in African Americans and Hispanics from the Caribbean, Central America, and parts of South America and less commonly in Mediterranean, Indian, and Middle Eastern populations. In African Americans, the incidence of Hgb SS is 1:350 and that of Hgb SC is 1:835. The two hallmark pathophysiologic features of sickle cell disorders are chronic hemolytic anemia and vaso-occlusion, resulting in ischemic tissue injury.

Pathophysiology

- Normal Hgb is a tetramer consisting of two alpha and two beta chains.. **Hgb S** results from the substitution of valine for glutamic acid at the sixth amino acid of the beta-globin gene. The change in the molecular structure of Hgb S results in the polymerization of the Hgb tetramers leading to the sickled shape of the RBC and increased whole-blood viscosity.
- **Factors that contribute to Hgb S polymerization** include decreased pH, RBC dehydration, and, most importantly, decreased O_2 tension. The poor deformability of the RBC containing Hgb S results in occlusion of the microvasculature and ischemic tissue injury.
- It is now appreciated that pro-inflammatory interactions among the sickled cell, the vascular endothelium, and circulating leukocytes and reticulocytes contribute to vaso-occlusion. Sickled RBCs adhere to and activate vascular endothelium, causing further up-regulation of endothelial adhesion molecules and recruitment and activation of WBCs. Adherent WBCs and sickled RBCs form aggregates in the microvasculature, impede blood flow, and lead to continued hypoxia. Abnormal vasomotor tone favoring vasoconstriction also contributes to vaso-occlusion. Organs prone to venous stasis such as spleen and bone marrow are susceptible to frequent vaso-occlusion and infarction.

DIAGNOSIS

Clinical Presentation

The hallmarks of SCD are **anemia** due to decreased RBC lifespan and chronic hemolysis, and **vaso-occlusion** leading to acute and chronic complications secondary to end-organ dysfunction.[2] The major causes of morbidity are acute vaso-occlusive pain crises, anemia, and infections. The clinical manifestations of SCD vary tremendously both within and among the major genotypes. Even within genotypes regarded as being the most severe for patients with SCD, some patients are entirely asymptomatic, whereas others are disabled by recurrent pain and chronic complications. SCD is associated with a shortened life expectancy due to multisystem failure from acute and chronic vaso-occlusion. One autopsy series[3] reported **causes of death in sickle cell patients,** in decreasing order of frequency, as infection, stroke, therapy complications, splenic sequestration, pulmonary emboli/thrombi, renal failure, pulmonary hypertension, hepatic failure, red cell aplasia, and left ventricular dysfunction. Of note, death was sudden in 40% of the cases. In 1973, the mean survival was only 14.3 years. Currently, the life expectancy is 42 years for men and 48 years for women with sickle cell anemia. **Risk factors for mortality in SCD** are frequent pain crises, acute chest syndrome (ACS), and renal and pulmonary disease.

• Sickle cell trait

Sickle cell trait (Hgb AS) has a prevalence of ~8% to 10% in African Americans. Sickle cell trait is a benign carrier condition with no hematologic manifestations. Red cell morphology, red cell indices, and the reticulocyte count are normal. Patients with sickle cell trait have a normal life expectancy. Clinical complications of sickle cell trait have been reported, most typically splenic infarction occurring at high altitudes; hematuria; increased frequency of urinary tract infection, especially in pregnancy; and a mild defect in ability to concentrate urine. Sickle cell trait is also associated with a 30-fold increased incidence of sudden death during basic training of African American military recruits, apparently related to exercise-induced vaso-occlusion and rhabdomyolysis. Risk factors include exertion under extreme conditions, and the risk of sudden death can be reduced with measures to prevent exertional heat illness. Sickle cell trait is not a contraindication to competitive sports and screening prior to participation is not required. In individuals who appear to have sickle cell trait but are symptomatic, the lab diagnosis must be verified. Hemoglobins other than S that polymerize may account for reports of "sickle cell trait" associated with clinical problems, and these patients should be further evaluated.

• Hemoglobin SC disease

Hgb SC disease is approximately one-fourth as frequent among African Americans as Hgb SS. Although deoxygenated Hgb C forms crystals, Hgb C does not participate in polymerization with deoxy–Hgb S. This results in a disease that is less severe than homozygous Hgb SS disease, and the degree of anemia and leukocytosis is frequently mild. Splenomegaly may be the only physical finding, and clinical complications may be less frequent than in sickle cell anemia. The lifespan of Hgb SC and Hgb SS red cells is 27 and 17 days, respectively. The predominant red cell abnormality on the peripheral smear is an abundance of target cells and crystal-containing cells. The frequency of acute painful episodes is approximately one-half that of sickle cell anemia, and the life expectancy is two decades longer. However, there is a higher incidence of peripheral retinopathy in Hgb SC disease than Hgb SS disease. These patients may present with splenic sequestration and infarct in adulthood.

Diagnostic Testing

- **Neonatal screening** resulting in timely definitive diagnosis and appropriate comprehensive care has been shown to reduce the morbidity and mortality of SCD in early childhood. Forty-four states and the District of Columbia provide universal screening for newborns, and screening upon request is provided in the other six states. When a screening test indicates SCD, a definitive diagnosis is established through further blood testing. SCD is identified through lab testing alone. There are no findings on physical exam that suggest the presence or absence of Hgb S.
- The **peripheral smear** is normal in sickle cell trait (Hgb AS), but sickle cells are seen in each of the major SCD syndromes. Solubility testing is abnormal in all syndromes having at least one sickle cell gene and thus detects all carriers of the Hgb S gene, as well as those with the SS phenotype.
- **Hgb electrophoresis** is able to provide the clinician with the exact phenotype of SCD. Typical electrophoretic profiles are listed in Table 11-1.

TREATMENT[4]

Chronic Management

- Many patients can live for long periods without experiencing acute or severe exacerbations of SCD. Increased awareness of the disease and its long-term complications is contributing to the prolonged survival seen in sickle cell patients today.
- All patients with SCD should have routine office appointments to establish baseline physical findings, lab data, and a relationship between the patient and the treating physician. Patients with Hgb SS should have regular medical evaluations every 3 to 6 months, depending on the symptoms or manifestations of the disease.
- **Preventive care** should be initiated and maintained. A vaccination history should also be maintained. Adults should have seasonal influenza vaccines. If the patient has never received the pneumococcal vaccination, it should be offered and given at intervals based on the recommendations of the American Association of Family Physicians. Daily **folic acid** (1 mg PO daily) is given for the prevention of folate deficiency in the chronic hemolytic state. Retinal evaluation by an ophthalmologist is begun at school age and should be continued to monitor for evidence of retinopathy. Patients with relative hypertension are at increased risk for stroke and should be monitored and treated. Patients should be counseled during routine clinic visits about red flags for which they should seek further medical attention (Table 11-2).
- **Hydroxyurea** is a cytotoxic drug that has been shown to decrease the frequency of acute pain crisis, ACS, hospital admissions, and blood transfusions and to decrease mortality in adults with Hgb SS. It is generally indicated in patients with more severe manifestations of SCD. The mechanism by which hydroxyurea influences sickle cells and vaso-occlusion is likely multifactorial, including increases in Hgb F synthesis, improved red cell deformability, modulation of sickle cell adherence properties, increased nitric oxide production, and effects on WBCs. Hydroxyurea causes a decrease in the reticulocyte, platelet, and WBC counts. The dose is titrated to achieve clinical effect with minimal toxicity. However, not all patients respond to hydroxyurea. Of note, hydroxyurea has been shown to be teratogenic in mice, and should be avoided

TABLE 11-1 CLINICAL AND HEMATOLOGIC FINDINGS IN THE COMMON VARIANTS OF SICKLE CELL DISEASE

		Hgb Electrophoresis (%)				Hematologic Value[a]		
Morphology	**Clinical Severity**	**S**	**F**	**A_2**	**A**	**Hgb (g/dL)**	**MCV (fL)**	**RBC**
SS	Usually marked	>90	<10	<3.5	0	6–11	>80	Sickle cells, target cells
SC	Mild to moderate	50	<5	—[b]	0	10–15	75–95	Sickle cells, target cells
AS	None	40–50	<5	<3.5	50–60	12–15	>80	Normal
S-beta^0	Marked to moderate	>80	<20	>3.5	0	6–10	<80	Sickle cells, target cells
S-beta$^+$	Mild to moderate	>60	<20	>3.5	10–30	9–12	<80	No sickle cells, target cells

Hgb, hemoglobin; MCV, mean corpuscular volume.

[a]Hematologic values are approximate.

[b]Fifty percent Hgb C.

TABLE 11-2 RED FLAGS THAT REQUIRE MEDICAL ATTENTION FOR PATIENTS WITH SICKLE CELL DISEASE

Fever >101°F
Lethargy
Dehydration
Worsening pallor
Severe abdominal pain
Acute pulmonary symptoms
Neurologic symptoms
Pain associated with extremity weakness or loss of function
Acute joint swelling
Recurrent vomiting
Pain not relieved by conservative measures or home medications
Priapism lasting >3 h

in pregnancy. Hydroxyurea has the potential to be carcinogenic, but the exact risk is unknown.

SPECIAL CONSIDERATIONS

Surgery and Anesthesia

Surgery and anesthesia are stress states that can provoke a painful sickle crisis. Currently, it is recommended that patients with SCD undergo simple transfusion to an Hgb of 10 mg/dL before elective surgery. Studies comparing aggressive transfusion (Hgb S levels <30%) versus conservative transfusion (Hgb S <60%, Hgb = 10 mg/dL) showed no benefit of the more aggressive regimen.[5] Intraoperative overexpansion of blood volume should be avoided, particularly in patients with decreased cardiac function. Hypothermia must also be avoided in the OR to prevent sickling. After surgery, IV fluid management must ensure adequate hydration, with the avoidance of volume overload and pulmonary complications. Incentive spirometry should also be employed.

Dental Procedures

Procedures requiring local anesthesia can be performed in the dentist's office. However, any dental procedure requiring general anesthesia warrants hospital admission.

Transfusion Therapy[6]

- Transfusion of RBCs has been used for almost every complication of SCD, although clinical trials have not been performed supporting efficacy for each complication. Indications for transfusion include the need to improve O_2-carrying capacity (as in aplastic crisis or ACS), increase blood volume (as in splenic sequestration), or improve blood rheology (to prevent stroke recurrence, prior to surgery). **Simple transfusion** can be sufficient to improve O_2-carrying capacity and blood volume and is generally indicated in aplastic crisis, acute splenic and hepatic sequestration, milder cases of ACS, and prior to surgery. **Partial exchange transfusion** has the advantage of decreasing the percentage of

Hgb S without increasing the blood volume or causing hyperviscosity. It is generally recommended for acute indications such as ACS, acute ischemic stroke, retinal artery occlusion, and multiple organ failure and may be recommended for chronic transfusion programs, in which avoiding hyperviscosity and iron overload is important.

- **Indications for chronic transfusion,** which may be either simple or exchange, are primary stroke prevention for at-risk children and secondary stroke prevention in children; of note, many clinicians apply the same principles to adults with stroke. Patients with pulmonary hypertension and recurrent ACS may also benefit from chronic transfusion. The goal of transfusion is to raise the Hgb to a level of ~10 g/dL. Levels >10 g/dL can lead to hyperviscosity and increased vaso-occlusion. Transfusion is not indicated for compensated anemia, uncomplicated acute painful crises, uncomplicated pregnancy, avascular necrosis, infection, or minor surgery without anesthesia. Transfusion is controversial for priapism and leg ulcers.
- **Transfusion complications** in sickle cell patients are common and include the following:
  - **Alloimmunization** in transfused sickle cell patients is due in part to minor blood-group incompatibilities (Rh, Kell, Duffy, and Kidd antigens) resulting from antigenic discrepancy in the donor (mostly Caucasian) and recipient (mostly African American) pool. Five to fifty percent of SCD patients who have received multiple transfusions develop alloimmunization, which is a risk for delayed hemolytic reactions and can make obtaining compatible blood difficult.
  - **Hyperviscosity syndrome** is characterized by a posttransfusion elevation in blood pressure and congestive heart failure, mental status change, or stroke. Treatment is exchange transfusion.
  - **Iron overload** and its complications of end-organ damage become a problem in those patients who are chronically transfused. Chelation is recommended when the total-body iron level is elevated, as measured by serum ferritin levels or, more reliably, serial liver biopsy. Chelation therapy with deferoxamine (Desferal), which requires subcutaneous overnight infusion, is an extremely time-consuming and inconvenient therapy for the patient, in addition to being very expensive. This is one of the motivating factors for a reduction in the number of transfusions and the use of exchange transfusion in patients with SCD. Oral iron chelators, such as deferasirox (Exjade), are now available, although not all patients can afford or tolerate this drug. Patients with iron overload on chelation therapy are at increased risk for infection with *Yersinia enterocolitica.*

COMPLICATIONS

Hematologic Complications

Acute exacerbations of anemia in the patient with SCD are a significant cause of morbidity and mortality. The most common causes of these exacerbations are splenic sequestrations and aplastic crises.

- **Acute splenic sequestration** of blood is characterized by an exacerbation of anemia, increased reticulocytosis, and a tender, enlarging spleen. Acute sequestration can progress to hypovolemic shock and death. It is associated with a 15% mortality rate, accounted for 6.6% of deaths in one autopsy series, and is common in children with SCD-SS. Patients susceptible to splenic sequestration are those whose spleens have not undergone fibrosis (i.e., young patients with sickle cell anemia and adults with Hgb SC disease or S-beta$^+$ thalassemia). Treatment is **simple transfusion to restore blood volume and red cell mass.** Transfusion can lead to release of sequestered cells, and overtransfusion and resulting hyperviscosity should be avoided. Because splenic sequestration recurs in 50% of cases, splenectomy is recommended after the event has abated. Acute sequestration can also occur in the liver.

- **Aplastic crises** are transient arrests of erythropoiesis characterized by abrupt falls in Hgb levels and decreased reticulocytosis. Given the decreased lifespan of RBC in SCD, aplastic crises place patients at risk for severe anemia that is frequently symptomatic. **Parvovirus B19** accounts for the majority of aplastic crises in children with SCD, but the high incidence of protective antibodies in adults makes parvovirus a less frequent cause of aplasia. Intravenous immune globulin can be used to treat parvovirus infection. Other infections have been reported to cause transient aplasia. Aplastic crisis can also be the result of bone marrow necrosis, which is characterized by fever, bone pain, reticulocytopenia, and a leukoerythroblastic response. The mainstay of treating aplastic crises is simple **transfusion to correct severe anemia.** SCD patients in the peri-infection period are at increased risk for complications, including pain crisis, ACS, and stroke. A useful guideline for transfusion is the reticulocyte count. In parvovirus B19 infection, reticulocytopenia lasts 7 to 10 days. A patient having an exacerbation of a chronic anemia with an elevated absolute reticulocyte count is less likely to require urgent transfusion than one with a normal or low absolute reticulocyte count.
- **Hyperhemolytic crisis** is the sudden exacerbation of anemia with increased reticulocytosis and elevated bilirubin level. The usual therapy for a hyperhemolytic crisis is **simple transfusion.** Most of these patients recover within 14 days. The diagnosis of a delayed hemolytic transfusion reaction should be considered in any patient receiving a recent blood transfusion.
- **Subacute anemia:** The gradual onset of worsening anemia may be due to developing renal insufficiency or folic acid deficiency. Chronic hemolysis results in increased use of folic acid stores and can lead to megaloblastic crises if nutritional supplementation is not used.

Acute Painful Crisis

- Acute pain is the first symptom of disease in >25% of patients. The acute painful episode is the most frequent reason for which patients with SCD seek medical attention. There is tremendous variability of painful episodes within genotypes and within the same patient over time. In one large study of patients with sickle cell anemia, one-third rarely had pain, one-third were hospitalized for pain approximately two to six times per year, and one-third had more than six hospitalizations per year. More frequent pain crises are associated with higher mortality rates. Pain episodes may be precipitated by temperature extremes, dehydration, infection, hypoxia, acidosis, stress, menses, and alcohol consumption. In addition, patients may cite that anxiety, depression, or physical exhaustion may be precipitants. In many instances, no precipitating factors can be identified. The painful episodes can occur in any area of the body, most commonly the back, chest, extremities, and abdomen. In ~50% of painful episodes, patients will present with objective clinical signs such as fever, joint swelling, tenderness, tachypnea, hypertension, nausea, and vomiting. There is no clinical or lab finding that is pathognomonic for painful crisis.

- In general, the management of acute painful crises includes the **identification and treatment of possible precipitating factors, IV fluid hydration,** and **analgesics.** When a patient presents complaining of pain, the physician is charged with ruling out etiologies other than vaso-occlusion. Acute painful episodes generally last 4 to 6 days but may vary in intensity and duration. The possibility that the pain is precipitated by a concurrent medical condition, such as an infection, should be considered, and the physician should search for a precipitating illness in every instance.
- Providing aggressive relief of pain often requires the use of parenteral narcotics. Patients will often be aware of the medications and dosages that have provided adequate relief in the past, and they are often undertreated for pain. Of note, **patients with SCD do not respond to conventional doses of analgesia.** They typically are on chronic oral narcotics and may have developed a tolerance to conventional doses of narcotics. **Patient-controlled anesthesia (PCA) pumps** are effective in the treatment of an acute painful crisis. Appropriate conversion between chronic PO medications and IV doses of narcotics must be used to ensure adequate and prompt pain relief. In cases in which there is no nausea or vomiting, patients are continued on the PO regimen prescribed for continuous relief at home, and PCA-demand-only doses can be added. Demerol may be used occasionally but should be avoided if possible. Patients should be monitored frequently and objective pain scores followed closely for titration of effective analgesia.
- Painful events are not commonly associated with changes in the patient's Hgb levels, and transfusions are not indicated for simple acute painful crises. **Hydroxyurea reduces the frequency of painful crises.**

Infections

Infections are a leading cause of morbidity and mortality in SCD patients. Outcomes for children improved with the use of prophylactic penicillin to prevent *Streptococcal pneumoniae* sepsis. Although adults are less susceptible, all patients should receive the **pneumonia vaccinations.** Adults with Hgb SS disease are functionally asplenic and fever should be worked up aggressively with the appropriate cultures, imaging studies, and consideration of prompt antibiotic coverage. Patients with other genotypes are also at risk for infection, although they are not always functionally asplenic. Sources of fever include sepsis, meningitis, ACS, osteomyelitis, and urinary tract infection. In meningitis, empiric coverage should include *Streptococcus pneumoniae* and *Haemophilus influenzae.* Coverage for acute chest syndrome and osteomyelitis are discussed below.

Neurologic Complications

- Neurologic complications are common in patients with SCD, including transient ischemic attacks, cerebral infarction, cerebral hemorrhage, seizures, spinal cord infarction or compression, CNS infections, vestibular dysfunction, and sensory hearing loss. The risk for cerebral infarction, including clinical and silent infarctions, is as high as 30%. The highest stroke rates occur in children, and the risk of stroke by age 20 is 11%. Ischemic strokes[7] are more common in children and those >30 years old, whereas hemorrhagic stroke is more common at between 20 and 30 years of age.

- **Risk factors** for strokes include severe anemia, low reticulocyte counts, low Hgb F levels, high WBC counts, the Hgb SS genotype, ACS within the previous 2 weeks, and systolic hypertension.
- Strokes are fatal in ~20% of initial cases, and 70% of patients will have a recurrence within 3 years. Patients with symptoms and signs of an acute stroke should be evaluated immediately. In those with hemorrhage, initial management depends on the site and amount of bleeding. In children with infarcts, prompt partial exchange transfusion is performed to reduce Hgb S to <30%.
- **Chronic exchange transfusion therapy** to maintain Hgb S levels below 30% has been shown to prevent recurrent thrombosis. At this time, it is unclear how long chronic transfusion should be maintained. Prophylactic transfusions to reduce Hgb S to <30% in children with abnormal transcranial Doppler velocity measurements in cerebral blood vessels have been shown to reduce the risk of first clinical stroke. Unfortunately, there are few systematic data on primary prevention of stroke in adults with SCD. It is unclear whether acute ischemic stroke in adults should be treated with immediate exchange transfusion as it is in children, or whether it should be approached as it is in adults without SCD (i.e., recombinant tissue plasminogen activator, aspirin, etc.) The role of chronic transfusion for secondary prevention in adults is unclear.

Pulmonary Complications

- One of the most feared acute pulmonary complications in SCD is **acute chest syndrome.**[8,9] ACS is defined as a **new infiltrate on chest x-ray (CXR) and one or more of the following: fever, cough, chest pain, dyspnea, tachypnea, and hypoxemia.** Of note, the initial CXR may be negative. The definitive etiology of ACS is not known but infection, vaso-occlusion and infarct, fat embolism from necrotic marrow or a combination of these factors have been implicated. It has been reported to occur in 29% of patients with SCD and can progress to respiratory failure and death. ACS is the second most frequent cause of hospitalization and the most frequent complication of surgery in SCD. It should be noted, however, that nearly 50% of cases occur during hospitalization for other causes.
- **Risk factors** include prior episodes of ACS, Hgb SS, leukocytosis, hospitalization for acute pain crisis, and high-baseline Hgb concentrations.
- Atypical and typical bacterial pathogens and viruses, especially respiratory syncytial virus (RSV), have been found in patients with ACS. **Antibiotics** are indicated as initial therapy, preferably a cephalosporin and a macrolide or fluoroquinolone.
- Hypoxemia should be corrected by **supplemental oxygen**.
- **Analgesics** and incentive spirometry to correct splinting from chest pain should be initiated. Bronchodilators should be considered.
- Either **simple or exchange transfusion** should be considered promptly if there is a change in oxygen status from baseline. Simple transfusion can be

used if there is a need for increased O_2-carrying capacity such as mild hypoxemia or worsened anemia. Severe hypoxemia, clinical deterioration, or impending respiratory failure should lead to urgent consideration of exchange transfusion.

- Care in an intensive care unit and ventilator support may be required. ACS has a mortality rate of ~10%. Chronic therapy with hydroxyurea can reduce the frequency of episodes.
- **Chronic pulmonary disease** is an important cause of morbidity and mortality in patients with SCD. SCD patients may have restrictive and obstructive lung diseases, pulmonary fibrosis, and pulmonary hypertension. Pulmonary disease is more common in those with a history of ACS. Pulmonary hypertension occurs in up to 32% of SCD patients and carries a poor prognosis, even with mean pulmonary pressure elevations in the mild to moderate range.[10] The etiology of pulmonary hypertension in SCD is unknown, although chronic intravascular hemolysis, which impairs normal vasodilation through its effects on the nitric oxide pathway, may contribute. Diagnosis is made with cardiac catheterization or echocardiogram-Doppler study. Patients presenting with exertional dyspnea and findings of right heart failure should be evaluated promptly. There are few data on the efficacy of different treatment modalities, and maximizing supportive care, treating comorbid conditions, and employing medications used in other patient populations with pulmonary hypertension may be of benefit. These patients may be considered for hydroxyurea, pulmonary vasodilators, anticoagulation, and home O_2 therapy.

Hepatobiliary Complications

- The prevalence of pigmented **gallstones** in SCD is directly related to the rate of hemolysis. In sickle cell anemia, gallstones occur in children as young as 3 to 4 years and are eventually found in ~70% of patients. Patients presenting with fever, nausea, vomiting, and right upper quadrant pain should be evaluated for acute cholecystitis. Cholecystectomy should be considered even for asymptomatic gallstones.
- **Hepatomegaly and liver dysfunction** in SCD can be caused by multiple etiologies, including intrahepatic blood sequestration, transfusion-acquired hepatitis, transfusion-related iron overload, and very rarely autoimmune liver disease. **Hepatic sequestration** is characterized by a rapidly enlarging liver, decreased hematocrit, and rising reticulocyte count. Diagnosis is difficult, as CT and ultrasound show only a diffusely enlarged liver, liver function tests may be normal to moderately elevated, and the liver is variably tender. Both simple and exchange transfusions have been used to treat hepatic sequestration. As in splenic sequestration, care must be taken not to overtransfuse.
- **Benign cholestasis of SCD** results in severe, asymptomatic hyperbilirubinemia without fever, pain, leukocytosis, or hepatic failure. Progressive cholestasis with right upper quadrant pain, marked elevations in bilirubin and alkaline phosphatase, and progression to liver failure have been reported. These patients are treated with exchange transfusion and supportive care. Another serious complication is the **hepatic crisis,** in which hepatic ischemia results in fever, right upper quadrant pain, leukocytosis, severe hyperbilirubinemia, and abnormal

liver function tests. It may progress to fulminant liver failure, which has a dismal prognosis. Because of the nearly uniform mortality of this type of hepatic crisis, exchange transfusion, plasmapheresis, and liver transplantation have been used as therapy, but no controlled data are available to support this approach.

Obstetric and Gynecologic Complications

- Delayed menarche, dysmenorrhea, ovarian cysts, pelvic infection, and fibrocystic disease of the breast are more common in women with SCD. However, the major reproductive concern in these patients is pregnancy. The improvement in fetal and maternal outcomes is largely due to improved prenatal and high-risk obstetric care. The incidence of spontaneous abortion, intrauterine growth retardation, pre-eclampsia, placental abruption, low birth weight, and intrauterine fetal death are higher in women with SCD.
- **Maternal complications during pregnancy** include increased rates of acute painful episodes, severe anemia, infections, and even death. The course of pregnancy is more benign in Hgb SC disease.
- Therapeutic interventions for painful crises in pregnant women should be identical to those in nonpregnant women, with IV hydration, attention to complications, and adequate pain control. Opiates can affect fetal movement and heart rate but are not teratogenic. Transfusions are generally reserved for patients with worsening anemia (Hgb <6 g/dL) and in anticipation of surgery. Hydroxyurea has been shown to be teratogenic in animals and should be stopped in pregnancy. There is a very high incidence of acute painful episodes associated with therapeutic abortions. Inpatient IV hydration immediately before the procedure and for the 24 hours after the procedure is recommended. Oral contraceptives containing low-dose estrogen are a safe, recommended method of birth control in women with SCD.

Renal Complications

- The kidney is particularly vulnerable to complications of SCD with manifestations that result from medullary, distal and proximal tubular, and glomerular abnormalities leading to the **inability to concentrate the urine**. Papillary infarction with hematuria, renal tubular acidosis, and abnormal potassium metabolism occur more commonly in patients with SCD or sickle cell trait. Patients with hematuria should be evaluated with ultrasound.
- Patients with SCD cannot excrete acid and potassium normally but usually do not develop systemic acidosis or hyperkalemia without an additional acid load, such as in the setting of renal insufficiency. **Chronic renal insufficiency** may be predicted by albuminuria and should be suspected in the setting of hypertension and worsening anemia.
- Risk factors for the development of chronic renal failure include hypertension and the use of anti-inflammatory drugs. The average age at onset of chronic renal failure is 23 years in sickle cell anemia and 50 years in Hgb SC disease.
- The use of ACE inhibitors was found to diminish proteinuria and pathological glomerular changes; it is unclear whether their use slows the progression of sickle nephropathy. Renal transplantation is recommended for patients with end-stage renal failure.

Priapism[11]

- Priapism affects 29% to 42% of males with SCD. It peaks in frequency at 1 to 5 and at 13 to 21 years of age. Priapism is most likely to develop in patients with lower Hgb F levels and reticulocyte counts, increased platelet counts, and the Hgb SS genotype.
- First-line therapy is conservative, including increasing PO fluid intake and analgesia. If the episode persists for 3 hours, the patient should seek medical care. IV fluids, parenteral narcotics, and a Foley catheter to promote bladder emptying are the initial treatments for acute priapism. If the episode lasts 4 to 6 hours, penile aspiration and irrigation as well as intracavernous injection of an alpha-adrenergic agonist by a urologist should be performed. Partial exchange transfusion can be considered, although efficacy has not been proved in randomized controlled trials and it can be associated with complications in this setting.
- ASPEN syndrome (*a*ssociation of *S*CD, *p*riapism, *e*xchange transfusion, and *n*eurologic events), which involves headache, mental status change, neurologic deficits, and stroke, has been described in SCD patients with priapism undergoing exchange transfusion. It is important that initiation of transfusion does not delay more definitive treatment.
- If detumescence does not occur with nonsurgical management, a spongiosum–cavernosum or cavernosaphenous vein shunt may be recommended.
- Despite interventions, impotence remains a frequent complication of priapism. There is a paucity of clinical trials for the secondary prevention of priapism, although chronic transfusion according to stroke protocol, hydroxyurea, and vasoactive agents such as pseudoephedrine are used at some centers.

Ocular Complications

- Anterior chamber ischemia, retinal artery occlusion, and proliferative retinopathy with the risk of subsequent hemorrhage and retinal detachment can lead to vision loss in SCD. Sickle retinopathy is found most frequently between 15 and 30 years of age. Although found in all SCD, it is most frequent in Hgb SC.
- All patients who sustain eye trauma must be evaluated by an ophthalmologist urgently because they are at increased risk of visual loss. Patients should undergo a yearly retinal exam performed by an ophthalmologist. Sickle cell retinopathy may require vision-improving therapy with laser photocoagulation.

Bone Complications

- Bone and joint problems are a common cause of both acute and chronic pain in SCD. Erythroid hyperplasia secondary to chronic hemolytic anemia leads to widening of the medullary space and thinning of the trabeculae and cortices. This results in bony distortion, especially in the skull, vertebrae, and long bones. Vaso-occlusion and subsequent bone and marrow infarct are common, especially in the spine, ribs, and long bones.
- **Dactylitis,** painful swelling of the hands and feet, is caused by microinfarcts of the phalanges and metatarsals and usually occurs in early childhood.
- **Osteonecrosis** occurs in all SCD phenotypes but most frequently in sickle cell anemia with coexistent alpha thalassemia. Osteonecrosis occurs in both the femoral and the humeral heads, as well as in the vertebral bodies. The femoral heads more commonly undergo **GS**progressive destruction as a result of chronic

weightbearing. MRI is the most accurate imaging study to diagnose avascular necrosis of the femoral head. Core decompression surgery to relieve increased intraosseous pressure can be used in early-stage osteonecrosis. A patient with more advanced disease is a candidate for total hip arthroplasty. This decision must take into account the likelihood that a second hip revision may be required and that there are more complications and a relatively high failure rate in patients with SCD compared to other patient populations. Vertebral infarction also occurs and leads to chronic back pain.

- **Osteomyelitis** must be differentiated from the more common bone infarction, because the two syndromes present with similar clinical and imaging findings but are treated very differently. Staphylococcus and salmonella are common pathogens for osteomyelitis in sickle cell patients. Increasing antibiotic resistance to salmonella is a major problem in SCD. Septic arthritis must also be distinguished from the more common joint effusion associated with acute painful episodes. Bone biopsy and culture are the most reliable tests to establish the diagnosis before starting long-term antibiotics.

Dermatologic Complications

Skin ulcers are major causes of morbidity in SCD. Ulcers occur commonly near the medial or lateral malleolus and are frequently bilateral. About 2.5% of patients age 10 and older develop leg ulcers. Ulcers may begin spontaneously or as a result of trauma. They are commonly infected with *Staphylococcus aureus, Pseudomonas,* streptococci, or *Bacteroides* species. Males have a threefold greater risk of developing leg ulcers. Therapy with gentle débridement, wet-to-dry dressings, and compression bandages is typically effective. Compression stockings may be used to prevent recurrence.

Cardiac Complications

An important cardiac consideration in the management of patients with SCD is the high cardiac output related to chronic anemia. Chronic high cardiac output can result in four-chamber enlargement and cardiomegaly. Age-dependent loss of cardiac reserve can lead to a greater risk of heart failure in adult patients during fluid overload, transfusion, or other reduced O_2-carrying capacity states. Acute myocardial infarction in the absence of coronary disease has been reported but is rare.

REFERENCES

1. Beutler E. Disorders of hemoglobin structure: sickle cell anemia and related abnormalities. In: Lichtman MA, Beutler E, Kipps TJ, et al., eds. *Williams Hematology.* 7th ed. New York: McGraw-Hill; 2006:667–700.
2. Stuart MJ, Nagel RL. Sickle cell disease. *Lancet.* 2004;364:1343–1360.
3. Manci EA, Culberson DE, Yang YM, et al. Causes of death in sickle cell disease: an autopsy study. *Br J Haematol.* 2003;123(2):359–365.
4. Bunn HF. Pathogenesis and treatment of sickle cell disease. *N Engl J Med.* 1997;337: 762–769.
5. Vichinsky EP, Haberkern CM, Neumayr L, et al. A comparison of conservative and aggressive transfusion regimens in the perioperative management of sickle cell disease. *N Engl J Med.* 1995;333:206–213.
6. Wanko S, Telen M. Transfusion management in sickle cell disease. *Hematol Oncol Clin North Am.* 2005;19(5):803–826.

7. Switzer J, Hess DC, Nichols FT, et al. Pathophysiology and treatment of stroke in sickle-cell disease: present and future. *Lancet Neurol.* 2006;5:501–512.
8. Johnson CS. The acute chest syndrome. *Hematol Oncol Clin North Am.* 2005;19(5):857–879.
9. Vichinsky E, Neumayr LD, Earles AN, et al. Causes and outcomes of the acute chest syndrome in sickle cell disease. *N Engl J Med.* 2000;342;1855–1865.
10. Gladwin MT, Sachdev V, Jison ML, et al. Pulmonary hypertension as a risk factor for death in patients with sickle cell disease. *N Engl J Med.* 2004;350:886–895.
11. Rogers Z. Priapism in sickle cell disease. *Hematol Oncol Clin North Am.* 2005;19(5): 917–928.

Drugs that Affect Hemostasis: Anticoagulants, Thrombolytics, and Antifibrinolytics

12

Amanda Cashen

GENERAL PRINCIPLES

Hemostasis is a regulatory process with two functions: (1) maintain clot-free blood flow and (2) aggressively respond to localized vascular injury with formation of a hemostatic plug. Aberrancies in this system can cause either thrombus formation or uncontrolled bleeding. When hemostasis is inappropriately or overexuberantly activated, **anticoagulants** or **thrombolytics** are used to moderate this process, with a potential risk of bleeding. **Procoagulants** are used to stop bleeding, reverse the effects of anticoagulation medications, or replenish factors required for clot formation and stabilization.

Normal Hemostasis

Endothelial cells line the inner surface of blood vessels. These cells produce vasodilators that prevent platelet aggregation and block the coagulation cascade, thrombus formation, and fibrin deposition. Disruption of endothelial cells bares the subendothelial extracellular matrix (ECM), which promotes platelet adherence and activation and exposes tissue factor, a membrane-bound procoagulant factor. Tissue factor, in conjunction with secreted platelet factors, induces platelet aggregation and activates the coagulation cascade. This converts prothrombin to thrombin (factor IIa), which forms the initial hemostatic plug. Thrombin converts fibrinogen to insoluble fibrin, which forms a permanent plug.

The **coagulation cascade** (Fig. 12-1) is a series of enzymatic reactions with feedback promotion and inhibition that regulate and restrict the process of hemostasis to the site of vascular injury. A deficiency of procoagulant factors or cofactors, such as vitamin K (necessary for the function of factors II, VII, IX, and X), can cause bleeding; whereas low levels or decreased function of factors involved in limiting coagulation can trigger thrombosis.

The **adhesion of platelets** (Fig. 12-2) to exposed collagen is mediated by von Willebrand factor (vWF), which links collagen fibrils to the surface of platelets. Activated platelets release factors such as thromboxane A_2 (TXA_2) and adenosine diphosphate (ADP), which bind to their respective receptors. This initiates a series of enzymatic reactions that decrease cyclic adenosine monophosphate (cAMP) levels and promote the release of the same factors to recruit additional platelets. Recruited platelets are connected by fibrin cross-linking of glycoprotein (GP) IIb/IIIa receptors.

ANTICOAGULANTS: AGENTS THAT PREVENT THROMBOSIS

Antiplatelet Drugs[1]

Aspirin

Mechanism of action. Aspirin (acetylsalicylic acid) irreversibly inhibits cyclo-oxygenase-1 (COX-1) in platelets, blocking the conversion of arachidonic acid to TXA_2, which is involved in the recruitment and aggregation of platelets. A minimum dose

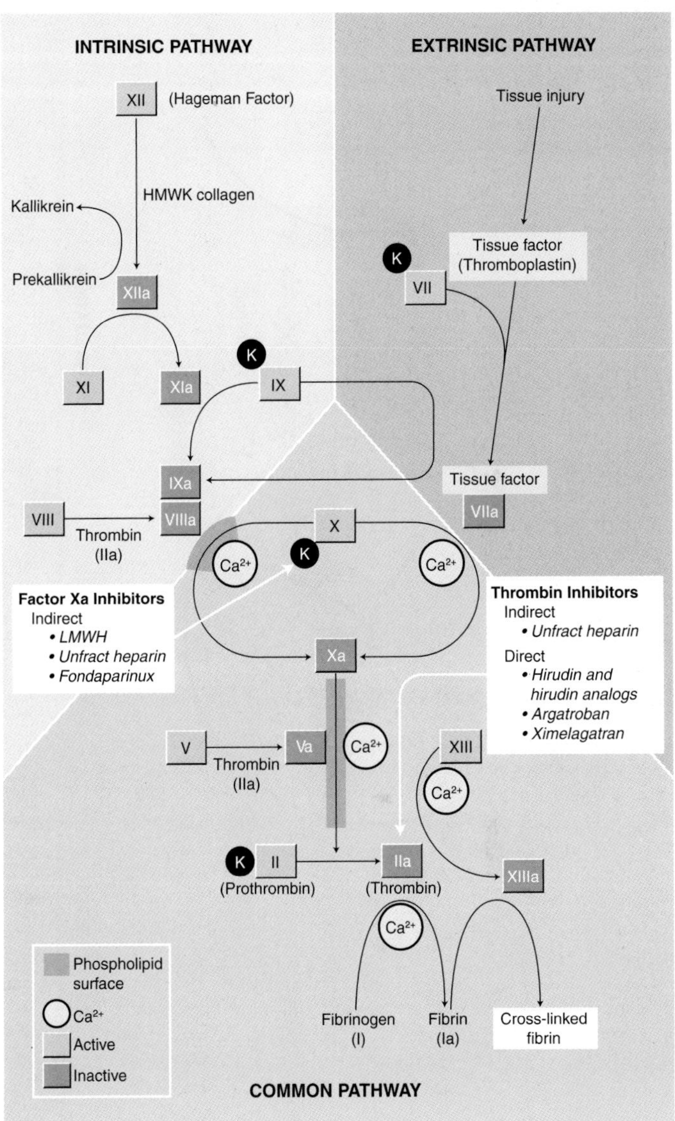

FIGURE 12-1. The coagulation cascade. The coagulation cascade is divided into two pathways: extrinsic and intrinsic, which converge at factor X, the start of the common pathway leading to thrombin formation and fibrin cross-linking. The extrinsic pathway is activated by tissue factor. Contact with subendothelial surfaces or a negatively charged surface activates factor XII (Hageman factor) and starts the intrinsic coagulation cascade. (Diagram modified from Kumar V. *Robbins & Cotran Pathologic Basis of Disease.* Philadelphia: W. B. Saunders; 2004: Fig. 4-9.)

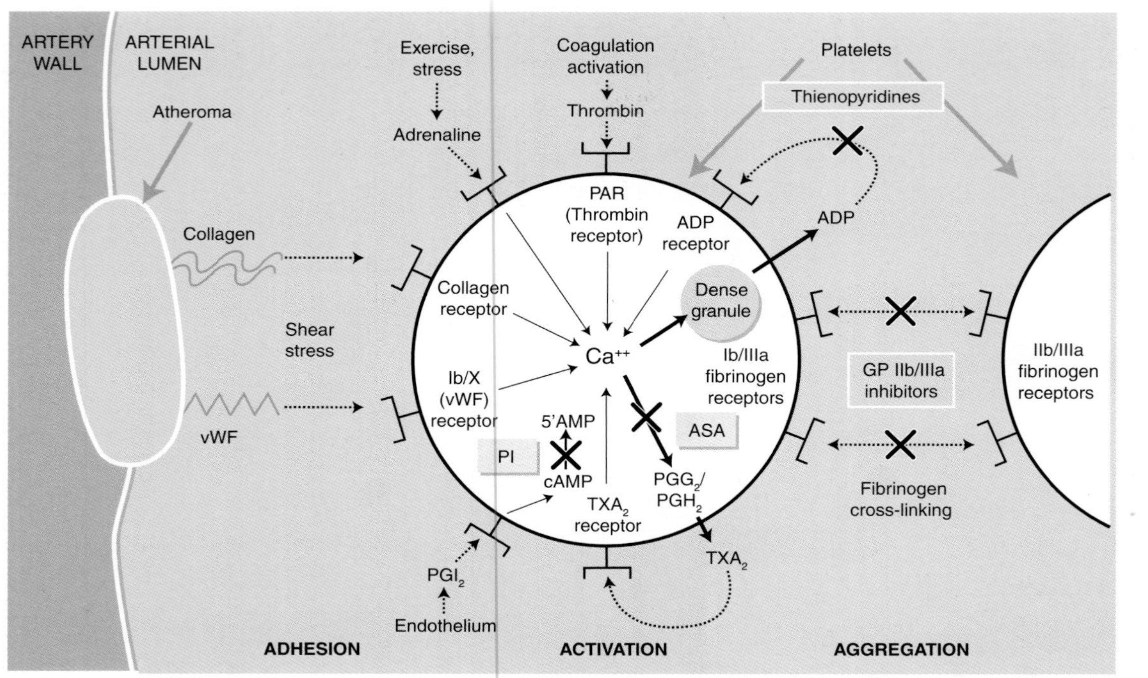

FIGURE 12-2. Mechanisms implicated in platelet adhesion, activation, and aggregation. Aspirin irreversibly inhibits thromboxane A_2 (TXA_2) synthesis, dipyridamole increases cAMP levels, clopidogrel irreversibly modifies the ADP receptor, and abciximab antagonizes the glycoprotein IIb/IIIa receptor. (Hankey GJ and Eikelboom JW. **Antiplatelet drugs.** *MJA* 2003;178:568–574. © Copyright 2003 *The Medical Journal of Australia*—reproduced with permission.)

of 160 mg of aspirin is required to maximally inhibit platelet function within 30 minutes. The effect of aspirin remains for the life span of the platelet (8 to 10 days). Normal hemostasis is regained when 20% of platelets have normal COX-1 activity.

Preparation and dosage. Aspirin is absorbed through the mucous membranes of the gastrointestinal tract, achieving peak levels between 30 and 60 minutes, depending on dosage, formulation, and physiologic factors. Aspirin is hydrolyzed in the plasma, conjugated in the liver, and then primarily cleared by the kidneys. In the United States, aspirin is available as 81- or 325-mg doses.

Clinical indications[2,3]

- **Ischemic stroke and transient ischemic attack (TIA).** In patients with a history of stroke or ischemia due to fibrin platelet emboli, aspirin therapy (50 to 325 mg daily) reduces the combined end point of TIA, stroke, and death by 13% to 18%.
- **Suspected acute myocardial infarction (MI).** Aspirin treatment in patients with acute coronary syndrome reduces vascular mortality by 23%. Patients are asked to chew the aspirin tablet(s) (160 to 325 mg) to enhance absorption due to formulation variability.
- **Prevention of recurrent MI and unstable angina.** Aspirin therapy (75 to 325 mg daily) in patients with a history of MI is associated with a 20% reduction in death and reinfarction. A 5% to 10% decrease in event rate is observed in patients with unstable angina.
- **Chronic stable angina.** Aspirin reduces the risk of nonfatal MI, fatal MI, and sudden death by 34%. The secondary end point for vascular events (first occurrence of MI, stroke, or vascular death) is decreased by 32%.
- **Revascularization procedure.** Lifelong aspirin is recommended for patients who undergo cardiac or peripheral revascularization, if there is a preexisting condition for which aspirin is already indicated.

Adverse effects. Common side effects of aspirin include stomach pain, nausea, vomiting, dyspepsia, and risk of gastrointestinal bleeding. Some of these effects can be moderated by enteric coating, which protects the gastric mucosa. Aspirin may cause urticaria, angioedema, and bronchospasm. It is contraindicated in patients with a known allergy to nonsteroidal anti-inflammatory drugs and in patients with the syndrome of asthma, rhinitis, and nasal polyps. Aspirin should not be used in children with viral illness because of the risk of Reye syndrome.

Overdose. The earliest sign of salicylate toxicity is tinnitus (ringing in the ears). Respiratory alkalosis occurs early but is quickly followed by metabolic acidosis. Treatment is supportive.

Dipyridamole

Mechanism of action. Dipyridamole (Aggrenox, Persantine) reversibly inhibits the uptake of adenosine into platelets and endothelial cells, increasing cAMP levels and, therefore, inhibiting platelet response to recruitment factors. Dipyridamole also inhibits tissue phosphodiesterase, augments the antiplatelet adhesion effects of nitric oxide, and stimulates prostacyclin release, thereby inhibiting TXA_2 formation.

Preparation and dosage. Peak levels of dipyridamole are generally achieved 2 hours after ingestion (range, 1 to 6 hours). Metabolism occurs by liver conjugation and excretion through the gastrointestinal tract. Aggrenox is available as a capsule containing 25 mg of aspirin and 200 mg of extended-release dipyridamole. Persantine is available as 25-, 50-, and 75-mg tablets.

Clinical indications.[4] In patients with a history of ischemic stroke or TIA, Aggrenox reduces the risk of subsequent stroke compared to therapy with aspirin alone.

Adverse effects. Aggrenox and Persantine have a gastrointestinal side-effect profile similar to that of aspirin, with twice the rate of headache and dizziness. Serious side effects include thrombocytopenia.

Clopidogrel

Mechanism of action. Clopidogrel (Plavix) irreversibly modifies the ADP receptor on platelets, inhibiting the binding of ADP to its receptor and the subsequent activation of the GPIIb/IIIa complex involved in platelet aggregation.

Preparation and dosage. Peak levels of clopidogrel occur 1 hour after tablet ingestion. Metabolism occurs by hydrolysis and renal excretion. Plavix is available as a 75-mg tablet.

Clinical indications

- **Recent MI, recent stroke, or established peripheral vascular disease.** The CAPRIE study compared a daily dose of 325 mg aspirin to 75 mg clopidogrel and demonstrated a relative risk reduction of 7% for fatal and nonfatal MI, stroke, and overall event rate in the clopidogrel-treated group.
- **Acute coronary syndrome.** The CURE study demonstrated that patients presenting with a non-ST-elevation MI within 24 hours of the onset of symptoms had a 20% relative risk reduction in cardiovascular death, MI, or stroke when treated with an oral load of clopidogrel in addition to standard therapies (aspirin and heparin, no GPIIb/IIIa-receptor blocker 3 days prior to randomization) compared to patients receiving only standard therapies.

Adverse effects. Clopidogrel is associated with a higher rate of rash, diarrhea, and gastrointestinal bleeding compared to aspirin. The combination of clopidogrel and aspirin versus aspirin alone increases the risk of major bleeding (3.7% vs. 2.7%, respectively). There is a rare association with thrombotic thrombocytopenic purpura after short exposure (<2 weeks). **Ticlopidine** (Ticlid) is chemically similar to clopidogrel and is associated with a 0.8% risk of severe agranulocytosis. There was no difference in the incidence of agranulocytosis between the clopidogrel- and the aspirin-treated groups.

Glycoprotein IIb/IIIa Antagonists

Mechanism of action. Abciximab (ReoPro), **tirofiban** (Aggrastat), and **eptifibatide** (Integrilin) are GPIIb/IIIa antagonists. Abciximab is the Fab fragment of the chimeric human-murine monoclonal antibody, which binds to and causes a conformational change in the GPIIb/IIIa receptor, preventing the binding of platelet "glue"—fibrinogen or vWF. Abciximab also blocks other procoagulant properties of platelets and leukocytes. Tirofiban (a nonpeptide) and eptifibatide (a cyclic heptapeptide) are reversible antagonists of the GPIIb/IIIa receptor. GPIIb/IIIa inhibitors are intended for use with aspirin and heparin.

Preparation and dosage. Following IV bolus administration, plasma levels of abciximab decrease rapidly, with a half-life of <10 minutes. The second half-life is about 30 minutes, likely related to dose-dependent reversible binding of the GPIIb/IIIa receptor. Platelet function recovers over 48 hours, although abciximab remains in the circulation for 15 days. Within 30 minutes of tirofiban infusion, >90% platelet inhibition is obtained. The half-life is ~2 hours, with clearance largely influenced by renal function; however, tirofiban can be dialyzed out of circulation, if needed. The pharmacokinetics of eptifibatide is essentially the same as that of tirofiban.

Clinical indications[3]

- **Abciximab.** Following percutaneous coronary intervention (PCI) or atherectomy, an IV abciximab bolus (0.25 mg/kg) followed by an infusion (0.125 μg/kg/min × 12 hours) decreases the composite of death, MI, and urgent intervention for recurrent ischemia in the first 48 hours postprocedure, a benefit that extended to 3 years. The CAPTURE trial demonstrated a lower preintervention and 30-day postintervention MI rate with IV abciximab. However, there was no mortality benefit at 1 or 6 months and no difference in event rate between the abciximab-treated and the placebo groups.
- **Tirofiban.** In a study of patients undergoing PCI or arthrectomy, tirofiban (with heparin therapy) decreased the composite end point (death, new MI, refractory ischemia, and repeat cardiac procedure) by 32%.
- **Eptifibatide.** Eptifibatide infusion prior to PCI decreased the composite end point of death, MI, and urgent intervention by 1% at 30 days, and this benefit extended to 1 year.

Adverse effects. GPIIb/IIIa receptor blockers are associated with thrombocytopenia, which can be severe.

Anticoagulation Drugs

Anticoagulants interfere with the coagulation cascade, reducing the generation of thrombin and the buttressing effects of fibrin.

Warfarin

Mechanism of action. Warfarin (Coumadin) is an anticoagulant that acts by inhibiting the synthesis of vitamin K-dependent coagulation factors (II, VII, IX, and X, proteins C and S). Since the half-lives of proteins C and S are about one-third the half-life of the other vitamin K-dependent procoagulation factors, patients are briefly hypercoagulable before anticoagulation effects take place. For this reason, patients are often bridged with heparin, as they become therapeutic on warfarin.

Preparation and dosage. The anticoagulation effects of warfarin occur within 24 hours of ingestion, peaking at 72 to 96 hours and lasting 2 to 5 days. Cytochrome P-450 is involved in the metabolism of warfarin. Drugs that affect P-450 expression will alter the metabolism of warfarin and affect International Normalized Ratio (INR) levels. Warfarin is available in multiple-dose tablets, and therapy requires periodic INR monitoring. For more detailed suggestions on dosage initiation for warfarin, visit www.WarfarinDosing.org.

Clinical indications

- **Deep venous thrombosis (DVT) and pulmonary embolism (PE).** Current recommendation for anticoagulation in patients with an initial event and reversible risk factor for DVT or PE is 6 to 12 months. Recurrent thromboembolic disease warrants a hypercoagulable workup, and studies suggest a benefit of lifelong anticoagulation therapy (goal INR, 2 to 3).
- **Atrial fibrillation.** Prospective trials of patients with atrial fibrillation show a risk reduction of 60% to 86% in systemic thromboembolism and less bleeding in the low INR range (1.4 to 3.0) compared to the high INR range (2.0 to 4.5).
- **MI.** Warfarin can be used postinfarction to reduce the risk of recurrent MI and stroke. Some cardiologists would consider discontinuing anticoagulation 2 to 3 months postinfarction if wall motion abnormalities on echocardiography have resolved.
- **Mechanical and bioprosthetic valves.** Anticoagulation with warfarin is generally not required in the management of bioprosthetic valves. A goal INR of 2.5

TABLE 12-1 REVERSAL OF WARFARIN

No bleeding	
INR >5	Hold warfarin
5 < INR <9	Vitamin K, 1–2.5 mg PO redose if INR high at 48 h
INR ≥9	Vitamin K, 2–10 mg PO or IV Follow INR q8h
Minor bleeding	Vitamin K, 1–5 mg PO or IV
Major bleeding	Vitamin K, 10 mg IV, and FFP or factor VII concentrate

FFP, fresh-frozen plasma.

to 3.5 is generally recommended for mechanical aortic and mitral valve replacements, with the following exceptions: aortic St. Jude's and other bileaflet aortic values can be maintained with an INR of 2 to 3. A subtherapeutic INR or need to change quickly the anticoagulation status is usually managed with IV heparin.

Adverse effects. Warfarin is associated with a significant risk of hemorrhage, which is associated with higher INR levels. The anticoagulation effects of warfarin can be reversed within 1 to 3 days with oral or IV vitamin K (Table 12-1). Immediate reversal of anticoagulation can be achieved with administration of fresh-frozen plasma (FFP). Warfarin is contraindicated in pregnancy due to teratogenic effects and the risk of fetal hemorrhage. **Warfarin-induced skin necrosis** (microthrombi due to earlier deficiency of proteins C and S compared to other vitamin K factors) is a rare complication of therapy; it occurs in areas of high-percentage adipose tissue and may become life threatening.

Unfractionated Heparin

Mechanism of action. Unfractionated heparin is a polysaccharide that binds to anti-thrombin III (ATIII) and increases the rate of ATIII inactivation of thrombin (II) and factor Xa.

Preparation and dosage. Heparin is administered IV or SC, based on patient lean body weight and clinical context (Table 12-2). IV heparin is monitored by

TABLE 12-2 HEPARIN NOMOGRAM

PTT (s)	Bolus (U)	Infusion Rate
<40	3000	↑3 U/kg/h
40–50	2000	↑2 U/kg/h
51–59	None	↑1 U/kg/h
60–94	None	No change
95–104	None	↓1 U/kg/h
105–114	Hold 30 min	↓2 U/kg/h
≥114	Hold 1 h	↓3 U/kg/h

PTT, partial thromboplastin time. Typical heparin bolus, 60 U/kg (80 U/kg for pulmonary embolus/deep venous thrombosis); maximum, 5000 U. Typical infusion, 14 U/kg/h. Monitor PTT q6h until two consecutive PTTs are therapeutic (60–96) and at least once daily thereafter. Monitor CBC q48h.

measuring the partial thromboplastin time (PTT). Discontinuation of IV heparin results in normalization of anticoagulation within 2 to 3 hours.

Clinical indications

- **Anticoagulation bridge therapy.** Heparin is used as bridge therapy to initiate and discontinue anticoagulation in patients with prosthetic heart valves (to prevent valve thrombosis) and thrombotic disease.
- **Prophylaxis.** Hospitalized patients at significant risk for developing DVT and associated sequelae are given SC heparin (5000 U bid or tid) to decrease the incidence of thrombotic disease.
- **Acute coronary syndrome and vascular surgery.** The advantage of heparin is immediate anticoagulation.
- **Invasive lines and catheters.** Invasive pressure catheters and lines are flushed with heparin to prevent catheter clotting.

Adverse effects. Heparin is associated with a risk of bleeding. Rapid reversal of heparin can be achieved by infusion of protamine sulfate (1 mg protamine reverses 100 units of circulating heparin). Heparin-induced thrombocytopenia (HIT) is a complication that results in a rapid fall in platelet number (see Chap. 4). Suspicion of HIT should prompt discontinuation of heparin; platelet counts generally recover within 1 to 2 weeks. Warfarin should be avoided in acute HIT, unless combined with another anticoagulant while the INR is subtherapeutic.

Low-Molecular-Weight Heparin

Mechanism of action. **Enoxaparin** (Lovenox) is a low-molecular-weight heparin that inhibits thrombin (factor IIa) and factor Xa.

Preparation and dosage. Enoxaparin is administered SC. Maximum activity occurs 3 to 5 hours after SC injection, and it is administered every 12 hours, except in patients with renal impairment, in whom once-daily dosing is sufficient for anticoagulation.

Clinical indications

- **Prophylaxis of deep venous thrombosis.** Enoxaparin is used to prevent thrombosis complications in patients with orthopedic, general surgical, or medical problems requiring prolonged immobilization (walking ≤10 m for ≤3 days). The prophylactic dose is 40 mg SC every 24 hours or 30 mg SC every 12 hours.
- **Prophylaxis of ischemic complications of unstable angina.** Dose is 1 mg/kg lean body weight SC every 12 hours.
- **Treatment of deep venous thrombosis and pulmonary embolism.** 1 mg/kg lean body weight SC every 12 hours.

Adverse effects. Bleeding is a complication of enoxaparin, and no therapy to reverse anticoagulation is available. Thrombocytopenia occurs in about 1% of patients. A drop in platelet count to $<100{,}000/mm^3$ should prompt discontinuation of this medication. Patients with HIT from heparin therapy are at risk for enoxaparin-induced thrombocytopenia; thus other anticoagulation drugs are preferred in these situations. The use of enoxaparin for thromboprophylaxis in pregnant women and in patients with mechanical valves has not been thoroughly studied.

Fondaparinux

Mechanism of action. Fondaparinux (Arixtra) binds to ATIII and selectively inhibits factor Xa.

Preparation and dosage. A therapeutic level of fondaparinux is achieved within 2 hours of SC injection and is eliminated by renal excretion. Multiple prefilled syringe doses are available. Dosing is based on body weight: 5 mg (<50 kg), 7.5 mg (50 to 100 kg), and 10 mg (>100 kg) SC daily.

Clinical indications

- **Prophylaxis.** Fondaparinux is indicated for DVT prophylaxis in patients undergoing orthopedic and general surgery procedures.
- **DVT and PE.** Fondaparinux is approved as bridge therapy for anticoagulation with warfarin.

Adverse effects. Fondaparinux carries a slightly higher risk of hemorrhage compared to enoxaparin (4% vs. 3%, respectively) and similar rates of thrombocytopenia. There is no antidote for fondaparinux.

Hirudin Derivatives

Mechanism of action. **Lepirudin** (Refludan) and **bivalirudin** (Angiomax) are recombinant hirudin polypeptides that directly inhibit thrombin. The hirudins were originally isolated from leech saliva but are now derived from recombinant DNA in yeast cells.

Preparation and dosage. The half-life of lepirudin is 10 minutes and that of bivalirudin is 25 minutes. Metabolism occurs by catabolic hydrolysis. The half-life is prolonged in patients with creatinine clearance ≤15 mL/min. Lepirudin and bivalirudin dosages are adjusted by PTT, checked 2 hours after the start or a change in infusion rate.

Clinical indications[5]

- **Lepirudin** is indicated for anticoagulation in patients with HIT and associated thromboembolic disease, at a dose of 0.5 mg/kg bolus, then 0.15 mg/kg/min (up to 110 kg), to target PTT of 45 to 70 seconds.
- **Bivalirudin.** In patients with HIT, dosing is 0.08 to 0.1 mg/kg/h for CrCl ≥30 mL/min or 0.04 to 0.06 mg/kg/h for CrCl <30 mL/min, to target PTT of 45 to 70 seconds. Bivalirudin can also be used in patients undergoing PCI (0.75 mg/kg bolus prior to intervention, then 1.75 mg/kg/h for the duration of the procedure, and up to 4 hours postprocedure); in acute coronary syndrome (0.1 mg/kg bolus, then 0.25 mg/kg/h); and as anticoagulation with streptokinase thrombolysis in ST-elevation MI and known HIT (0.25 mg/kg bolus 3 minutes before streptokinase, followed by 0.5 mg/kg/h × 12 hours, then 0.25 mg/kg/h × 36 hours).

Adverse effects. Antihirudin antibodies are observed in 40% of HIT patients treated with lepirudin. Back pain and nausea are common side effects of hirudin derivatives. There are reports of hypersensitivity and allergic reactions and liver function test abnormalities.

Argatroban

Mechanism of action. Argatroban is a synthetic derivative of L-arginine that directly inhibits thrombin by reversibly binding to the thrombin active site.

Preparation and dosage. Argatroban is 54% protein bound and is metabolized by the liver. Its half-life is 39 to 51 minutes. No dosage adjustment is necessary in renal dysfunction; however, the dosage should be adjusted in hepatic impairment (0.5 μg/kg/min). The INR may be falsely elevated with therapy.

Clinical indications.[5] Argatroban is used for prophylaxis or treatment of thrombosis in patients with HIT (0.5 to 2 μg/kg/min until PTT is 1.5 to 3 × baseline) or as anticoagulation in patients with HIT undergoing PCI.

Adverse effects. Argatroban prolongs the INR with warfarin and should be discontinued when the INR is >4 on combined therapy. Fever and diarrhea are frequent side effects. Hypotension can occur with infusion.

Dabigatran

Mechanism of action. Dabigatran is an oral direct thrombin inhibitor.

Preparation and dosage. The approved dose is 150 mg PO bid. Dose reduction to 75 mg bid is indicated in patients with renal insufficiency (creatinine clearance 15 to 30 mL/min).

Clinical indications. Dabigatran is indicated to reduce the risk of stroke in patients with atrial fibrillation. In a randomized trial, dabigatran was as effective as warfarin in the treatment of acute DVT.[6]

Adverse effects. The primary risk is bleeding. Dabigatran should be discontinued 1 to 2 days before an invasive procedure or surgery (3 to 5 days in patients with renal insufficiency). No INR monitoring is required.

THROMBOLYTICS AND FIBRINOLYTICS: AGENTS THAT DISINTEGRATE CLOT

Thrombolytics and fibrinolytics convert plasminogen to the active enzyme plasmin, which digests fibrin clots (Table 12-3). Allergic reactions to these agents have been reported, particularly streptokinase and urokinase. The most commonly reported reactions to streptokinase are fever and shivering (1% to 4%). Anaphylactic shock is much rarer, occurring in <0.1% of patients. To anticipate allergic reaction to streptokinase, an intradermal test dose of 100 IU has been suggested. Hypersensitivity reactions should be treated with adrenergic, corticosteroid, and/or antihistamine agents as needed.

The major risk of thrombolytics and fibrinolytics is bleeding. Relative **contraindications** to their use include the following:

- Recent surgery (within 10 days)
- Gastrointestinal bleeding
- Trauma, including intracranial or intraspinal trauma or surgery within the previous 3 months
- Known intracranial neoplasm, arteriovenous malformation, or aneurysm
- Known bleeding diathesis or INR >1.7
- Platelet count <100,000/mm^3
- Systolic blood pressure >180 mm Hg or diastolic pressure >110 mm Hg
- Subacute bacterial endocarditis
- Pregnancy
- Cerebrovascular disease

In these situations, the bleeding risk must be weighed against the benefits of thrombolysis.

COAGULANTS: AGENTS THAT TREAT BLEEDING

Desmopressin

Mechanism of action. Desmopressin (DDAVP) is a synthetic version of the naturally occurring pituitary hormone vasopressin (ADH). In patients with type 1 von

TABLE 12-3 THROMBOLYTICS AND FIBRINOLYTICS

Drug	Mechanism of Action	Indication	Dose[a]
Streptokinase	Binds plasminogen, increases conversion to plasmin	Acute MI[3]	1,500,000 IU
		PE	250,000 IU, then 100,000 IU/h × 24 h
		DVT	250,000 IU, then 100,000 IU/h × 72 h
Urokinase	Same as streptokinase	PE	4,400 IU/kg, then 4,400 IU/kg/h × 12 h
Alteplase	Tissue plasminogen activator (tPA)	Acute MI[3]	15 mg; then 0.75 mg/kg over 30 min; then 0.5 mg/kg over 1 h
		PE	100 mg over 2 h
		Acute stroke	0.9 mg/kg over 60 min
		PAD	Given intra-arterially for limb-threatening ischemia
Reteplase	Recombinant tPA that binds fibrin with less affinity than alteplase, allowing it to penetrate clots better	Acute MI[3]	10 U × 2 doses, 30 min apart
Tenecteplase	Recombinant tPA with decreased plasma clearance and increased binding to fibrin	Acute MI[3]	One-time, weight-based dose

[a]All doses are IV; MI, myocardial infarction; PE, pulmonary embolus; DVT, deep vein thrombosis; PAD, peripheral arterial disease.

Willebrand disease (vWD) and mild hemophilia A, desmopressin transiently increases plasma levels of vWF and factor VIII.

Preparation and dosage. Desmopressin can be administered intranasally, SC, IV, or orally. The dose and route of administration depend on the clinical context. The half-life of desmopressin given IV is 3 hours, and the drug is metabolized primarily by the kidney.

Clinical indications

- **Hemophilia A.** Desmopressin is used in patients with hemophilia A prior to surgery or patients who have spontaneous bleeding.
- **vWD (type 1).** Studies have demonstrated that patients with type 1 vWD have a qualitatively normal vWF and respond to desmopressin, unlike patients with type 2 vWD, who synthesize a qualitatively abnormal vWF.[7]

Adverse effects. Desmopressin has been associated with headaches, tachycardia, and facial flushing. Other side effects include rhinitis, stomach cramps, vulvar pain, and vomiting. In patients receiving repeated doses of the medication, tachyphylaxis can occur. Patients taking desmopressin should be educated to limit fluid intake to satisfaction of thirst only, as hyponatremia may occur via the ADH effect of the drug. Consequently, children taking this medication should have their body weight routinely monitored. Rarely, water intoxication and coma can occur.

Vitamin K

Mechanism of action. Phytonadione (vitamin K) is a fat-soluble vitamin required by the liver for synthesis of clotting factors II, VII, IX, and X. Vitamin K is derived from green, leafy vegetables and is also produced by bacteria in the digestive tract. It is given to reverse the effects of warfarin.

Preparation and dosage. Vitamin K can be taken orally from 2.5 mg to a maximum dose of 25 mg. Alternatively, the drug can be given SC, IM, or IV at doses ranging from 1 to 10 mg. Vitamin K is metabolized in the liver and excreted in the bile.

Clinical indications.[8] Vitamin K can be administered to reverse the effects of warfarin. See section on warfarin (above) for more details.

Adverse effects. Reactions to vitamin K include taste changes, flushing, dizziness, and hypotension. Severe anaphylaxis reactions and death have been reported following parenteral administration of the drug. Hyperbilirubinemia can be seen in infants, following administration of the drug.

Aminocaproic Acid

Mechanism of action. Aminocaproic acid (Amicar) inhibits fibrinolysis by inhibiting plasminogen activators. It is often used to treat excessive postoperative bleeding, as well as gingival bleeding in hemophiliacs undergoing dental work.

Preparation and dosage. Aminocaproic acid can be administered orally or IV. The drug comes in 500- or 1000-mg tablets and 250-mg syrup or injectable vials. Aminocaproic acid is metabolized in the liver and is primarily excreted in urine. For treatment of acute bleeding, dosing is 5 g IV or PO over 1 hour, followed by 1 g/h IV or PO for 8 hours or until bleeding is controlled.

Clinical indications. Aminocaproic acid can improve hemostasis when hemorrhage is due in part or whole to fibrinolysis, including the following situations: after cardiac surgery, thrombocytopenic hematologic disorders, severe abruption placentae, hepatic cirrhosis, and various malignancies. Studies have shown aminocaproic acid to be safe and efficacious as an adjunctive therapy for hemophiliacs undergoing dental procedures.

Adverse effects. Side effects include abdominal pain, diarrhea, pruritus, headache, malaise, allergic reactions, thrombocytopenia, hypotension, convulsions, dyspnea, rash, and tinnitus. Rarely, rhabdomyolysis and acute renal failure can occur with this medication. **Creatinine phosphokinase (CPK) monitoring** should occur regularly in patients undergoing long-term therapy, and the drug should be discontinued if elevations of the enzyme are noted.

Protamine

Mechanism of action. Protamine sulfate is a parenterally administered medication used to treat heparin overdose. It binds heparin and forms a stable complex, which negates the anticoagulation effects of heparin. When given alone, protamine has a mild anticoagulant effect.

Preparation and dosage. Protamine has a rapid onset of action, and the reversal of heparin occurs within 5 minutes after administering the drug. One milligram of protamine neutralizes approximately 100 units of heparin. It is given at a rate of 5 mg/min IV over 10 minutes, and the dose should not exceed 50 mg at one time.

Clinical indications. Protamine is used to treat heparin overdose. It can also be used to treat bleeding complications in patients undergoing PCI.

Adverse effects. Following administration of protamine, patients may experience hypotension and bradycardia. Other effects include nausea, vomiting, dyspnea, flushing, and fatigue. Severe reactions to protamine include anaphylaxis and anaphylactoid reactions. Some penicillins and cephalosporins have been shown to be incompatible with protamine. Protamine overdoses may cause bleeding.

Humate-P

Mechanism of action. Humate-P (antihemophilic factor/vWF complex) is a product pooled from human plasma, which contains factor VIII and vWF. Administration of Humate-P promotes coagulation. It is approved for the treatment of (1) bleeding in hemophilia A patients, (2) bleeding in patients with severe vWD, and (3) patients with mild to moderate vWD in whom desmopressin is ineffective.

Preparation and dosage. Dosage of Humate-P depends on patient weight, severity of bleeding, and vWF:RCo (ristocetin cofactor) activity. Dosage is calculated as (patient's weight [kg] × desired % increase in VFW activity) ÷ 1.5. The dose can be adjusted for the extent of bleeding.

Clinical indications. Humate-P has >95% efficacy when used to control bleeding in patients with vWD (types 1, 2A, 2B, and 3).[9]

Adverse effects. As Humate-P is derived from human plasma, it carries a risk of transmission of infectious agents. Common side effects include flushing, chills, fever, dizziness, and headache. Although allergic reactions have been reported, severe anaphylaxis is rare.

Recombinant Coagulation Factor VIIa

Mechanism of action. Coagulation factor VIIa (NovoSeven) is a recombinant human coagulation factor approved for bleeding in patients with hemophilia A or B with inhibitors or in patients with congenital factor VII deficiency. NovoSeven works by activating the extrinsic pathway of coagulation.

Preparation and dosage. NovoSeven is administered IV, and the dosage depends on the clinical context. For hemophiliacs with bleeding episodes, 90 μg/kg is given every 2 hours until bleeding stops. In patients with congenital factor VII deficiency, NovoSeven is given at 15 to 30 μg/kg every 4 to 6 hours until cessation of bleeding.

Clinical indications. NovoSeven has been shown to be at least partially effective in 85% of serious bleeding episodes.[10]

Adverse effects. As with any recombinant product, anaphylaxis is a potential side effect. NovoSeven is contraindicated in patients who have a known allergic reaction to mouse, hamster, or cow products. Common side effects include bleeding, fever, and hypertension. There is a slightly increased risk of thrombosis after administration of the medication.

REFERENCES

1. Patrano C, Baigent C, Hirsh J, et al. Antiplatelet drugs: American College of Chest Physicians evidence-based clinical practice guidelines (8th edition). *Chest.* 2008;133(6 Suppl): 199S–233S.
2. US Preventive Services Task Force. Aspirin for the prevention of cardiovascular disease: U.S. Preventive Services Task Force recommendation statement. *Ann Intern Med.* 2009;150: 396–404.
3. Goodman SG, Menon V, Cannon CP, et al. Acute ST-segment elevation myocardial infarction: American College of Chest Physicians evidence-based clinical practice guidelines (8th edition). *Chest.* 2008;133(6 Suppl):199S–233S.
4. ESPRIT Study Group, Halkes PH, van Gijn J, et al. Aspirin plus dipyridamole versus aspirin alone after cerebral ischemia of arterial origin (ESPRIT): randomized controlled trial. *Lancet.* 2006;367:1665–1673.
5. Warkentin TE, Greinacher A, Koster A, et al. Treatment and prevention of heparin-induced thrombocytopenia: American College of Chest Physicians evidence-based clinical practice guidelines (8th edition). *Chest.* 2008;133(6 Suppl);340S–380S.
6. Schulman S, Kearon C, Kakkar AK, et al. Dabigatran versus warfarin in the treatment of acute venous thromboembolism. *N Engl J Med.* 2009;361:2342–2352.
7. Castaman G, Lethagen S, Federici AB, et al. Response to desmopressin is influenced by the genotype and phenotype in type 1 von Willebrand disease (VWD): results from the European Study MCMDM-1VWD. *Blood.* 2008;111:3531–3539.
8. Dezee KJ, Shimeall WT, Douglas KM, et al. Treatment of excessive anticoagulation with phytonadione (vitamin K): a meta-analysis. *Arch Intern Med.* 2006;166:391–397.
9. Auerswald G, Kreuz W. Haemate P/Humate-P for the treatment of von Willebrand disease: considerations for use and clinical experience. *Haemophilia.* 2008;14(Suppl 5):39–46.
10. Hardy JF, Bélisle S, van der Linden P. Efficacy and safety of recombinant activated factor VII to control bleeding in nonhemophiliac patients: a review of 17 randomized controlled trials. *Ann Thorac Surg.* 2008;86:1038–1048.

Plasma Cell Disorders

13

Kristen M. Sanfilippo

INTRODUCTION TO PLASMA CELL DISORDERS

Plasma cell disorders encompass a group of hematologic malignancies characterized by neoplastic clonal proliferation of plasma cells producing a monoclonal protein. The range and severity of diseases are broad and include multiple myeloma (MM), monoclonal gammopathy of undetermined significance (MGUS), Waldenström macroglobulinemia (WM), and amyloidosis. The monoclonal protein (M protein) varies by disease entity; MM generally produces IgG and IgA, whereas WM is caused by IgM gammopathy.

MULTIPLE MYELOMA

GENERAL PRINCIPLES

Multiple myeloma (MM) results when there is neoplastic clonal proliferation of plasma cells resulting in production of a monoclonal immunoglobulin (Ig), also known as the M protein, which is present in the blood and/or urine. Lytic bone lesions in MM result from disruption of the normal bone remodeling process, caused by upregulation of osteoclasts, inhibition of osteoblasts, and interactions with bone marrow stromal cells. Even with adequate therapy, the lytic lesions remain, and new bone formation does not occur.

Epidemiology

In the United States, ~5.6 of 100,000 people are diagnosed with MM each year. In 2010, 20,180 new cases were diagnosed and 10,650 deaths occurred.

DIAGNOSIS

Clinical Presentation

Presentation of MM can be nonspecific, including complaints of fatigue, bone pain, weight loss, parasthesias/neuropathy, and recurrent bacterial infections. The hallmark of the disease is bone destruction, and 85% of patients have **lytic lesions** or **diffuse osteopenia** at diagnosis. Approximately 60% of patients develop **pathologic fractures** and 66% have symptomatic **bone pain.** MM can be associated with **plasmacytomas** that invade vertebrae which may result in vertebral fracture or neurologic emergencies such as cord compression.

Diagnostic Criteria

The International Myeloma Working Group and Mayo Clinic developed **diagnostic criteria** for MM, refined in 2003. **All three criteria must be met:**

- Presence of a serum and/or urine monoclonal protein (except in patients with true nonsecretory MM)
- Presence of clonal bone marrow plasma cells ≥10%
- Presence of end-organ damage attributed to the plasma cell disorder such as hypercalcemia; renal insufficiency; normochromic/normocytic anemia; or bone lesions (lytic lesions, osteopenia, or fracture)

A diagnosis of **smoldering MM** (SMM), sometimes called asymptomatic MM, is made by meeting both of the following criteria:

- Serum monoclonal protein ≥3 g/dL and/or clonal bone marrow plasma cells ≥10%
- Absence of end-organ damage attributed to the plasma cell disorder

Smoldering MM progresses to MM at a rate of approximately 10% per year.[1]

Diagnostic Testing

Laboratories

All patients suspected of having MM should undergo an extensive workup. Initial laboratories should include CBC, electrolytes, BUN, creatinine, and calcium. Examination of the peripheral blood smear may reveal presence of rouleaux formation. A serum protein electrophoresis (SPEP) with immunofixation, quantitative immunoglobulins, and measurement of serum-free light chains should be performed. Once the diagnosis of a plasma cell disorder is established, 24-hour urine, urine protein electrophoresis (UPEP) and immunofixation are needed. LDH can be measured to reflect tumor burden, while serum β_2-microglobulin and albumin serve as important prognostic indicators. An M protein is detectable in the serum of ~90% of patients with MM, with 50% of patients having IgG and 20% having IgA. Sixteen percent of patients secrete light chains only.

Imaging

A **skeletal survey** to assess for lytic lesions should be performed. CT/MRI can be considered in patients with bone pain not explained by skeletal survey to assess for occult fracture.

Diagnostic Procedures

A **bone marrow aspirate and biopsy** should be done with immunophenotyping, cytogenetics, and fluorescence in situ hybridization (FISH), as certain translocations have prognostic significance.

TREATMENT

The decision of when to treat typically depends on presence of symptoms from the disease. A Cochrane review compared chemotherapy at the time of diagnosis to chemotherapy at the time of disease progression and found that early treatment effectively delayed progression of the disease; however, there were no significant effects on mortality or on response rate to initial therapy.[2] Patients with SMM may remain stable for years before requiring therapy, and should be followed every 3 months to monitor for disease progression.

- **Initial therapy.** Patients with symptomatic disease on presentation should undergo treatment as survival without therapy is a median of 6 months. The goals of induction therapy include decreasing tumor burden and symptoms, improving end-organ damage, and prolonging survival. The preferred induction regimen has not been clearly defined, and the upfront therapy of myeloma is rapidly evolving.[3,4] **Melphalan and prednisone** (MP) is a well tolerated regimen with a response rate that approaches 50%. However, in those who are expected to proceed to stem cell transplantation (SCT), MP should be avoided because the alkylating agent compromises stem cell reserve. **Thalidomide/dexamethasone** (TD) was commonly used in the recent past, but recent studies have demonstrated superiority of alternate regimens. **Lenalidomide/dexamethasone** (LD) has shown superiority over TD, with increased partial response rate (PR) of 80% versus 61%, in addition to increasing time to progression (TTP), progression-free survival (PFS), and overall survival (OS).[5] The toxicity profile for thalidomide includes venous thromboembolism (VTE) and peripheral neuropathy, while that for lenalidomide includes myelotoxicity and VTE. **Bortezomib,** a proteasome inhibitor, has high activity in MM, and, in combination with dexamethasone, it has an overall response of 65% in untreated patients.[6] Toxicity profile for bortezomib includes peripheral neuropathy. An older regimen consisting of vincristine, doxorubicin, and dexamethasone (VAD) has comparable RR to newer therapy; however, its use has fallen out of favor due to a cumbersome administration schedule and requirement for central line. Combination therapies that incorporate lenalidomide, bortezomib, steroids, and alkylators, as well as various consolidation and maintenance approaches, are under active investigation.

- **Hematopoetic stem cell transplant.** Autologous SCT has been shown to extend disease-free survival in patients with myeloma; although its role may evolve given improvements in induction therapy. Currently, most patients deemed suitable for autologous SCT proceed to harvesting of stem cells after several cycles of induction therapy. Response rates to SCT approach 90%, with one-third of patients experiencing a complete response. The main deciding factors for who is eligible to undergo autologous SCT include age, performance status, and presence of comorbidities. Allogeneic transplants are also occasionally performed, although they are generally reserved for young patients with a matched sibling donor who have failed autologous SCT. Initial response to induction therapy has not been shown to predict outcome after autologous SCT. Maintenance therapy with lenalidomide or other active agents may extend disease-free survival post-SCT.
- **Adjunctive therapy.** Given advancements in overall survival of MM, the role of adjunctive therapy is increasing. Bisphosphonates play a role in decreasing skeletal events (i.e., fractures, lytic lesions, and osteoporosis) and in decreasing bone pain due to lytic lesions. Radiation therapy is effective in decreasing bony pain from distinct lesions and can be used during complications such as spinal cord compression. Patients on thalidomide or lenalidomide should be on prophylactic anticoagulation because of increased risk of thrombotic events.

FOLLOW-UP

Follow-up of MM should be done by following the M-protein level and other markers of disease progression including serum-free light chains, CBC, and serum creatinine. Skeletal surveys are not used to follow disease response as lesions may not show healing on x-rays.

PROGNOSIS

- **International Staging System (ISS).** The ISS was developed in 2005 and is based on a database of more than 10,000 patients. The staging system also serves as an important prognostic tool. Median survivals are 62, 44, and 29 months for stages I, II, and III, respectively.[7]
  - Stage I: β_2-Microglobulin <3.5 mg/L and serum albumin ≥3.5 g/dL
  - Stage II: Neither stage I nor stage III
  - Stage III: β_2-Microglobulin ≥5.5 mg/L
- **Durie–Salmon staging system.** The older staging system is called the Durie–Salmon criteria published in 1975, also consist of three stages. This system was developed based on total tumor cell mass but has not been shown to correlate with prognosis. A designation of A or B was added to the clinical stage for patients with or without a serum creatinine ≥2 mg/dL, respectively.
  - Stage I: All of the following: hemoglobin >10 g/dL, normal serum calcium, normal skeletal survey or a solitary plasmacytoma, serum IgG <5 g/dL and IgA <3 g/dL and urine light chain excretion <4 g/24 h.
  - Stage II: Neither stage I nor stage III.
  - Stage III: One or more: hemoglobin <8.5 g/dL, serum calcium >12 mg/dL, ≥3 lytic bone lesions, serum IgG >7 g/dL or IgA >5 g/dL, and urine light chain excretion >12 g/24 h.
- **Cytogenetics.** While utilization of this information has yet to lead to alterations in clinical management, identification of certain cytogenetic abnormalities can aid in prognostication.
  - Cytogenetics: Poor prognosis with deletion of chromosome 13 or hypodiploidy.
  - FISH: Poor prognosis with t(4;14), t(14;16), 13q-, and 17p-.

SOLITARY PLASMACYTOMAS

GENERAL PRINCIPLES

Solitary plasmacytoma is a collection of monoclonal plasma cells localized in tissue without evidence of a systemic plasma cell dyscrasia. There are two types of solitary plasmacytomas; solitary plasmacytoma of bone (SBP) and solitary extramedullary plasmacytoma (SEP). Plasmacytomas in the bone are more common than in extramedullary sites, with both constituting less than 10% of all plasma cell dyscrasias.

Epidemiology

The incidence of solitary plasmacytoma occurs at an annual rate of approximately 0.34 per 100,000 person-years in the United States. The average age of diagnosis is 55 years, with incidence for both higher in males than in females.

DIAGNOSIS

Clinical Presentation

Solitary plasmacytomas of bone often present with bony pain, pathological fracture, or cord compression. Bones undergoing increased hematopoiesis are more commonly involved in SBP, with the three most common involved sites including vertebrae, pelvis, and upper extremities. While SEP has a predilection for the aerodigestive tract, the most common location tends to be in the head and neck area.

Diagnostic Criteria

Diagnostic criteria for solitary plasmacytoma **must encompass each of the following:**

- presence of biopsy proven plasmacytoma showing a population of clonal plasma cells;
- absence of clonal plasma cell population on bone marrow biopsy and aspiration;
- absence of end-organ damage that can be attributed to an underlying plasma cell disorder such as hypercalcemia; renal insufficiency; or anemia; and
- absence of other lytic lesions on skeletal survey or MRI of the spine/pelvis.

Diagnostic Testing

Laboratories

Diagnostic testing for solitary plasmacytoma should contain tests to exclude alternate diagnoses. Initial laboratory workup includes CBC, electrolytes, BUN, creatinine, and calcium. An SPEP and UPEP with immunofixation should be performed as up to 74% of cases may have presence of a small M protein. The presence of M protein tends to be higher in patients with SBP as oppose to SEP.[8] Serum free light chains as well as immunoglobulin levels should also be done.

Imaging

A **skeletal survey** should be done to exclude presence of multiple lytic lesions. Also, **MRI of the spine and pelvis** should be performed to exclude lesions that may have been missed on x-ray.

Diagnostic Procedures

Biopsy of the suspected solitary lesion should be performed at the onset of work up to establish the working diagnosis. To exclude a significant population of clonal plasma cells in the bone marrow, a bone marrow biopsy and aspiration should be performed.

TREATMENT

The mainstay of therapy for solitary plasmacytoma is **localized radiation therapy** at a dose of 40 to 50 Gy over 20 to 25 treatments from which response exceeds 90%.[9] Surgery is an alternative if immediate tumor debulking is needed for complications such as fracture or spinal cord compression; with adjuvant radiation therapy considered. There is controversial data on the use of adjuvant chemotherapy, mainly with melphalan and prednisone.

PROGNOSIS

More than 50% of patients with SBP will progress to MM, compared to fewer than 30% with SEP, with median time to progression of 2 to 4 years. Recently, two prognostic indicators have been identified to predict who will develop MM. A study at

Mayo Clinic identified that patients with SBP who have an abnormal serum-free light chain (FLC) ratio or presence of a urinary M protein at diagnosis have higher risk of progression at 5 years (44% vs. 25%).[10] Patients whose serum M protein is still elevated 1 year after treatment also have an increased risk of progression. Overall survival is higher in SEP than SBP (10 year survival 70% vs. 50%).

MONOCLONAL GAMMOPATHY OF UNDETERMINED SIGNIFICANCE

GENERAL PRINCIPLES

Monoclonal gammopathy of undetermined significance (MGUS) is a clinically asymptomatic, premalignant condition characterized by the presence of a small neoplastic clonal population of plasma cells in the bone marrow. The pathophysiology of the clonal population is the same as in MM; however, definitive criteria of MGUS are the absence of end organ damage caused by the clonal population. It is estimated that the prevalence of MGUS is approximately 3.2% in Caucasian patients over the age of 50 and reaching 7.5% in those patients of age ≥85.[11]

DIAGNOSIS

Clinical Presentation

Patients with MGUS are clinically asymptomatic. It is typically diagnosed during routine workup of elevated total serum protein or proteinuria.

Diagnostic Criteria

The International Myeloma Working Group developed diagnostic criteria for MGUS in 2003. **All three criteria must be met:**

- presence of a serum monoclonal protein (M protein) IgA, IgG, or IgM <3 g/dL;
- presence of fever that 10% clonal bone marrow plasma cells; and
- absence of end-organ damage attributed to the underlying plasma cell disorder such as hypercalcemia; renal insufficiency; normochromic normocytic anemia; or lytic bone lesions.

Diagnostic Testing

Laboratories

All patients should undergo similar testing as with a workup for MM. Initial laboratory workup should include a CBC, serum electrolytes, BUN, serum creatinine, and serum calcium. A serum and urine protein electrophoresis (SPEP) with immunofixation, quantitative immunoglobulins, and measurement of serum free light chains should be performed.

Imaging

A **skeletal survey** to assess for lytic lesions should be performed on all patients.

Diagnostic Procedures

A **bone marrow aspirate and biopsy** should be done with immunophenotyping, cytogenetics, and fluorescence in situ hybridization (FISH).

TABLE 13-1 RISK OF PROGRESSION TO MM IN PATIENTS WITH MGUS

Risk	No. of Risk Factors	Absolute Risk of Progression at 20 y
Low	0	5%
Low-intermediate	1	21%
Intermediate-high	2	37%
High	3	58%

Risk factors: M protein >1.5 g/dL, non-IgG MGUS, abnormal serum free light chain ratio (<0.26 or >1.65).

TREATMENT

There is currently **no treatment indicated for MGUS.** As it is generally a slowly progressing disorder, the majority of patients will not progress to a malignant disease. Generally, it is accepted practice to follow these patients annually with evaluation including SPEP, UPEP, CBC, and creatinine. If patients develop symptoms concerning for progression to myeloma, they should undergo more extensive evaluation.

PROGNOSIS

In general, the rate of progression for all patients diagnosed with MGUS is approximately 1% per year. However, prognostic indicators have recently been defined that indicate patients at higher risk of progression (Table 13-1).[12]

WALDENSTRÖM MACROGLOBULINEMIA

GENERAL PRINCIPLES

Waldenström macroglobulinemia (WM), also known as lymphoplasmacytic lymphoma, is a rare malignant lymphoproliferative disorder characterized by the production of an IgM paraprotein. It differs from IgM MM in that it is characterized by the presence of excess lymphoplasmacytoid cells in the bone marrow.

Epidemiology

There are approximately 1500 new cases of WM annually in the United States. The rate is higher in men than women, and higher in Caucasians than African Amerians.

DIAGNOSIS

Clinical Presentation

Presentation of WM is generally vague and can be attributed to infiltration of lymphocytes or plasmacytoid cells into tissue and organs, secondary to the monoclonal IgM protein, or paraneoplastic neuropathy. Infiltration into organs can lead to hepatosplenomegaly, lymphadenopathy, or dermatologic findings. At high quantities, the IgM protein can lead to hyperviscosity of the blood causing signs of stasis including stroke, transient ischemic attacks, and venous thromboembolism. There is a correlation between hepatitis C and increased incidence of WM, and 10% of patients with WM will have cryoglobulinemia.

Diagnostic Criteria

Two diagnostic criteria must be fulfilled to establish a diagnosis of WM:

- IgM monoclonal protein of any value in the serum
- ≥10% lymphocytes with plasmacytoid differentiation in the bone marrow in an intertrabecular pattern

Diagnostic Testing

Diagnostic testing should include **SPEP and UPEP with immunofixation and bone marrow biopsy with aspiration** to establish the diagnosis. Ancillary testing should include CBC, LDH, β_2-microglobulin, and serum viscosity.

TREATMENT

Treatment of WM should **only be initiated when symptoms develop or there is evidence of significant end organ damage.**[13] Those without these findings are termed to have smoldering WM. While there is no set standard of therapy, treatment generally includes alkylating agents, nucleoside analogues, and rituximab. Patients with symptoms of hyperviscosity should be treated with emergent plasmapheresis to decrease the burden of the IgM monoclonal protein. In qualifying patients with refractory or relapsed disease, high dose chemotherapy followed by autologous HCT should be offered. No treatment has been shown to cure, with median survival from time of diagnosis ~5 years.

AMYLOIDOSIS

GENERAL PRINCIPLES

Amyloidosis is characterized by the tissue deposition of amyloid fibrils in a beta-pleated sheet configuration which is resistant to proteolysis.

Epidemiology

It is a rare disorder, affecting 5.1 to 12.8 per million people each year.

DIAGNOSIS

Clinical Presentation

Clinical presentation of amyloid is heterogeneous and depends on type of amyloid. The majority of symptoms are defined by the predominant organ affected and can include nephrotic syndrome, cardiomyopathy, neuropathy, hepatic dysfunction, and bleeding diatheses. Specific physical exam findings may include hepatomegaly, periorbital ecchymoses, macroglossia, and edema.

Diagnostic Criteria

Diagnostic criteria depend on the type of amyloid being diagnosed.

- **Primary amyloid (AL amyloid)** is a plasma cell dyscrasia in which monoclonal Ig light chain fragments lead to deposition of protein. As such, a majority of patients will have a monoclonal light chain detected in the serum or urine. It can occur alone or in conjunction with another plasma cell dyscrasia.
- **Secondary amyloid (AA amyloid)** occurs in conjunction with chronic diseases such as rheumatoid arthritis (RA), in which the chronic inflammatory state of the disease leads to deposition of acute phase reactant serum amyloid A. Senile systemic amyloid has a predilection to affect the heart and is due to deposition of transthyretin. Dialysis associated amyloid occurs in patients on long term hemodialysis and is the result of β_2-microglobulin fibril deposition. There are numerous other heritable forms of amyloidosis.

Diagnostic Testing

- Regardless of the type of amyloid, **tissue biopsy** is required to establish the diagnosis. In general, biopsy should be derived from the organ most affected. However, if this is unattainable, abdominal fat pad aspiration is recommended. Presence of amyloid is revealed with use of **Congo red staining** which shows a **characteristic apple green birefringent appearance on polarized microscopy.**
- When AL amyloid is suspected in a patient without underlying known plasma cell dyscrasias, SPEP and UPEP with immunofixation should be performed. Bone marrow biopsy and aspiration can confirm presence of a plasma cell dyscrasia. Serum-free light chains may also be useful in diagnosis.
- Ancillary testing as needed should be performed to determine the extent of end organ damage.

TREATMENT

Treatment varies with the type of amyloid. If amyloid is felt to be secondary to a plasma cell dyscrasia or another chronic medical condition, then treatment of the underlying disorder is required. Treatment of a hereditary amyloidosis may require organ transplantation in those who are candidates. Overall, prognosis in those with amyloid is poor and novel treatments continue to be investigated.

REFERENCES

1. Kyle RA, Remstein ED, Therneau TM, et al. Clinical course and prognosis of smoldering (asymptomatic) multiple myeloma. *N Engl J Med.* 2007;356:2582–2590.
2. He Y, Wheatley K, Glasmacher A, et al. Early versus deferred treatment for early stage multiple myeloma. *Cochrane Database Syst Rev.* 2003;1:CD004023.
3. Morabito F, Gentile M, Mazzone C, et al. Therapeutic approaches for newly diagnosed multiple myeloma patients in the era of novel drugs. *Eur J Haematol.* 2010;85:181–191.
4. Engelhardt M, Kleber M, Udi J, et al. Consensus statement from European experts on the diagnosis, management, and treatment of multiple myeloma: from standard therapy to novel approaches. *Leuk Lymphoma.* 2010;51:1424–1443.
5. Gay F, Hayman SR, Lacy MQ, et al. Lenalidomide plus dexamethasone versus thalidomide plus dexamethasone in newly diagnosed multiple myeloma: a comparative analysis of 411 patients. *Blood.* 2010;115:1343–1350.

6. Rosinol L, Oriol A, Mateos MV, et al. Phase II PETHEMA trial of alternating bortezomib and dexamethasone as induction regimen before autologous stem-cell transplantation in younger patients with multiple myeloma: efficacy and clinical implications of tumor response kinetics. *J Clin Oncol.* 2007;25:4452–4458.
7. Greipp PR, San Miguel J, Durie BG, et al. International staging system for multiple myeloma. *J Clin Oncol.* 2005;23:3412–3420.
8. Dimopoulos MA, Moulopoulos LA, Maniatis A, et al. Solitary plasmacytoma of bone and asymptomatic multiple myeloma. *Blood.* 2000;96:2037–2044.
9. Soutar R, Lucraft H, Jackson G, et al. Guidelines on the diagnosis and management of solitary plasmacytoma of bone and solitary extramedullary plasmacytoma. *Br J Haematol.* 2004;124:717.
10. Dingli D, Kyle RA, Rajkumar SV, et al. Immunoglobulin free light chains and solitary plasmacytoma of bone. *Blood.* 2006;108:1979.
11. Kyle RA, Therneau TM, Rajkumar SV, et al. Prevalence of monoclonal gammopathy of undetermined significance. *N Engl J Med.* 2006;354:1362–1369.
12. Rajkumar SV, Kyle RA, Therneau TM, et al. Serum free light chain ratio is an independent risk factor for progression in monoclonal gammopathy of undetermined significance. *Blood.* 2005;106:812–818.
13. Ansell SM, Kyle RA, Reeder CB, et al. Diagnosis and management of Waldenström macroglobulinemia: Mayo stratification of macroglobulinemia and risk-adapted therapy (mSMART) guidelines. *Mayo Clin Proc.* 2010;85:824–833.

Introduction and Approach to Oncology

14

Gayathri Nagaraj

GENERAL PRINCIPLES IN THE APPROACH TO A CANCER PATIENT

There have been enormous advances in our understanding of cancer biology over the past few decades. The novel treatment approaches, including newer targeted agents, immunotherapies, and advancement in supportive care strategies have given rise to increasing optimism in the fight against cancer. Yet a new diagnosis of cancer raises emotional and spiritual issues in a manner that few other diagnoses do, giving the medical oncologist a unique role in caring for the patient. While caring for a cancer patient, it is important to individualize management to his/her needs and disease state. Listening and taking the time to explain terminology, prognosis, and treatment options are key components in the relationship between the oncologist and the patient. Given the oncologist's knowledge of and experience with the behavior of advanced malignancies, combined with the use of complex medical regimens often lead to the oncologist serving as the primary care physician during active treatment. Oncologists are central in providing palliative care for symptom relief as well as assisting in the role of end-of-life discussions and care. A trusting relationship thus builds between the patient and the treating physician. This chapter provides an overview of this widely expanding field and provides a platform to understand the basics oncology terminologies and approaches. The chapters following this will provide further details in the management of specific cancers and associated clinical conditions.

Definition

Cancer or malignant tumors is defined as an uncontrolled growth of cells with potential for local invasion and distant metastases.

Classification

- Classification of tumors in medical oncology is primarily based on site or organ of origin of the malignancy. Tumors are further classified based on the histopathologic characteristics of the tissue of origin. A pathologic diagnosis is one of the most important steps in management of the cancer, along with the identification of the primary site. Improvement in immunohistochemical (IHC) staining techniques has aided in uniform identification and classification of tumors in general. It is important to remember that the individual characteristics and biology of the tumor, their ability to invade and metastasize, and their response to various therapies varies widely across the tumor types.
- The two important terminologies used to refer tumor characteristics are stage and grade.
  - **Staging** describes the extent of the disease in an individual patient. Staging is used for most solid tumors, unlike hematological malignancies. Staging is essential to the oncologist to plan optimal treatment strategies and prognosis

discussions. Stage is also the most important predictor of survival. In research studies, staging is used for comparison between cancer trials. The most commonly used staging systems are the **TNM classification system** developed by the **American Joint Committee on Cancer (AJCC).** "T" represents the primary tumor characteristics. "N" represents the presence and extent of nodal sites of the disease. "M" represents metastasis or distant sites of spread. It is recommended that the reader consult an up-to-date staging manual when evaluating a patient because of frequent revisions for each individual malignancy. **Clinical staging** primarily uses radiographic data to describe the extent of gross disease. **Pathologic staging** on the other hand provides additional information gained by the pathologist through microscopic examination of the tumor.

- ○ The **grade** of a tumor is a pathologic description of the cellular characteristics of a given malignancy. It is a measure of the degree of anaplasia or deviation of the growth and differentiation characteristics of a cancer from the parental cell type. Thus a **low-grade tumor** retains many of the characteristics of the originating cell type and they tend to be associated with a less aggressive behavior and more favorable prognosis. A **high-grade tumor** is characterized by loss of the characteristics of the originating cell type as evidenced by a higher mitotic activity. High grade tumors are often associated with a poorer prognosis, given the more aggressive behavior of the cells.

Epidemiology

Cancer is the second leading cause of death in the United States after heart disease. The lifetime risk of developing cancer in the United States is one in two for men and one in three for women. In the United States, the surveillance, epidemiology and end results (SEER) program has been collecting population based data including cancer related data since 1975 and provides an important source of cancer trends in the population.

Terminologies Used in Cancer Epidemiology and Statistics

It is important to make a distinction between cancer incidence and prevalence.

- The **cancer incidence rate** is the number of newly diagnosed cancers in a set population in a finite amount of time. It is usually expressed as number of new cancer diagnoses per 100,000 people in 1 year.
- **Cancer prevalence** is the number or percentage of people alive with a cancer diagnosis on any given date. This includes new cases and existing cases and is therefore a function of incidence and survival. Cancer prevalence cannot differentiate persons with cured cancer from those with active cancer.
- **Cancer mortality rate** as expected is the number of cancer related deaths, in a specified population over a defined period of time.
- **Survival is described in three broad terms: relative 5-year survival, median survival, and overall survival.** These statistics are based on observational studies.
  - ○ **Relative 5-year survival rates** compare the survival among cancer patients with survival among the general population matched in age, gender, and race, adjusted for comorbidities. This statistic method is used in monitoring the progress of cancer detection and treatment in the population.
  - ○ **Overall survival** is the percentage of people in a study or treatment group who are alive for a specific period of time, usually 5 years, after being diagnosed with or treated for a cancer. This is also referred to as the **cancer survival rate.**

- The **median survival** is more indicative of prognosis and is the statistic that is most commonly quoted to cancer patients. According to the National Cancer Institute, median survival is the time from diagnosis or treatment at which half of the patients with a given disease are found to be alive. In a clinical trial, the median survival time is one way to measure the effectiveness of a given treatment.
- **Progression-free survival** is another terminology that is often used in clinical studies, which refer to the duration of time during and after treatment when the cancer has not worsened in a patient.

Epidemiologic Factors

The risk of developing cancer is affected by important demographic and geographic factors in addition to other specific risk factors associated with individual cancers.

- **Age is both an important epidemiologic factor and a risk factor.** The highest incidence of certain cancers varies with age, for example, acute lymphoblastic lymphoma and neuroblastomas have their highest incidence in young children, while testicular cancers and Hodgkin's lymphoma have their peak incidence in young adulthood. On the other hand, the risk of common adult cancers increases with age, likely from combination of accumulating effects of environmental carcinogens and internal factors such as genetic mutations, hormonal influences and immune system impairments.
- Cancer affects both **sexes** with some cancers being gender specific. While overall incidence of cancer is higher in men than women, the gender distribution of individual cancers varies.
- **Race and ethnicity** are other important epidemiologic factors that influence both cancer incidence and death rates. Although it is not completely understood at this time, it is possibly related to interaction of the genetic and biologic characteristics of the individual patient with environmental factors such as exposure to certain dietary products or infectious agents.
- **Socioeconomic factors** such as lack of education and unemployment also plays a very intricate role with the above factor. Societies with lower socioeconomic status are at a higher risk that is attributable to inadequate use of screening tests, high-risk behavior such as alcohol use and smoking, and delays in seeking medical attention.
- **Geographic location** influences certain cancers primarily from the environmental exposure to certain carcinogens and indirectly by the socioeconomic status and racial and ethnic background of its population composition.

Cancer Statistics

According to American Cancer Society, a total of 1,529,560 new cancer cases and 569,490 deaths from cancer are projected to occur in the United States in 2010. Overall **cancer incidence rates decreased** in the most recent period in both men (1.3% per year from 2000 to 2006) and women (0.5% per year from 1998 to 2006). There was also noted **decrease in the death rates** in both sexes. Among men, death rates for all races combined decreased by 21% between 1990 and 2006. Among women, the overall cancer death rates between 1991 and 2006 decreased by 12.3%. The reduction in the overall cancer death rates translates to the avoidance of approximately 767,000 deaths from cancer over the 16-year period. See Table 14-1 for the gender specific cancer incidence and mortality rates.[1]

TABLE 14-1 INCIDENCE AND MORTALITY RATES OF CANCER

	Men	Women
Incidence rates	• Prostate (28%) • Lung and bronchus (15%) • Colon and rectum (9%) • Urinary bladder (7%)	• Breast (28%) • Lung and bronchus (14%) • Colon and rectum (10%) • Uterine corpus (6%)
Mortality rates	• Lung and bronchus (29%) • Prostate (11%) • Colon and rectum (9%)	• Lung and bronchus (26%) • Breast (15%) • Colon and rectum (9%)

Pathophysiology

Few concepts in medicine are as complex as the pathophysiology of cancer. Chapter 15 deals with the molecular basis of carcinogenesis.

Risk Factors

Certain risk factors have been associated with specific cancers, such as tobacco use in lung and head and neck cancers, cytotoxic therapy with secondary hematological malignancies, HPV infection and risk of cervical dysplasia and head and neck cancers. There is however still several unknown risk factors that contributes to the natural history of cancer. The individual risk factors for specific cancers are elucidated in the remaining chapters.

DIAGNOSIS

Common Clinical Presentation

Lymphadenopathy

Lymphadenopathy may cause a patient to seek medical attention, may be found incidentally on physical examination, or found by imaging. The differential diagnosis is broad, including infectious etiologies, autoimmune diseases, sarcoidosis, drug hypersensitivity, benign or clonal lymphoproliferative disorders, and malignancy. Malignant causes of lymphadenopathy include lymphoma and metastatic solid tumors. Features that suggest a malignant etiology of lymphadenopathy include lymph nodes >2 cm in size, lymph nodes that are hard or fixed to adjacent structures, and supraclavicular or epitrochlear lymphadenopathy. Lymphadenopathy may be localized or generalized, and the differential diagnosis varies depending on the location and distribution of the enlarged lymph nodes. When biopsy is indicated, an open biopsy is preferred over a core biopsy or aspiration as it allows for evaluation of the lymph node architecture, which is often necessary for classification of lymphoma.[2]

Brain Mass

- The differential diagnosis for a brain mass includes metastatic disease, primary brain tumors, CNS lymphoma, hamartoma, AV malformation, demyelination, cerebral infarction or bleeding, and infection.

- Brain **metastases** are the most common intracranial tumors in adults, accounting for 50% of all brain tumors. The presence of blood-brain barrier prevents penetration of chemotherapeutic agents into the CNS, thus providing a sanctuary site for metastatic tumor cells. The incidence of brain metastases is increasing, perhaps due to the increasing sensitivity of MRI. Lung, kidney, colorectal, and breast carcinomas and melanoma frequently metastasize to the brain. Cancer of the prostate, esophagus, oropharynx and nonmelanoma skin cancers rarely metastasize to the brain.
- Signs and symptoms of a brain mass include headache, focal neurological deficits, altered mental status, seizures, and stroke.
- The imaging study of choice is a contrast-enhanced MRI, which will delineate the location, presence of other lesions, margins of the lesion, and presence of vasogenic edema. Brain metastases are usually located in the gray and white matter junction and have a large amount of vasogenic edema.
- A brain biopsy should be preformed whenever the diagnosis is in doubt. This is particularly important in patients who have a single lesion or have a cancer that rarely metastasizes to the brain. Often, a brain lesion is the primary presentation of a malignancy. Evaluation for a source of a metastatic focus, particularly lung and breast cancer, should precede biopsy.
- Basic initial workup includes staging CT of the chest, abdomen and pelvis, colonoscopy, comprehensive skin exam, and mammogram.

Liver Metastases

- The differential diagnosis of a focal liver lesion includes primary malignant liver tumors (such as hepatocellular carcinoma, cholangiocarcinoma, lymphoma, and sarcoma), metastatic liver lesions, benign hepatic cysts, cavernous hemangioma, hepatic adenoma, and abscesses.
- Before proceeding to diagnostic testing, it is important to assess the clinical scenario. For example, is this an incidental finding? Does the patient have any risk factors such as hepatitis C/cirrhosis, oral contraceptive use, travel history, history of malignancy, or constitutional symptoms?
- Diagnostic modalities include liver ultrasound, triphasic CT of the liver, and MRI of the liver. If there is a likelihood of malignancy, a fine-needle biopsy can be done. It is important to note that if a patient has a remote history of cancer, one cannot assume that a new liver lesion is due to metastases. A new liver lesion has to be definitively diagnosed, as a second unrelated malignancy cannot be ruled out.

Bone Lesions

- Bone lesions can be the initial presentation of metastatic cancer or can present later in advanced malignancy. Bone metastases are commonly due to multiple myeloma, breast cancer, or prostate cancer, but almost any solid malignancy can metastasize to the bone. They are classified as osteolytic or osteoblastic lesions. Osteolytic lesions refer to the destruction of normal bone, whereas osteoblastic lesions are the result of deposition of new bone. Multiple myeloma lesions are purely osteolytic. Metastases from prostate cancer are usually osteoblastic. Breast cancer metastases are usually a combination of both. Bone is a preferential site for metastasis because tumor cells express and produce various chemokines and adhesive molecules that bind corresponding molecules on the stromal cells of the bone. For example, expression of RANKL (receptor activator of nuclear factor kappa B ligand) in bone facilitates development of metastasis by binding RANK (receptor activator of nuclear factor kappa B) on the surface of tumor cells. Also, tumor cells can express bone sialoprotein and bind collagen type I in the extracellular matrix in the bone, thus becoming more adhesive.

- Signs and symptoms of bone involvement include focal pain, pathologic fractures, hypercalcemia, and cord compression.
- Diagnosis is usually made by radiological testing, including plain films, which diagnose osteolytic lesions, and bone scans, which detect osteoblastic lesions only.
- Treatment includes systemic chemotherapy and hormone therapy. Local radiation can be used to palliate symptoms and prevent pathological fractures. Bisphosphonates are used to treat hypercalcemia, treat bone pain, prevent fractures, and prevent further destruction of the normal bone.

History

The importance of a thorough history taking cannot be stressed enough. The duration of symptoms can provide some insight into the aggressiveness of the malignancy. The associated symptom complex can provide information on the extent of the disease, especially organ specific symptoms which can point toward metastatic involvement by the disease. For example, new onset neurologic symptoms in a lung cancer patient should prompt imaging of the head. In a patient with metastatic disease, it may be important to first address the most bothersome symptom(s) for the purpose of palliation before starting definitive treatment for the cancer. Assessment of nutritional status and weight changes is an integral part of cancer management. Performance scales as mentioned below are used to assess the functional status of the patient either before starting treatment or during ongoing treatment. While evaluating a patient on active treatment, it is important for the treating physician to first familiarize with the most common side effects of that treatment in order to dose adjust or change treatment if necessary.

Evaluation of Performance Status

Performance status describes the functional abilities of the oncology patient. It is frequently used to provide a standardized assessment of patients considered for inclusion in protocols or to characterize patients at diagnosis or during treatment or follow-up. The initial performance status score predicts survival. The Karnofsky Performance Status and the Eastern Cooperative Oncology Group (ECOG) performance status scale (Table 14-2) are two of the most frequently used scales.

Physical Examination

A complete physical examination is warranted in any newly diagnosed cancer patient with particular attention to the organ involved. In metastatic cancers where the **primary site** is not yet identified, a physical examination may provide the first clue as to the diagnosis. This should include a breast and pelvic examination in women, a genital examination in men, and rectal examination in both men and women. In other instances, a good physical examination may provide clue as to the **extent** of the primary malignancy. They may also point toward **metastatic spread** of tumors, for example enlargement of the liver in a patient with colon cancer or bone tenderness in a breast cancer patient. A good physical examination can also aid in **following response** to treatment, such as the decreasing size of the breast mass or lymph nodes.

TABLE 14-2 KARNOFSKY AND EASTERN COOPERATIVE ONCOLOGY GROUP (ECOG) PERFORMANCE STATUS SCALES

The ***Karnofsky scale*** *runs in increments of 10 from 0 (death) to 100 (no impairment) and can be divided into three broad ranges.*

100–80:	Normal activity without the need for special assistance and no or minimal symptoms of disease
50–70:	Unable to work but able to live at home and capable of self-care, although varying levels of assistance may be required
10–40:	Incapable of self-care, requiring acute or chronic care in a hospital or institutional setting, with rapidly progressive disease process
0:	Death

The ***ECOG scale*** *runs in increments of 1 from 0 (no impairment) to 5 (death).*

0: Full activity, without symptoms
1: Ambulatory, able to carry out light activity, minimal symptoms
2: Unable to work, ambulatory for >50% of daytime activity
3: In bed or chair for >50% of daytime activity, limited self-care
4: Completely disabled, confined to bed or chair, unable to do any self-care
5: Death

Diagnostic Testing

Pathology Diagnosis

The treatment of a malignancy requires a **diagnosis based on tissue pathology.** In only rare emergent situations is treatment started without a diagnosis. Consultation from the surgical, medical, and radiation oncology team members is essential. These oncology professionals are crucial to include in cases in which prompt therapy should be delivered to the patient to reduce the risk of morbidity or mortality in certain oncologic emergencies.

- **Light microscopy** is central to diagnosis. It delineates the microscopic structure of the malignancy, such as nuclear-to-cytoplasm ratio in leukemia, invasion into the microvasculature, or extent of glandular crowding in adenocarcinoma. Additional studies, including immunohistochemical staining, flow cytometry, cytogenetics, and molecular studies for gene rearrangements can corroborate a suspected diagnosis and assist in further subclassification.
- **Immunohistochemical staining** identifies specific proteins in the tissue based on the principle of antigen-antibody complex. The development of fluorescent and nonfluorescent chromogens along with various amplification techniques has increased the sensitivity and specificity of this procedure. This technique is widely used in surgical pathology for typing tumors based on the principle of differential expression of proteins in different biologic tissues. They help provide such fundamental information as: is this a tumor? Is it benign or malignant? What type of tumor is it? They also provide information on the tissue of origin of the tumor. For example, cytokeratin stains are used to identify carcinomas from sarcomas, CD20 for B-cell lymphoma, etc. Others provide prognostic information such as Ki67, which is a marker of proliferation.

- **Flow cytometry** characterizes and sorts individual cells suspended in liquid as they flow in a narrow stream that pass through a beam of laser light. It is most frequently applied in hematologic malignancies where certain antigen profiles are diagnostic (e.g., CD5/CD23 coexpression in chronic lymphocytic leukemia). In **cytogenetic testing,** chromosomes from blood, bone marrow, or solid tissue can be isolated to identify deletions, translocations, trisomies, or insertions into the genome. In this process, chromosomes of 20 cells are counted in metaphase. The bands within the chromosomes are studied to identify any of the aforementioned abnormalities. Cytogenetic testing has been taken one step further with the advent of **FISH** (fluorescence in situ hybridization). The cellular DNA from the biopsy specimen prepared on glass and mixed with a known DNA probes that are fluorescently labeled, such as 9;22 rearrangement for chronic myeloid leukemia. If the DNA contains that translocation, the probe light up under fluorescent microscopy will align differently than if the translocation is not present. The advantage of this test is that it can identify subtle changes in the chromosome. However, it can only identify one abnormality at a time (unlike cytogenetic testing) so the investigator must know which abnormality to look for.

Laboratory Testing

Routine evaluation with complete blood counts and a comprehensive metabolic panel is important for baseline information about organ function. Any abnormal laboratory data may provide additional information on organ infiltration by the tumor, for example, an elevated alkaline phosphatase may provide indication on bony metastasis, transaminitis may be indicative of liver involvement, and low blood counts may point toward bone marrow infiltration. **Tumor markers** may provide additional information in some cases. Tumor markers are useful in **diagnostic workup** of certain germ cell tumors, such as testicular and neuroendocrine tumors. The majority of tumor markers, however, **lack** sensitivity and specificity for cancer diagnosis. Some tests may provide **prognostic information** as they reflect tumor burden, such as an LDH in lymphoma, and LDH, HCG, and AFP in testicular germ cell tumors. Most tumor markers are used in clinical practice for the purpose of **monitoring treatment** response and progression of cancer. The only tumor marker that is part of **screening** in the United States is prostate-specific antigen (PSA) for prostate cancer, which is now controversial.

Imaging Modalities[3]

- **CT** (computed tomography) allows cross-sectional imaging of the patient. Additional applications of CT include three-dimensional reconstructions and CT angiography. Intravenous radiocontrast medium is frequently utilized to enhance the sensitivity of the imaging. Risks of radiocontrast media include allergic reaction and nephrotoxicity.
- **MRI** (magnetic resonance imaging) is widely used in imaging the brain for either primary CNS tumors or metastases. MRI also has an emerging role in evaluation of breast cancer with breast MRI. MRI of the liver has a role in hepatocellular carcinoma as well as evaluation of solitary liver metastases in colon cancer. Absolute contraindications to MRI scanning include pacemakers, aneurysm clips, certain metallic cardiac prosthetic valves, and intraocular metal fragments.
- **PET** (positron emission tomography) is a functional imaging modality that images the distribution of intravenously administered radiolabeled tracers.

18-Fluorodeoxyglucose (FDG) is the most widely utilized metabolic tracer. PET is most sensitive in aggressive and metabolically active tumors such as melanoma, head and neck, breast, lung, esophageal, cervical, and colorectal cancer, as well as aggressive subtypes of lymphoma. FDG-PET has a lower sensitivity in slower-growing tumors such as low-grade lymphomas, neuroendocrine tumors, and bronchioalveolar cell lung carcinoma. PET scans can be performed with concurrent CT (PET-CT) to merge both functional and anatomic imaging.

- **Radionuclide bone scans** are frequently used to detect bone metastases. They are less sensitive to purely osteolytic lesions, such as in multiple myeloma.
- **Skeletal survey** includes plain x-rays of the skull, spine, pelvis, and extremities. It is utilized in multiple myeloma to survey for osteolytic bone lesions.

Utilization of other forms of medical imaging including volumetric (3D) anatomical imaging, dynamic contrast imaging and functional (molecular) imaging are in the process of being tested and validated in clinical trials. If successful, the use of medical imaging may serve as surrogate endpoint in clinical trials and aid clinicians in making earlier treatment decisions.

Diagnostic Procedures

An array of diagnostic procedures is available to establish a cancer diagnosis in a given patient. This may range from simple blood tests or bone marrow biopsies obtained by the treating physician in hematological malignancies to a multispecialty approach. Tissue for pathologic evaluation can be obtained by surgical approaches, such as lymph node biopsy or surgical resection specimen. Image guided such as CT or USG guided biopsy of target lesion is gaining popularity, as they are less invasive. Evaluations of luminal tumors are aided by the use of various endoscopic procedures. Some clinical situations may, however, pose special clinical challenges requiring more than one attempt and involvement of more than one specialty. Other diagnostic procedures such as lumbar puncture, pleural fluid thoracentesis or ascitic fluid paracentesis are done as part of diagnostic workup or for palliation of symptoms. Other sophisticated techniques such as chemo-embolization are discussed in relevant chapters.

TREATMENT

Approach to Oncology Treatment

The majority of adult solid malignancies are best managed through a multidisciplinary approach involving surgeons, radiation oncologists, and medical oncologists. There are often multiple different treatment options, and patients should be an active part of the decision-making process. An important element in the treatment of cancer patients is to define the goals of treatment, addressing the possibilities of cure, prolongation of survival, or improvement in quality of life in individual cases. Treatment recommendations should be carefully tailored to the individual patient, taking into account comorbid conditions, performance status, and other psychosocial issues.

Principles of Surgical Approach in Cancer

Surgery still remains the most effective modality for curing cancer confined to a local site. In many instances, the surgical removal of the primary cancer also involves the removal of a regional lymph node area. Appropriate patients can be identified for **definitive or curative surgery.** The goal is for the surgeon to remove all neoplastic cells, including the resection of a complete margin of normal tissue around the primary tumor. Depending on the primary tumor, patients with a solitary or limited number of metastases to sites such as the brain, liver, and lung can be cured by the surgical resection of the metastatic disease. **Cytoreductive surgery or tumor debulking** can facilitate subsequent radiation and/or chemotherapy in some malignancies such as ovarian cancer. Surgery may also be necessary in the **palliative setting** to relieve symptoms, such as intestinal obstruction from colon cancer.

Principles of Radiation Therapy

Radiation therapy is the treatment of choice for some cancers. The use of this treatment modality is based on the responsiveness of the cancer to ionizing radiation. Some cancers are extremely sensitive, including lymphomas and seminomas, whereas others are relatively resistant. Radiation therapy can be the sole **curative local modality** in malignancies such as cervical cancer and prostate cancer. It is also useful in the **adjuvant setting** to increase the likelihood of local or regional control after surgery. Radiation therapy also plays a key role in the **palliation of symptoms** from primary or metastatic tumor masses, including spinal cord compression and bone metastases. Further details of the principles and uses of radiation therapy are elucidated in Chapter 17. See Table 14-3 for list of radiosensitive tumors.

Principles of Systemic Therapy

In contrast to surgery or radiation therapy, which has only local effects on the tumor, the role of systemic therapy is geared at treating both the local tumor and potential or actual areas of metastatic disease throughout the body. Systemic therapy for treatment of cancers refers to traditional cytotoxic chemotherapy, immunotherapy and newer targeted therapy. The uses of different systemic therapy in various cancers and the side effects are discussed in subsequent chapters. **Clinical trials** are important tools in medical oncology to test novel treatment approaches in the management of cancer. Important clinical trials in the past decade have paved the way for more effective and less toxic regimens. Trials have also added multiple new agents and important biologic information in the fight against cancer. It is important to screen the individual patient for eligibility for the clinical trials available at your institution.

TABLE 14-3 SENSITIVITY OF MALIGNANT TUMORS TO RADIATION

Very Responsive	Moderately Responsive	Poorly Responsive
Hodgkin lymphoma	Head and neck cancer	Melanoma
Non-Hodgkin lymphoma	Breast cancer	Glioblastoma
Seminoma, dysgerminoma	Prostate cancer	Renal cancer
Neuroblastoma	Cervical cancer	Pancreatic cancer
Small-cell cancers	Esophageal cancer	Sarcoma
Retinoblastoma	Rectal cancer	Hepatoma
	Lung cancer	

TABLE 14-4 CANCERS CURABLE OR OCCASIONALLY CURABLE WITH CHEMOTHERAPY ALONE

Curable with chemotherapy alone
- Gestational choriocarcinoma
- Hodgkin lymphoma
- Germ cell cancer of the testis
- Acute lymphoid leukemia
- Non-Hodgkin lymphoma (some subtypes)
- Hairy cell leukemia

Occasionally curable with chemotherapy alone
- Acute myeloid leukemia
- Ovarian cancer
- Small-cell lung cancer

Chemotherapy

Before the initiation of chemotherapy, the **goal of treatment** must be clearly defined and discussed with the patient. Not all patients are candidates for chemotherapy. Potential risks and benefits must be considered when deciding to treat a patient with cytotoxic agents. The performance status and overall nutritional state of the cancer patient is extremely important when making the decision to use chemotherapy. Patients with performance status scores of 3 to 4 on the ECOG scale are usually not candidates for systemic therapy unless they have previously untreated tumors known to be especially responsive to chemotherapy. See Table 14-4 for list of chemosensitive tumors.

Immunotherapy

Immunotherapy refers to the use of pharmacologic agents that are intrinsic to the immune system. High concentrations of these biologic response modifiers stimulate the immune system to kill cancer cells. Examples include interferon-alpha, interleukin-2, and monoclonal antibodies. Toxicities can range from fevers and flulike symptoms to anaphylaxis and adult respiratory distress syndrome–like manifestations. Development of tumor vaccines and other potent immunotherapies are gaining momentum with increasing understanding of cancer immunology.

Targeted Therapies

These therapies interfere with specific pathways needed for the growth and survival of cancer cells. These therapies may include monoclonal antibodies or small molecule inhibitors, which target specific receptors or kinases such as the epidermal growth factors receptor, the vascular endothelial growth factor receptor, and the Bcr-Abl tyrosine kinase. The past decade has seen the approval of several targeted agents in the treatment of various cancers either as single agent or in combination with chemotherapy. Endocrine therapies used in the treatment of prostate and breast cancer are among the oldest form of targeted agents. They are very effective treatment strategies in these hormone sensitive cancers and used widely in multiple clinical settings.

Systemic chemotherapy has been used in various clinical settings.

- **Adjuvant therapy** refers to the use of systemic therapy following complete surgical resection to improve both disease-free and overall survival. The goal is to **eliminate undetected local and micrometastatic foci of tumor.** There is no way to measure or follow response to therapy, and thus duration of treatment is determined empirically by clinical trials. Cancers for which adjuvant chemotherapy has proved to benefit survival include colorectal, breast, lung, ovarian cancers, rhabdomyosarcoma, Ewing's sarcoma, and osteosarcoma. Similarly, adjuvant hormonal therapy is effective in improving survival in breast cancer patients who are estrogen receptor positive.

- **Neoadjuvant therapy** refers to systemic therapy that is administered before surgery. The goal of neoadjuvant therapy is to decrease the tumor burden for the definitive surgical procedure, thus minimizing complications and making **organ preservation** more feasible. In addition, the clinician can monitor the **tumor responsiveness** to the systemic agent and able to deliver systemic treatment without delay to eliminate micrometastatic disease. Neoadjuvant chemotherapy is used in breast, esophageal, rectal, lung, and bladder cancers, as well some sarcomas.
- **Combined modality therapy** refers to the combination of chemotherapy and radiotherapy used to treat bulky disease, especially when curative resection is not possible or less effective or when **organ preservation** is considered. For example, combination therapy can be curative and organ preserving in certain tumors such as laryngeal and anal cancers. Combined modality therapy improves survival for some patients with locally advanced lung, esophageal, head and neck, pancreatic, and cervical cancers. The combined modality therapy can also be used to decrease the size of the tumor for either a curative or a salvage surgical procedure later.
- **Palliative chemotherapy** is typically administered in metastatic setting or advanced stage of malignancy. This treatment modality is not intended for cure, but for **slowing progression of disease and prolongs life.** The chemotherapy agents are either administered as combination or single agents sequentially in this setting.
- **Induction chemotherapy** is used as the initial treatment of a malignancy to achieve complete remission or significant cytoreduction. It is commonly used in the treatment of acute leukemia and lymphoma. **Consolidation chemotherapy** is given after a patient is in remission to prolong the duration of remission and overall survival in patients with acute leukemia. **Maintenance chemotherapy** is the use of prolonged, low-dose chemotherapy to prolong the duration of remission and achieve a cure in those patients; it is currently only utilized in certain leukemias. **Salvage chemotherapy** is given with the intent to control disease or palliate symptoms after the failure of initial treatments.
- **High-dose chemotherapy** is typically used in the treatment of hematologic malignancies. High doses of chemotherapy are used to ablate the bone marrow requiring rescue with **allogeneic** or **autologous** bone marrow or stem cell replacement to repopulate the marrow. Allogeneic transplants have been curative in selected patients with chronic myelogenous leukemia and acute leukemias. Autologous stem cell transplants have been most successful for aggressive lymphomas and multiple myeloma. The use of bone marrow transplant in solid organ malignancies remains controversial.

MONITORING/FOLLOW-UP

Response to Therapy

In general, responses to therapy are measured by objective changes in tumor size and increases in disease-free and overall survival. The RECIST (response criteria in solid tumors) is a widely utilized tool for describing changes in solid tumor size in response to therapy. RECIST criteria are a voluntary, international standard that is not an NCI standard. They are based on a simplification of former methods (WHO, ECOG) and based on measurable disease.[4] Other response criteria are utilized in hematologic malignancies. The single most important indicator of the effectiveness of chemotherapy is the complete response rate. No patient with advanced cancer can be cured without attaining a complete remission. There are frequent changes in the definitions of response criteria assessment. The reader is advised to look for updated guidelines in this regard. The present information is currently available and defined on the NCI website.[5]

- **Complete response** is defined as the disappearance of all target lesions on imaging studies of at least one month of duration.
- **Partial response** is when there is at least a 30% reduction in the sum of the longest diameter of a target lesion when compared to the baseline study.
- **Progressive disease** is when there is at least a 20% increase in the sum of the longest diameter of target lesions, appearance of new lesions, or the death of the patient as a result of the tumor. Chemotherapy is discontinued in the setting of progression, and the patient is reevaluated.
- The term **stable disease** is used when the measurable disease does not meet the criteria for complete response, partial response, or progression. Stable disease represents a difficult challenge to oncologists. If therapy is tolerated with no significant side effects, it is often continued, provided it is recognized that progressive disease will eventually occur.

OUTCOME/PROGNOSIS

Goals of Care

When a patient is diagnosed with cancer, one of the first questions an oncologist will be asked is: "How long do I have?" It is not the oncologist's place to assign a life expectancy to any one patient. Each clinical scenario is different; to speculate on life expectancy can have serious emotional ramifications. An individual's prognosis is based on staging, comorbidities, performance status, and response to treatment. Although it is possible to predict curability or median survival, long-term follow-up is essential to get a more accurate sense of prognosis for any given patient. Even when the overall prognosis is poor, an honest and compassionate discussion with the patient and family members is essential. The role of the medical oncologist is to provide upfront and honest answers to even the most difficult questions and to allow the patient and family to set realistic goals that will help guide future health care decisions.

Palliative Care

Palliative care of cancer patients entails the management of all of the symptoms related to the cancer itself and the toxicities of treatment. It also includes the multidisciplinary care of psychosocial issues, with the primary goal of optimizing the quality of life and minimizing the morbidity and symptoms related to cancer and its treatments. Prolongation of survival is a secondary goal, which may or may not be achieved, but cure is not the primary intent in palliative care. Chemotherapy, hormonal therapy, radiation, and surgery are still useful in palliation. Patient selection for interventions is crucial. For patients with advanced cancer and poor performance status, aggressive treatment may be detrimental rather than beneficial.

Hospice

Hospice is a philosophy of care based on a coordinated program of support services for terminally ill patients and their families. Palliative care is provided with the aim to improve quality of life and allow a comfortable death. Any patient with a limited life expectancy (≤6 months) may be eligible for hospice care. The interdisciplinary hospice team consists of nurses trained in pain and symptom management, physicians, home health aides, social workers, chaplains, and volunteers. Care is generally given in the home but may be imparted in nursing homes or hospitals if necessary. Medicare hospice benefits also include complete coverage for all medications pertaining to the hospice diagnosis, durable medical equipment, and oxygen. Most hospice agencies provide 24-hour on-call service, brief respite care, and bereavement counseling for up to one year after the patient dies.

REFERENCES

1. Jemal A, Siegel R, Xu J, et al. Cancer statistics, 2010. *Ca Cancer J Clin.* 2010;60:277–300.
2. Brown JR, Skarin AT. Clinical mimics of lymphoma. *Oncologist.* 2004;9:406–416.
3. Torigian DA, Huang SS, Houseni M, et al. Functional imaging of cancer with emphasis on molecular techniques. *Ca Cancer J Clin.* 2007;57:206–224.
4. Jaffe CC. Measures of response: recist, who, and new alternatives. *J Clin Oncol.* 2006;24:3245–3251.
5. http://imaging.cancer.gov/clinicaltrials/imaging.

Cancer Biology

15

Kian-Huat Lim

INTRODUCTION

Since the discovery of oncogenes in the 1970s, our understanding of cancer biology has expanded exponentially. Cancer is a product that evolves from cumulative genetic or epigenetic changes that progressively drive the transformation of normal cells into malignant derivatives.[1] These changes result in alterations of various signaling pathways that are now being intensively studied and increasingly used in aiding diagnosis and guiding cancer therapy. Our current understanding of cancer biology is too broad to be review comprehensively here. In this chapter, we try to highlight the general mechanisms of tumorigenesis and metastasis.

HALLMARKS OF CANCER

Proliferation of normal cells is constantly held in check and intricately regulated both by the cellular intrinsic signaling mechanisms and the extrinsic microenvironment. In contrast, failure of these regulatory mechanisms is the general basis for uncontrolled cellular proliferation and tumorigenesis. Cancer cells acquire several intrinsic pathologic traits that not only liberate them from the homeostatic signaling from neighboring cells, but that endow them with the ability to subvert the surrounding tissues into supporting their proliferation. It is now widely accepted that several hallmarks, each originating from aberrations of distinct signaling pathways, are acquired during tumorigenesis.[2,3] These are:

- **Self-sufficiency in growth signals.** Tumor cells can generate their own growth factors, stimulate the release of growth factors bound to the extracellular matrix, enhance their sensitivity to growth signals by overexpression of receptors, or proliferate independently of growth signals by constitutive activation of signaling pathways.
- **Insensitivity to antigrowth signals.** Aberrant cell proliferation is normally constrained by growth inhibitors such as transforming growth factor beta (TGFβ) that is secreted by other cells in the microenvironment. These factors help maintain cells in the quiescent phase (G0) or inhibit uncontrolled progression from the G1 to S phase. Tumor cells can evade TGFβ inhibition by downregulating TGFβ receptors, displaying mutant receptors, or inactivating downstream signaling proteins.
- **Evasion of apoptosis.** Signals evoked by oncogenes, DNA damage, detachment from basement membrane or hypoxic tumor environment often triggers apoptosis, a form of programmed cell death that involves p53 and the Bcl-2 family proteins such as Bad and Bax. Such control mechanisms are usually impaired in cancer cells by loss of p53 or overexpression of antiapoptotic proteins such as Bcl-2.
- **Limitless replication potential.** Telomere is a structure consisting of highly repetitive DNA sequence and specialized proteins at the ends of chromosomes that protects the chromosomes from degradation. During each cycle

of DNA replication, a small section of telomere is normally lost. When the length of the telomere reaches a critically low threshold, cells undergo senescence or apoptosis. On the other hand, cancer cells acquire the ability to maintain telomere length, either by reactivation of telomerase, an enzyme that elongates telomere or by another mechanism called ALT (alternative-lengthening of telomeres). This allows cancer cells to replicate indefinitely.

- **Angiogenesis.** Tumors cannot grow larger than 0.2 mm in diameter, the diffusion limit of oxygen, without access to blood vessels. Tumor cells are capable of inducing formation of new blood vessels, termed angiogenesis to support their growth. Angiogenesis is often induced by hypoxia and requires upregulation of proangiogenic factors, such as vascular-endothelial growth factor (VEGF) and fibroblast growth factor (FGF)-1 and -2, with simultaneous inhibition of antiangiogenic factors such as angiopoietin-1 and thrombospondin-1. Targeting angiogenesis by anti-VEGF agents, such as bevacizumab, is now a common strategy in cancer treatment.[4]
- **Tissue invasion and metastasis.** A defining feature of malignant as opposed to benign tumor is the ability to invade its surrounding tissue and metastasize. Cancer cells acquire the ability to disrupt the basement membrane by upregulating matrix metalloproteases (MMPs) and invade after undergoing epithelial–mesenchymal transition (EMT). An extremely few number of cancer cells which acquire the ability to intravasate, survive in bloodstream/lymphatic system, evade immune destruction and extravasate into distal organs will subsequently form metastatic clones.
- **Evasion of the immune system.** In order to survive, cancer cells must escape the immune response, particularly cytotoxic T lymphocytes and natural killer cells, by either preventing immune recognition or inducing immune tolerance. Escape from immune recognition is mediated by downregulating mechanisms necessary for antigen presentation. Examples include downregulation of MHC molecules and inhibition of costimulatory molecules on tumor cells. Generation of immune tolerance involves altering the complex cellular and cytokine network of antigen presentation. Examples include production of inhibitory cytokines, suppression of stimulatory cytokines, and induction of formation of T-regulatory cells.
- **Reprogramming of metabolism.** Unlike normal cells in which energy is generated mainly from oxidative phosphorylation in the mitochondria, cancer cells are often reprogrammed to derive their energy from glycolysis in the cytoplasm (Warburg effect). Such transformation not only helps the cancer cells to adapt to the hypoxic microenvironment, but also provides the essential substrates for synthesis of macromolecules such as amino acids and nucleosides required for rapid proliferation.[5] Such reprogramming is usually driven by oncoproteins such as AKT1, mTOR, and myc. Clinically, the high dependence of cancer cells on glucose metabolism provides the basis for [^{18}F] fluorodeoxyglucose positron emission tomography (FDG–PET) imaging, a powerful tool to detect and monitor tumorigenic growth.

ROOT CAUSE OF CANCER: GENETIC AND EPIGENETIC ALTERATIONS

Mechanisms underlying the above-mentioned phenotypes typically originate from sequential gain or loss of gene functions that can occur within the gene (genetic alterations) or the regulatory process that control gene expression (epigenetic alterations).[6]

Etiologies of Genetic Alterations Include the Following

- **Inherited defects.** Germline mutation in certain genes can predispose one to developing cancer over time, and is the cause of most familial cancer syndromes.
- **Exogenous damage.** Chemicals, especially aromatic hydrocarbons, heavy metals, and substances such as asbestos fibers can damage the DNA are all potential carcinogens. UVA induces production of reactive oxygen species (ROS), while UVB causes cyclobutane pyrimidine dimers and pyrimidine pyrimidone photoproducts. Platinum and alkylating chemotherapeutic agents are known to cause DNA crosslinks.
- **Oncogenic viruses.** Cells infected with certain DNA viruses and retroviruses can ultimately become tumorigenic. This can be caused by aberrant expression of oncogenes (transduction) or through enhanced expression of cellular proto-oncogenes (proviral insertion). Examples include HPV in cervical cancer, EBV in Burkitt's lymphoma and nasopharyngeal carcinoma, HBV and HCV in hepatocellular carcinoma, and HTLV-1 and -2 in T-cell leukemia.
- **Genomic instability.** DNA replication is not 100% fail-safe. Replication errors such as point mutation, chromosomal translocation, amplification or rearrangement can occur and are normally rectified through specified DNA repair mechanisms. If the error cannot be repaired, DNA damage response is triggered and cells are programmed to undergo apoptosis. However, certain errors such as point mutations, small insertions/deletions or reciprocal translocation can sometimes escape DNA repair mechanisms and be passed onto daughter cells. Importantly, cells with defects, either inherited or acquired, in DNA repair mechanism (such as BRCA1/2 mutation) or DNA damage response (such as ataxia-telangiectasia, germline p53 mutation or inhibition by viral proteins such as HPV E6 and E7) are much more likely to accumulate and propagate replication errors. The result is genomic instability and increased chance of cancer formation.

Epigenetic Changes

Other than changes in primary nucleotide sequence, gene expression is also regulated by epigenetic mechanisms such as methylation/demethylation of gene promoters/enhancers and histone modifications.[7] In the last decade, control of gene expression at posttranscriptional level by micro-RNAs was discovered and will also be discussed in this section.

DNA Methylation

Methylation of cytosines in CpG dinucleotides by DNA methyltransferases generally leads to transcriptional silencing. Repetitive CpG dinucleotides (or CpG islands) are often found within the upstream promoters of most genes. When methylated, these regions become inaccessible to transcription factors and can attract histone modifying proteins that lead to formation of compact, inactive chromatin. DNA methylation is essential in normal developmental processes such as genomic imprinting and cellular differentiation. However, when the promoter of a tumor suppressor gene is hypermethylated, transcription is shut down and cells are propelled toward malignant transformation. For example, hypermethylation of the promoter for *MLH1,* a gene involved in DNA mismatch repair, has been implicated in the pathogenesis of hereditary nonpolyposis colorectal cancer. Two DNA methyltransferase inhibitors, 5-azacytadine and decitabine (2′-deoxy-5-azacytidine), are approved therapy for the treatment of myelodysplastic syndrome and also have activity in acute myeloid leukemia.

Histone Deacetylation

Acetylation/deacetylation of lysine residues on histones by histone acetyltransferases (HATs) and histone deacetylases (HDACs), respectively, is another mode of epigenetic modification which can alter gene expression. Deacetylation causes histones to wrap more tightly around DNA, which blocks access of transcription factors to DNA. In cancer, tumor suppressor genes that are silenced by histone deacetylation can theoretically be reactivated by HDAC inhibitors. Currently, HDAC inhibitors such as Vorinostat and Romidepsin are approved for treatment of cutaneous T-cell lymphoma.

Posttranscriptional Regulation: Micro-RNAs

Micro-RNAs, an important discovery of the last decade, are a species of short, single-stranded, noncoding RNAs that can bind to the complementary sequences within target mRNAs and generally lead to their degradation. More than half of human genes are now believed to be regulated by micro-RNAs. Aberrant expression of micro-RNAs is found in many human cancers.[8] For example, miR-15a and miR-16–1, which negatively regulate Bcl-2, an antiapoptotic gene, are often deleted or downregulated in B-cell CLL. On the other hand, miR-9, which is overexpressed in breast cancer, promotes metastasis by downregulating E-cadherin. Therapies targeting micro-RNAs are still under investigation.

Outcome of Genetic/Epigenetic Alterations: Oncogenes and Tumor Suppressor Genes

The two major classes of genes are that are subject to these changes are the oncogenes and tumor suppressor genes. In principle, tumorigenic changes involve gain of oncogene function and loss of tumor suppressor function.

- **Oncogenes** are altered versions of normal genes (termed proto-oncogenes) that have acquired gain-of-function point mutations, gene copy amplifications or translocations. The results are cellular proliferation, growth, survival, invasion, and angiogenesis. Several categories of oncogenes have been described and these include:
    1. Growth factors: sis, trk
    2. Growth-factor receptors: EGFR, HER2/neu, c-kit, PDGFR, VEGFR
    3. Tyrosine kinases: bcr-abl, src, Syk-ZAP-70, BTK
    4. Serine-threonine kinases: Raf, Akt, MAPK, cyclin-dependent kinases, Aurora kinases
    5. GTPases: K-Ras, N-Ras, H-Ras, Cdc42, Rac, Ral
    6. Cytoplasmic proteins: Bcl-2, survivin
    7. Transcription factors: c-myc, jun, fos, Nf-kB
- **Tumor suppressor genes** or gate-keeper genes function to restrain cellular proliferation and/or maintain cellular homeostasis. Classic examples include ***PTEN, NF1, NF2, and APC*** which are negative regulators of proliferation; ***INK4a-ARF*** which controls cell cycle, ***p53*** which is the master switch of apoptosis, ***BRCA1/BRCA2*** which are key players in DNA damage response and ***VHJ*** which negatively regulates angiogenesis. In cancer cells, expression of tumor suppressor genes is usually lost by biallelic gene deletion, loss-of-function mutations or transcriptionally silenced by epigenetic mechanisms. While loss of tumor suppressor genes alone is not sufficient for malignant transformation, it does predispose cells to accumulate further genetic changes and cooperates with oncogenes to complete

TABLE 15-1 GENE LOSS AND FAMILIAL CANCER SYNDROMES

Syndrome	Genes Lost	Common Cancers
Ataxia-telangiectasia	*ATM*	Non-Hodgkin lymphoma, ALL, CLL
Basal cell nevus syndrome (Gorlin's syndrome)	*PTCH*	Basal cell carcinoma
Bloom syndrome	*BLM*	Lymphoid malignancies, Wilms' tumor, head and neck, lung, esophagus, colon, cervix
Carney syndrome	*PRKAR1A*	Testicular tumors (Sertoli and Leydig cell tumors) benign tumors: nevi, atrial myxoma
Cowden syndrome	*PTEN*	Breast, thyroid
Hereditary breast/ ovarian cancer	*BRCA1 and BRCA2*	Breast, ovarian, fallopian tube, pancreatic
Hereditary nonpolyposis colon cancer (Lynch syndrome)	*MLH1, MSH2, MSH6, and PMS2*	Colorectal, endometrial, gastric
Li–Fraumeni syndrome	*p53*	Skin, soft tissue sarcoma, breast, GBM, leukemias, lymphomas, adrenocortical carcinoma
Neurofibromatosistype1	*NF1*	Malignant peripheral nerve sheath tumor, astrocytoma, carcinoids
Neurofibromatosistype2	*NF2*	Glioma, ependymoma
Peutz–Jeghers syndrome	*STK11*	Gastrointestinal, pancreatic, lung
Retinoblastoma	*Rb*	Retinoblastoma, osteosarcoma
Tuberous sclerosis complex	*TSC1/TSC2*	Subependymal giant cell astrocytomas, renal cancer
von Hippel–Lindau syndrome	*VHJ*	Renal cell carcinoma

cellular transformation. Clinically, germline mutations/deletions of tumor suppressor genes are associated with several familial cancer syndromes (See Table 15-1).

- ***p53*** **mutations.**

The tumor suppressor ***p53*** is the most frequently mutated gene in human cancer and therefore warrants further discussion. ***p53*** is normally activated in response to stresses such as DNA damage, hypoxia, and oncogene activation. It encodes a transcription factor that primarily activates genes responsible for cell cycle arrest and apoptosis by several mechanisms. It activates cell cycle inhibitors such as ***p21*** and upregulation of proapoptotic genes such as ***Bax.*** Inactivating mutations of ***p53*** are found in more than 50% of all cancers. The majority of ***p53*** mutations (~75%) are missense mutations, usually within the DNA-binding domain that results in an abnormal tertiary structure with impaired ability to regulate transcription of target genes. Hypermethylation of the promoter for p53 and upregulation of its inhibitors, such as HDM-2 are also found in human cancers. Patients with **Li–Fraumeni** syndrome have germline mutations in the *p53* gene and are at high risk for early-onset cancers of multiple tissues types, including breast, bone, soft tissue, head and neck, and brain and, less commonly, lung, stomach, colon, and blood (leukemia). In sporadic cancers, the timing of *p53* loss can differ. p53 alterations are usually early events in lung, esophageal, head and neck, breast, cervical, bladder, and stomach cancers, but are late events in brain, thyroid, prostate, and ovarian cancers. There is no consistent pattern in p53 alterations in colon, bladder, and liver cancers. Delivery of p53 by gene therapy is currently in clinical trials.[9]

TUMOR METASTASIS

Tumor metastasis warrants more detailed discussion because it accounts for more than 90% of cancer deaths. In most cancers, metastatic trait is acquired late in the multistep oncogenic process. However, clinically the natural history, route and site of metastasis vary with different cancers, which underscore the complex signaling mechanisms behind metastasis. In fact, metastasis in itself is a consummation of multiple distinct properties that an extremely small number of cancer cells acquire during evolution from a genetically heterogeneous population.[10] These properties include:

- **Detachment from the primary tumor.** Adherence of tumor cells to adjacent cells and extracellular matrix is almost always altered. Intercellular adhesion is greatly diminished by downregulation of normal adhesion proteins such as E-cadherin and interactions with extracellular matrix is augmented by expression of specific integrins such as α6β4. These changes facilitate detachment of tumor cells from their primary locus.
- **Invasion, migration, and intravasation.** Expression of integrins such as α6β4 can greatly augment the invasion of cancer cells through stroma. Disruption of basement membrane is usually achieved via activation of metalloproteases. By undergoing epithelial-to-mesenchymal transition, cancer cells of epithelial origin acquire a mesenchymal cell phenotype that allows for motility and invasion.[11] Migration is further directed by various growth factors such as EGF, FGF, HGF and insulin-like growth factor. Subsequently, cancer cells are able to penetrate vascular endothelial lining (intravasation) and enter the bloodstream or lymphatic system.
- **Survival in the vasculature or lymphatic system.** Once in the circulation or lymphatic system, cancer cells must evade immune recognition as described before. Also, by abrogating their major apoptotic machinery, cancer cells are able to avoid anoikis, a type of apoptosis triggered by loss of contact with extracellular matrix. Nonetheless, most cancer cells succumb to the high-velocity shear stress within the circulation and only a tiny number of cells survive to reach target organs.
- **Arrest at the metastatic site and extravasation.** The anatomy of blood and lymphatic vasculature, as well as presence of specific chemokines is an important determinant of the site of metastasis. For example, breast cancer cells have high expression of the chemokine receptor, CXCR4, while its ligand, CXCL12, is highly expressed in organs to which it most commonly metastasizes: lung, liver, bone, and regional lymph nodes. Once at the target organ site, cells must

arrest in the vasculature and extravasate, which again involves alterations in cell adhesion molecules and proteases.

- **Survival in the metastatic microenvironment.** Once at the target organ, tumor cells (seeds) must successfully interact with their microenvironment (soil) in order to initiate colonization. In addition, angiogenic "switch" must be triggered by secretion of various angiogenic factors to sustain metastatic growth.

FUTURE

The discovery of important signaling pathways propelling certain cancer has led to successful stories of targeted agents such as imatinib, and currently more targeted agents are being developed and tested. However, most cancers consist of highly heterogeneous subpopulations of transformed cells that are driven by complex network of signaling mechanisms. Therefore, it is highly unlikely that targeting one or two signaling pathways is sufficient in curbing cancer growth in most cases. The advent of new, high-throughput techniques such as microarray, genomic sequencing (termed oncogenomics) and recently functional proteomics, in conjunction with bioinformatics and system biology now allow broader view into the signaling lesions underlying every type of cancer, with the potential of allowing combinations of targeted agents.[12] Importantly, these techniques are beginning to redefine or reclassify many cancers based on their molecular profile rather than histology alone. Application of these techniques in aiding diagnosis and treatment decision will likely become more common in the future and become a crucial part in personalizing cancer management.

REFERENCES

1. Fearon ER, Vogelstein B. A genetic model for colorectal tumorigenesis. *Cell.* 1990;61: 759–767.
2. Hanahan D, Weinberg RA. The hallmarks of cancer. *Cell.* 2000;100:57–70.
3. Hanahan D, Weinberg RA. Hallmarks of cancer: the next generation. *Cell.* 2011;144: 646–674.
4. Folkman J. Angiogenesis: an organizing principle for drug discovery? *Nat Rev Drug Discov.* 2007;6:273–286.
5. Cairns RA, Harris IS, Mak TW. Regulation of cancer cell metabolism. *Nat Rev Cancer.* 2011;11:85–95.
6. Harris TJ, McCormick F. The molecular pathology of cancer. *Nat Rev Clin Oncol.* 2010; 7:251–265.
7. Jones PA, Baylin SB. The epigenomics of cancer. *Cell.* 2007;128:683–692.
8. Inui M, Martello G, Piccolo S. MicroRNA control of signal transduction. *Nat Rev Mol Cell Biol.* 2010;11:252–263.
9. Brown CJ, Lain S, Verma CS, et al. Awakening guardian angels: drugging the p53 pathway. *Nat Rev Cancer.* 2009;9:862–873.
10. Chiang AC, Massague J. Molecular basis of metastasis. *N Engl J Med.* 2008;359: 2814–2823.
11. Polyak K, Weinberg RA. Transitions between epithelial and mesenchymal states: acquisition of malignant and stem cell traits. *Nat Rev Cancer.* 2009;9:265–273.
12. Bild AH, Potti A, Nevins JR. Linking oncogenic pathways with therapeutic opportunities. *Nat Rev Cancer.* 2006;6:735–741.

Chemotherapy

16

Kristan M. Augustin, Lindsay M. Hladnik, Sara K. Butler, Ali McBride, and Leigh M. Boehmer

GENERAL PRINCIPLES

- The management of malignancy with chemotherapy is the specific specialty of hematologist and medical oncologists. The appropriate and safe use of chemotherapy requires an understanding of various factors including, but not limited to, principles of the cell cycle and tumor growth kinetics, timing of chemotherapy administration, chemotherapy response assessment, and pharmacology of chemotherapy agents, including mechanisms of action, pharmacokinetic/pharmacodynamic properties, adverse effects, and mechanisms of drug resistance. Therefore, the prescribing and administration of these agents should only be done by those specifically trained and experienced healthcare professionals. The intent of this chapter is to provide a brief overview of some of the general principles of chemotherapy, various classes of chemotherapy agents, their respective mechanisms of action, and selected adverse effects.[1,2] See Table 16-1 for chemotherapy agent classification, mechanisms of action, selected toxicities, and other pertinent information relating to these agents.
- Endocrine-related tumors are often affected by hormone therapy (e.g., antiestrogens in breast cancer, thyroid hormone to suppress thyroid cancer, and antiandrogens to inhibit prostate cancer). These agents are not discussed here, and the reader is referred to Chapters 18, 25, and 26 for more information regarding those tumors. In addition, please see Chapter 34 for a discussion of nonchemotherapeutic medications and symptomatic and supportive treatments for patients with cancer.
- Most chemotherapy agents are toxic to cells of the human body. The justification for using substances that are toxic to normal cells is that malignant cells are preferentially sensitive to the effects of chemotherapy. A balance must be struck between toxicity to malignant and harm to benign, normal tissues that are intended to be spared. This concept is described as the therapeutic index, which is the ratio of toxicity to tumor cells to that of normal cells. The therapeutic index is quite narrow for many antineoplastic agents. Traditional chemotherapeutic agents interfere with normal cell processes, typically DNA synthesis or repair. However, it should be appreciated that these agents may act in methods other than simple cell killing (e.g., as initiators of apoptosis or cellular maturation agents).
- Several newer agents have been developed that depart from the traditional concept of cell killing as their primary action. These agents are targeted to specific receptors in or on the cancer cell, often in signal transduction pathways that regulate tumor cell growth, proliferation, migration, angiogenesis, and apoptosis.

TABLE 16-1 PHARMACOLOGIC AGENTS IN ONCOLOGY

Drug Classification/ Subclassification/Agents	Mechanism of Action	Selected Toxicities	Other Pertinent Information
Covalent DNA-binding agents			
Alkylating agents	Produce DNA-DNA crosslinks; non-cell cycle specific		
Bendamustine		Myelosuppression, N/V, infusion reactions/anaphylaxis, TLS, rash (SJS and TEN reported), diarrhea, stomatitis, constipation, secondary malignancies	Monitor for drug interactions with inhibitors/inducers of CYP1A2. Contains mannitol—caution or avoid with hypersensitivity reactions. Consider premeds for previous mild infusion reactions.
Busulfan		Myelosuppression, N/V, diarrhea, constipation, anorexia, VOD, pulmonary fibrosis, seizures	Seizure prophylaxis should be used with high-dose regimens.
Carmustine		Myelosuppression, N/V, elevated LFT, VOD, alopecia, renal insufficiency	Diluent for intravenous preparation contains ethanol.
Chlorambucil		Myelosuppression, pulmonary fibrosis, rash, elevated LFT	
Cyclophosphamide		Myelosuppression, N/V, hemorrhagic cystitis, SIADH, alopecia, cardiomyopathy, VOD, secondary malignancies, facial flushing, headache	The inactive metabolite, acrolein, may cause direct bladder toxicity resulting in hemorrhagic cystitis. May prevent this with brisk hydration and Mesna in the setting of high dose therapy.
Dacarbazine		Myelosuppression, N/V	

Ifosfamide		Myelosuppression, N/V, hemorrhagic cystitis, nephrotoxicity, SIADH, alopecia, neurotoxicity (somnolence, confusion, and hallucinations)	The inactive metabolite, acrolein, may cause direct bladder toxicity resulting in hemorrhagic cystitis. May prevent this with brisk hydration and Mesna.
Lomustine		Myelosuppression, N/V	
Mechlorethamine		Myelosuppression, N/V, diarrhea, mucositis, alopecia	
Melphalan		Myelosuppression, N/V, diarrhea, mucositis, alopecia	
Procarbazine		Myelosuppression, N/V, neurotoxicity, hallucinations	
Streptozocin		N/V, elevated LFT, nephrotoxicity, hypoalbuminemia	
Temozolomide		Myelosuppression, peripheral edema, headache, fever, fatigue, seizures, N/V, diarrhea	
Thiotepa		Myelosuppression, alopecia, rash	Cystitis may occur when given intravesically.
Platinum agents	Produce DNA-DNA adducts and crosslinks resulting in inhibition of DNA replication and synthesis; non-cell cycle specific		
Carboplatin		Nephrotoxicity, myelosuppression, peripheral neuropathy, hypomagnesemia, hypokalemia, hypocalcemia, hypophosphatemia, N/V, diarrhea, mucositis, alopecia	

(*continued*)

TABLE 16-1 PHARMACOLOGIC AGENTS IN ONCOLOGY (*Continued*)

Drug Classification/ Subclassification/Agents	Mechanism of Action	Selected Toxicities	Other Pertinent Information
Cisplatin		Nephrotoxicity, N/V, myelosuppression, peripheral neuropathy, hypomagnesemia, hypokalemia, hypocalcemia, hypophosphatemia, diarrhea, ototoxicity	May induce acute and delayed N/V, which can be severe.
Oxaliplatin		Myelosuppression, peripheral neuropathy, fatigue, N/V, diarrhea, constipation, anorexia, fever, elevated LFT, alopecia	Acute and chronic neurotoxicity may occur. Peripheral sensory neuropathy, exacerbated by cold, is seen in acute settings. Chronic toxicity is dose-dependent proprioception and neurosensory deficits.
Antimetabolites	Interfere with normal synthesis pathways of tumor cells; often inhibit DNA or RNA synthesis; S phase specific		
Pyrimidine antagonists			
5-Azacitidine	Hypomethylation of DNA	Myelosuppression, N/V, diarrhea, fever, renal tubular acidosis, elevated LFT, alopecia, fatigue	

Capecitabine	Inhibits thymidylate synthase	Palmar-plantar erythrodysesthesia, diarrhea, stomatitis, N/V, fatigue, fever, abdominal pain, anorexia, elevated bilirubin, myelosuppression	
Cytarabine		Myelosuppression, fever, cerebral and cerebellar toxicity, N/V diarrhea, mucositis, conjunctivitis, rash, alopecia, abnormal LFT, flulike syndrome	May be given intrathecally. High-dose regimens are toxic to the cerebellum and need to be monitored closely. Conjunctivitis associated with high-dose cytarabine may be prevented with prophylactic corticosteroid eye drops.
Decitabine	Hypomethylation of DNA	Myelosuppression, edema, fever, headache, N/V, diarrhea, constipation, anorexia, elevated LFT, cough	
Floxuridine	Inhibits thymidylate synthase	Myelosuppression, diarrhea, stomatitis, peptic ulcer disease	
5-Fluorouracil	Inhibits thymidylate synthase	Myelosuppression, N/V, mucositis, diarrhea, palmar-plantar erythrodysesthesia	
Gemcitabine		Myelosuppression, N/V, diarrhea, constipation, stomatitis, elevated LFT, flulike syndrome, alopecia, rash, hemolytic uremic syndrome, pain, dyspnea	

(continued)

TABLE 16-1 PHARMACOLOGIC AGENTS IN ONCOLOGY (*Continued*)

Drug Classification/ Subclassification/Agents	Mechanism of Action	Selected Toxicities	Other Pertinent Information
Purine antagonists			
Cladribine	Inhibits ribonucleotide reductase and DNA synthesis; cell cycle nonspecific	Myelosuppression, opportunistic infections, fever, fatigue	
Clofarabine	Inhibits ribonucleotide reductase and DNA polymerase	Myelosuppression, opportunistic infections, N/V, diarrhea, constipation, headache, fatigue, cardiotoxicity, dyspnea, renal tubular acidosis, elevated LFT, rash	
Fludarabine	Inhibits ribonucleotide reductase, DNA polymerase, primase, and ligase I	Myelosuppression, opportunistic infections, neurotoxicity	
6-Mercaptopurine	Inhibits purine synthesis	Myelosuppression, elevated LFT	
Pentostatin	Inhibits adenosine deaminase	Myelosuppression, fever, acute renal failure, elevated LFT	
6-Thioguanine	Inhibits purine synthesis	Myelosuppression	
Folate antagonists	Inhibit dihydrofolate reductase, which inhibits synthesis of thymidylate and purines		
Methotrexate	S phase specific	Myelosuppression, stomatitis, N/V, diarrhea, nephrotoxicity, abnormal LFT, neurotoxicity	May be given intrathecally. Leucovorin administration and following methotrexate levels should be performed with high-dose therapy.

Pemetrexed	Inhibits dihydrofolate reductase, thymidylate synthase, and glycinamide ribonucleotide formyltransferase, which are folate-dependent enzymes involved in the de novo biosynthesis of thymidine and purine nucleotides; G_1-S phase specific	Myelosuppression, rash, chest pain, fatigue, N/V, neuropathy, nephrotoxicity, dyspnea	Rash may be painful and generalized. Premedicate with corticosteroids. Supplement with folic acid and vitamin B_{12}.
Pralatrexate	Also an inhibitor for polyglutamylation by folylpolyglutamyl synthetase	Myelosuppression, mucositis, N/V, fever, dehydration, SOB, nephrotoxicity, hepatotoxicity, fatigue, dermatologic reactions	Vitamin B_{12} and folic acid supplementation should be initiated prior to the first pralatrexate and continued thereafter.
Antitumor antibiotics			
Anthracyclines	Inhibit topoisomerase II, produce free radicals, and intercalate adjacent DNA base pairs		
Daunorubicin		Myelosuppression, alopecia, cardiotoxicity, mucositis	Recommended lifetime cumulative dose is 400–600 mg/m^2.
Doxorubicin		Myelosuppression, cardiotoxicity, mucositis, N/V, diarrhea, alopecia	Recommended lifetime cumulative dose is 450–550 mg/m^2.
Epirubicin		Myelosuppression, cardiotoxicity, mucositis, N/V, diarrhea, alopecia	Recommended lifetime cumulative dose is 750–900 mg/m^2.

(*continued*)

TABLE 16-1 PHARMACOLOGIC AGENTS IN ONCOLOGY (*Continued*)

Drug Classification/ Subclassification/Agents	Mechanism of Action	Selected Toxicities	Other Pertinent Information
Idarubicin		Myelosuppression, N/V, cardiotoxicity, mucositis, diarrhea, alopecia, elevated LFT	Recommended lifetime cumulative dose is unknown.
Mitoxantrone		Myelosuppression, elevated LFT, alopecia, mucositis, N/V, anorexia, cardiotoxicity, diarrhea	
Other antitumor antibiotics			
Bleomycin	Inhibits DNA synthesis; S and G_2 phase specific	Pulmonary fibrosis, stomatitis, fever, skin changes, hypersensitivity reactions, Raynaud phenomenon	A test dose is recommended for patients with lymphoma, but may produce false negative results.
Dactinomycin	Intercalates into DNA resulting in inhibition of DNA and RNA synthesis	Myelosuppression, N/V, pulmonary fibrosis, elevated LFT, alopecia, mucositis, diarrhea, fatigue	
Mitomycin C	Produces DNA crosslinks; non-cell cycle specific, but maximal effects in late G and early S phases	Myelosuppression, hemolytic uremic syndrome, acute bronchospasm, alopecia, congestive heart failure, nail banding, fever	May be given intravesically.
Topoisomerase inhibitors			
Topoisomerase I inhibitors	Active in the unwinding of DNA, causing DNA strand breaks; S phase specific		

Irinotecan		Acute and delayed diarrhea, abdominal pain/cramping, N/V, myelosuppression, dyspnea, alopecia, elevated transaminases, fatigue, fever, weakness	Acute diarrhea may be treated with atropine and delayed diarrhea may be treated with loperamide.
Topotecan		Myelosuppression, N/V, diarrhea, alopecia, rash, elevated transaminases, fatigue, headache, fever, stomatitis, dyspnea, weakness	
Topoisomerase II inhibitors	Inhibit the ability to restore the structure of cleaved DNA, resulting in double-strand breaks; S and G_2 phase specific		
Etoposide		Myelosuppression, N/V, mucositis, anorexia, diarrhea, HOTN, disorientation, alopecia	Etoposide formulation contains ethanol, 30.3% (v/v). Etoposide phosphate 113.5 mg = etoposide 100 mg and dosages should always be calculated and expressed as the desired **etoposide** dose.
Teniposide		Myelosuppression, N/V, mucositis, diarrhea, anorexia, alopecia, HOTN	
Vinca alkaloids	Bind to tubulin and inhibit microtubule assembly; M and S phase specific		

(*continued*)

TABLE 16-1 PHARMACOLOGIC AGENTS IN ONCOLOGY (*Continued*)

Drug Classification/ Subclassification/Agents	Mechanism of Action	Selected Toxicities	Other Pertinent Information
Vinblastine		Myelosuppression, stomatitis, alopecia, SIADH	
Vincristine		Peripheral neuropathy, constipation, paralytic ileus, alopecia	
Vinorelbine		Myelosuppression, peripheral neuropathy, constipation, stomatitis, fatigue, elevated LFT	
Taxanes	Bind to microtubules and prevent their disassembly; G_2-M phase specific		
Cabazitaxel	Poor affinity for MDR proteins confers activity in taxane-resistant disease.	Myelosuppression, diarrhea, fatigue, N/V, peripheral neuropathy, weakness, hematuria, hypersensitivity reaction	Hypersensitivity reaction due to cabazitaxel and/or its vehicle, Polysorbate 80. Premedicate with corticosteroids and H_1- and H_2-blockers.
Docetaxel		Myelosuppression, hypersensitivity reaction, peripheral neuropathy, elevated LFT, rash, alopecia, stomatitis, fluid retention	Hypersensitivity reaction (dyspnea, fluid retention, tachycardia, flushing, HOTN, chest pain), due to docetaxel or its vehicle, Polysorbate 80, occurs in 2% of patients despite premedication with dexamethasone.

Paclitaxel		Myelosuppression, hypersensitivity reaction, peripheral neuropathy, HOTN, bradycardia, alopecia, elevated LFT	Hypersensitivity reaction due to paclitaxel or its vehicle, Cremophor EL. Premedicate with corticosteroids and H_1- and H_2-blockers.
Epothilone B analog			
Ixabepilone	Bind to the beta-tubulin subunit of the micro-tubules and prevent their disassembly	Myelosuppression, peripheral and sensory neuropathy, hypersensitivity reaction, myalgia/arthralgia, N/V, mucositis, diarrhea, alopecia	Hypersensitivity reaction due to ixabepilone and/or its vehicle, Cremophor EL. Premedicate with H_1- and H_2-blockers; add corticosteroids if history of reaction. BSA is capped at 2.2 m^2 for dose calculation.
Halichondrin B analog			
Eribulin	Non-taxane microtubule dynamics inhibitor that inhibits the growth phase of microtubules without affecting the shortening phase, sequesters tubulin	Myelosuppression, peripheral neuropathy, headache, fatigue, constipation, N/V, cough, arthralgia, elevated LFT	QTc prolongation has been demonstrated; monitor closely in patients with CHF, on antiarrhythmics, or have electrolyte abnormalities.
Histone deacetylase (HDAC) inhibitors	HDAC inhibitor, induces cell cycle arrest and apoptosis.		
Romidepsin		N/V, fatigue, QT prolongation, hypocalcemia, hypokalemia, hyper/hypomagnesemia, hyperglycemia, myelosuppression, dysgeusia, elevated LFT	Monitor for drug interactions (via CYP450), May enhance the anticoagulant effect of Vitamin K antagonist; monitor closely.

(*continued*)

TABLE 16-1 PHARMACOLOGIC AGENTS IN ONCOLOGY (*Continued*)

Drug Classification/ Subclassification/Agents	Mechanism of Action	Selected Toxicities	Other Pertinent Information
Vorinostat		Diarrhea, fatigue, N/V, myelosuppression, anorexia, dysgeusia, hyperglycemia, hypomagnesemia, hypocalcemia, hypokalemia, xerostomia, QT prolongation, PE, DVT	May enhance the anticoagulant effect of Vitamin K antagonists; monitor closely.
Mammalian target of rapamycin (m-TOR) inhibitors			
Everolimus	m-TOR inhibitor with antiproliferative and antiangiogenic properties	Elevated cholesterol and triglycerides, rash, cough, hyperglycemia, stomatitis, hypophosphatemia, myelosuppression, peripheral edema, fever, elevated LFT, elevated creatinine, fatigue, diarrhea	Approved medication guide must be dispensed with this medication.
Temsirolimus	m-TOR inhibitor with antiproliferative and antiangiogenic properties	Edema, chest pain, rash, hyperglycemia, hypercholesterolemia, hyperlipidemia, hypophosphatemia, hypokalemia, mucositis, stomatitis, cough	Monitor for drug interactions as it undergoes hepatic metabolism via CYP3A4.

Miscellaneous agents			
Bortezomib	26S proteasome inhibitor (enzyme complex that regulates cellular protein homeostasis)	Peripheral neuropathy, edema, HOTN, myelosuppression, fever, rash, N/V, diarrhea, constipation, infection, CHF, QT prolongation, pulmonary toxicities, elevated LFT	Monitor for drug interactions, as it undergoes hepatic metabolism via CYP450.
Hydroxyurea	Inhibits ribonucleotide reductase and DNA synthesis; S phase specific	Myelosuppression	
L-Asparaginase	Inhibits protein synthesis by converting asparagine to aspartic acid and ammonia; G_1 phase specific	Fever, chills, hyperglycemia, acute pancreatitis, hypofibrinogenemia, elevated LFT, hypersensitivity reactions, nephrotoxicity	A test dose is recommended.
Differentiating agents			
Arsenic trioxide	Apoptosis of leukemia cells	QT prolongation, tachycardia, fatigue, fever, electrolyte abnormalities, N/V, dyspnea, leukocytosis, APL differentiation syndrome	
Tretinoin	Terminal differentiation and apoptotic cell death	Headache, fever, weakness, fatigue, N/V, bleeding, leukocytosis, dyspnea, elevated cholesterol and triglycerides, APL differentiation syndrome	

(*continued*)

TABLE 16-1 PHARMACOLOGIC AGENTS IN ONCOLOGY (*Continued*)

Drug Classification/ Subclassification/Agents	Mechanism of Action	Selected Toxicities	Other Pertinent Information
Targeted therapies			
Monoclonal antibodies	May affect cellular signaling pathways by inhibiting ligand-receptor interactions, may stimulate host defense mechanisms causing antitumor activity, or may be combined with protein toxins or cytotoxic agents that disrupt protein synthesis		
Alemtuzumab	Binds to CD52 resulting in complement-mediated and/or ADCC	HOTN, HTN, peripheral edema, tachycardia, fever, fatigue, rash, N/V, diarrhea, myelosuppression, rigors, myalgias, infection, serious and potentially fatal infusion-related reactions	Prophylactic therapy against *Pneumocystis carinii* pneumonia and herpes viruses needed. Premedicate. Dose escalation is required at initiation and after therapy interruption for ≥7 days.
Bevacizumab	Binds to and neutralizes VEGF	HTN, N/V, diarrhea, constipation, leukopenia, proteinuria, nephrotic syndrome, GI perforations, intra-abdominal abscesses, impaired wound healing, hemorrhage, thromboembolic events, CHF, infusion reactions, reversible posterior leukoencephalopathy	

Cetuximab	Recombinant human/mouse chimeric monoclonal antibody that binds to EGFR and inhibits ligand binding	Dermatologic toxicities, hypomagnesemia, N/V, diarrhea, constipation, infusion reactions, peripheral edema, cardiopulmonary arrest (in combination with radiation therapy), elevated LFT, interstitial lung disease, photosensitivity	Risk of infusion-related reactions. Premedications and monitoring during infusion and for at least 1 h after infusion is complete are required. Efficacy in colon cancer only seen with KRAS wild type tumors.
Denileukin diftitox	Recombinant fusion protein (diphtheria toxin + IL-2), which delivers a cytotoxic dose of diphtheria toxin after interacting with IL-2 receptors on malignant cells	Vascular leak syndrome, flulike illness, rash, N/V, diarrhea, myelosuppression, elevated LFT, hypersensitivity reactions, infection, loss of visual acuity or color	Serum albumin levels should be ≥3 g/dL before and during therapy.
Eculizumab	MAb against the complement protein C5, blocks the cleavage of C5 to C5 convertase and inhibits the process of complement-mediated cell destruction	Headache, myalgia, nasopharyngitis, pain, nausea, fatigue, cough, viral infections, anemia, pyrexia	Meningococcal vaccination must be administered to all patients at least 2 wk prior to the first dose.
Ofatumumab	Binds to small and large extracellular loops of CD20; induces complement-dependent cytotoxicity and ADCC	Infusion reactions, cytopenias, progressive multifocal leukoencephalopathy, hepatitis B infection/reactivation, nausea, diarrhea, intestinal obstruction, infections	Premedications and infusion rate titration are required. Screen patients at high risk of hepatitis B virus before initiation of therapy and close monitoring of carriers is required during and after therapy.

(*continued*)

TABLE 16-1 **PHARMACOLOGIC AGENTS IN ONCOLOGY (*Continued*)**

Drug Classification/ Subclassification/Agents	Mechanism of Action	Selected Toxicities	Other Pertinent Information
Panitumumab	Recombinant human IgG2 monoclonal antibody that binds to EGFR and inhibits ligand binding	Dermatologic toxicities, acne-form rash, fissures, peripheral edema, fatigue, hypomagnesemia, cough, stomatitis, eyelash growth, infusion reactions	Lower risk of infusion reactions since not chimeric antibody. Premedication not required. Efficacy in colon cancer only seen with KRAS wild type tumors.
Rituximab	Binds to CD20; induces complement-dependent cytotoxicity and ADCC	Cytokine release syndrome, rash, nausea, myelosuppression, infection, tumor lysis syndrome, severe and potentially fatal mucocutaneous reactions, infusion reactions (may be severe or fatal)	Premedications and infusion rate titration are required.
Trastuzumab	Binds to the HER2 coreceptor protein and inhibits HER-family receptor dimerization, inhibiting signal transduction; induces ADCC against cells that overproduce HER2; internalizes the HER2 receptor; down regulates surface HER2	Infusion-related reactions, diarrhea, CHF, left ventricular dysfunction, cardiomyopathy, myelosup-pression, severe hypersensitivity reactions, pulmonary events	

Tyrosine kinase inhibitors	Inhibit signal transduction within cellular signaling cascades affecting DNA synthesis, cell growth, proliferation, migration, angiogenesis, and apoptosis		
Dasatinib	Multitargeted TKI; inhibits BCR-ABL tyrosine kinase; targets most imatinib-resistant BCR-ABL mutations except the T315I and F317V mutants	Myelosuppression, fluid retention/ edema, N/V, diarrhea, constipation, mucositis, rash, QTc prolongation, arrhythmia, elevated LFT, arthralgia/ myalgia, neuropathy, infection, CHF, alopecia, photosensitivity	Monitor for drug interactions (via CYP450). Antacids, H_2-blockers, and PPIs may decrease dasatinib absorption.
Erlotinib	EGFR TKI	Edema, fatigue, dermatologic toxicities, GI toxicities, hyperbilirubinemia, pulmonary toxicities, infection, MI, cerebrovascular events, pancreatitis	Monitor for drug interactions (via CYP450). Administer on an EMPTY stomach at least 1 h before or 2 h after meals.
Imatinib	BCR-ABL TKI; inhibitory effects on other receptor tyrosine kinases (SCF/c-KIT, PDGFRα, PDGFRβ)	N/V, diarrhea, dyspepsia, rash, fluid retention/edema, hepatotoxicity, hemorrhage, myelosuppression, arthralgia/ myalgia, left ventricular, dysfunction, CHF, photo-sensitivity, Stevens-Johnson syndrome	Monitor for drug interactions (via CYP450).

(*continued*)

TABLE 16-1 PHARMACOLOGIC AGENTS IN ONCOLOGY (*Continued*)

Drug Classification/ Subclassification/Agents	Mechanism of Action	Selected Toxicities	Other Pertinent Information
Lapatinib	EGFR and HER2 TKI	In combination with capecitabine: GI toxicities, dermatologic toxicities, fatigue, decrease in LVEF, QT prolongation, abnormal LFT, myelosuppression	Monitor for drug interactions (via CYP450). Administer at least 1 h before or 1 h after meals; once daily dosing only.
Nilotinib	BCR-ABL TKI; also inhibits c-KIT and PDGFR; overcomes imatinib-resistant BCR-ABL kinase mutations	Myelosuppression, QT prolongation, sudden deaths, elevated lipase/amylase/ pancreatitis, abnormal LFT, electrolyte abnormalities, N/V, abdominal pain, diarrhea, rash, myalgias/arthralgias, headache, constipation	Administer on an EMPTY stomach at least 1 h before or 2 h after meals. Avoid QT interval prolonging drugs, strong CYP3A4 inhibitors/inducers, and grapefruit/grapefruit juice. Use PPIs, H_2-blockers, and antacids with caution. Obtain ECGs at baseline, 7 d after initiation, periodically thereafter, and following dose adjustments. Correct hypokalemia and hypomagnesemia prior to administration.

Pazopanib	Multi-TKI of VEGFR 1, VEGFR 2, VEGFR3, PDGFRα, PDGFRβ, FGFR1, FGFR 3, Kit, Itk, Lck, c-Fms TKI	Elevated LFT, jaundice, fatigue, abdominal pain, N/V, diarrhea, headache, HTN, anorexia, depigmentation of hair and skin, myelosuppression, hyper/hypoglycemia, hypophosphatemia, hyponatremia, hypomagnesemia, elevated lipase, proteinuria, hypothyroidism, QT prolongation, arterial thrombosis,	Use with caution in patients with history of QT prolongation, taking antiarrhythmics, or other medications that may prolong QT interval, and those with relevant preexisting cardiac disease. Baseline and periodic monitoring of ECGs and maintenance of electrolytes should be performed. Coadministration with CYP3A4 inhibitors results in increased pazopanib plasma concentrations. Take at least 1 h before or 2 h after a meal.
Sorafenib	Raf kinase TKI; effects on other receptor tyrosine kinases (VEGFR 2, VEGFR 3, PDGFRβ, Flt-3, c-KIT)	Rash, hand-foot syndrome, N/V, diarrhea, constipation, HTN, fatigue, neuropathy, alopecia, pruritus, dry skin, hypophosphatemia, elevated amylase/lipase, myelosuppression, cardiac ischemia/infarction, wound healing complications	Monitor for drug interactions (via CYP450). Administer on an EMPTY stomach at least 1 h before or 2 h after meals.

(*continued*)

TABLE 16-1 PHARMACOLOGIC AGENTS IN ONCOLOGY (*Continued*)

Drug Classification/ Subclassification/Agents	Mechanism of Action	Selected Toxicities	Other Pertinent Information
Sunitinib	VEGF TKI; effects on other receptor tyrosine kinases (SCF/c-KIT, PDGFRα, PDGFRβ, Flt-3)	HTN, edema, fatigue, rash, hyperpigmentation, dry skin, hair color changes, hand-foot syndrome, alopecia, N/V, diarrhea, mucositis, constipation, increased amylase/lipase, myelosuppression, increased LFT, arthralgia/myalgia, decreased left ventricular ejection fraction, deep vein thrombosis, pulmonary embolism, MI, peripheral neuropathy, hemorrhagic events, adrenal function abnormalities	Monitor for drug interactions (via CYP450). Avoid grapefruit juice, as it increases sunitinib concentrations.

ADCC, antibody-dependent cell-mediated cytotoxicity; APL, acute promyelocytic leukemia; BCR-ABL, breakpoint cluster region-Abelson; BSA, body surface area; CD, cluster of differentiation; c-Fms, macrophage colony stimulating factor receptor; CHF, congestive heart failure; CYP, cytochrome P450; DNA, deoxynucleic acid; DVT, deep vein thrombosis; ECG, electrocardiogram; EGFR, epidermal growth factor receptor; FGFR, fibroblast growth factor receptor; Flt-3, FMS-like tyrosine kinase 3; GI, gastrointestinal; H_1, histamine 1; H_2, histamine 2; HDAC, histone deacetylase inhibitor; HER2, human epidermal growth factor receptor 2; IL-2, interleukin 2; HOTN, hypotension; HTN, hypertension; KRAS, V-Ki-ras2 Kirsten rat sarcoma viral oncogene homolog; Itk, IL2-inducible T-cell kinase; Lck, lymphocyte specific protein tyrosine kinase; LFT, liver function tests; LVEF, left ventricular ejection fraction; MDR, multidrug resistance; MI, myocardial infarction/ischemia; m-TOR, mammalian target of rapamycin; MAb, monoclonal antibody; N/V, nausea/vomiting; PDGFR, platelet-derived growth factor receptor; PE, pulmonary embolism; PPIs, proton pump inhibitors; RNA, ribonucleic acid; SCF, stem cell factor; SIADH, syndrome of inappropriate secretion of antidiuretic hormone; SJS, Stevens-Johnson syndrome; SOB, shortness of breath; TEN, toxic epidermal necrolysis; TKI, tyrosine kinase inhibitor; TLS, tumor lysis syndrome; VEGF, vascular endothelial growth factor; VOD, veno-occlusive disease.

Recent advances in cancer have led to the identification of several specific molecular targets for drug therapy.

Cell Cycle

- The growth and division of cells can be conceptualized by the cell cycle. There are several phases to the life cycle of the dividing cell, including the **g**rowth (G) phase, **s**ynthesis (S) phase, and **m**itosis (M) phase. There also is a "rest" phase, or G_0, in which cells are not actively participating in the cell cycle. Cells can then undergo terminal differentiation or re-enter the cell cycle.
- One of the factors that influence the development of chemotherapy regimens is the phase at which the chemotherapy agent works in the cell cycle. Many chemotherapeutic agents are cell cycle specific (e.g., they have activity only in certain phases of the cell cycle). Those that are non-cell cycle specific may cause damage to a cell during any phase of the cell cycle.

REFERENCES

1. DeVita VT, Rosenberg SA, Hellman S. *Cancer: Principles and Practice of Oncology.* 8th ed. Philadelphia: Lippincott Williams & Wilkins; 2008.
2. Pazdur R, Wagman LD, Camphausen KA, et al. *Cancer Management: A Multidisciplinary Approach.* 12th ed. New York: CMP Healthcare Media; 2009.

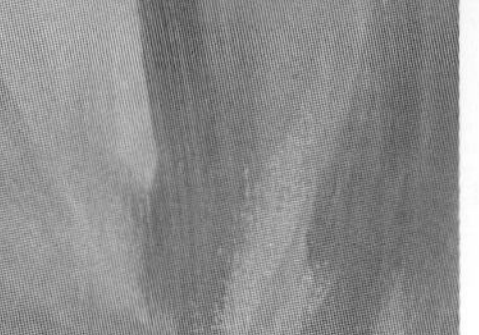

Introduction to Radiation Oncology

17

Daniel J. Ma, Parag J. Parikh, and Imran Zoberi

INTRODUCTION

Radiation oncology unifies the study of cancer with the therapeutic use of radiation. The radiation oncologist is the medical specialist who decides when and how to best use radiation. Under the supervision of the radiation oncologist, an array of nonmedical specialists, including physicists, dosimetrists, and technicians, assist in the planning and delivery of radiation to patients. This chapter introduces some of the basic principles of radiation oncology, some common treatment strategies, and an overview of the common toxicities that may be encountered in the inpatient setting.

PHYSICAL AND BIOLOGIC PRINCIPLES

- **Ionizing radiation** is energy that causes the ejection of an orbital electron. It may be either electromagnetic (photons or gamma rays) or particulate (electrons, protons, or other atomic particles). The energy of photons that can be generated in the clinic has increased over the years, which allows more doses to be delivered to internal malignancies while respecting the tolerance of the skin to radiation. **Radiation dose** is measured as energy per unit mass, where 1 joule (J)/kg is 1 gray (Gy). The previously used term, **rad,** is equal to 1 centigray (cGy).
- Radiation causes DNA damage in both normal tissues and tumor cells. In general, cells are most susceptible in the G1, G2, and M phases of the cell cycle. Susceptible cells may enter apoptotic cell death by a variety of mechanisms or undergo necrosis. Hypoxic cells are thought to be less susceptible to radiation than well-oxygenated cells, owing to preferential free radical formation. **Fractionated radiotherapy** (radiation given in multiple small doses over a given period instead of a single large dose) allows normal tissue to repair sublethal damage and repopulate while the tumor cells re-sort themselves in the cell cycle and become better oxygenated. A great deal of current research involves the cell cycle–signaling pathways involved in each aspect of the damage, repair, and reoxygenation pathways.[1]

RADIATION TREATMENT GOALS AND METHODS

- Radiation can be given by directing x-rays from a treatment machine to the patient (**external beam radiotherapy**) or by placing a radioactive source in close proximity to the patient (**brachytherapy**). Brachytherapy is most often used in gynecologic cancers, prostate cancer, and head and neck cancer. Sometimes both techniques are used to provide the optimal dose distribution.[2]

- Advances in imaging and external beam delivery now allow for ablative radiation techniques (**stereotactic radiotherapy**). These techniques require very precise immobilization and deliver large doses of highly focused radiation in a few (i.e., 1 to 5) fractions. Stereotactic radiotherapy works best for smaller, well-defined lesions such as limited brain/liver metastases or early-stage lung cancer.
- Radiation can be given for curative or palliative intent and commonly is the definitive treatment. Often, it is combined with chemotherapy and surgery in the complete cancer care of the patient. It can be given before (neoadjuvant) or after (adjuvant) the definitive therapy. Many solid tumors are treated with radiation and chemotherapy at the same time (concurrent chemoradiation).
- Accurate tumor **localization** is essential for optimum delivery of radiation. This can be done clinically (e.g., in palliative cases and gynecologic cancers) or using radiographic studies. Clinical localizations are quick and allow the patient to start treatment immediately but do not allow for conformal delivery of radiation. To plan most radiotherapy, the patient needs to have a **simulation** ("sim") in which he or she is brought to the radiation oncology department to make a treatment plan. This plan will aid in delivering the maximal dose of radiation to tumor tissue while attempting to avoid healthy tissue. Often, specialized immobilization devices are constructed for the patient during simulation to reduce intertreatment variation in patient position. After the simulation, the radiation oncologist develops a treatment plan. Because the time between the initial consultation and the first treatment is often 2 to 3 weeks, patients are best served by early radiation oncology consultation.
- In general, for external-beam radiotherapy, a patient will be placed on a flat, mobile treatment table each day during the course of radiation therapy. Marks on the patient's skin and any immobilization devices are used to obtain accurate and precise patient positioning. Each treatment may last 10 to 30 minutes. The total course of radiation therapy can vary from 1 day (prostate brachytherapy, some stereotactic treatments) to several weeks (fractionated external-beam radiotherapy). Most fractionated treatment is given once a day, 5 days per week, although some treatments are given more frequently.

INDICATIONS FOR URGENT RADIATION THERAPY

Urgent radiation therapy is useful in certain oncologic emergencies. **Spinal cord compression** is the only true radiation oncology emergency and is described further in Chapter 35. It is imperative that radiation oncology and surgical services are consulted early and that an MRI of the entire spine is obtained as soon as possible. **Brain metastases** can be treated with radiation therapy, with timing based on symptoms and performance status. **Uncontrolled bleeding** of tumors (commonly breast, gynecologic, lung, colon, or bladder) often responds well to radiation therapy. **Superior vena cava (SVC) syndrome,** in which the SVC is compressed by tumor (typically small-cell lung cancer), can be palliated by radiation, with resolution after weeks of therapy. Although SVC syndrome by itself is rarely fatal, these tumors frequently encase other critical structures of the mediastinum.

LATE EFFECTS AND TISSUE TOLERANCE

Radiation therapy balances side effects to normal tissue with the need to deliver adequate doses to the tumor. Side effects are considered to be either **late** (months to years after completion of radiation therapy) or **acute** (during radiation therapy). The radiation tolerance of normal tissue varies from patient to patient and depends on dose, fractionation scheme, and exposed tissue volume. The most common fractionation scheme is 1.8 to 2 Gy/d. Table 17-1 briefly summarizes the best available human data. These data represent only general parameters, and a radiation oncologist may elect to exceed these dose levels or be more conservative based on individual patient considerations.

COMMON TREATMENT GUIDELINES AND ASSOCIATED ACUTE EFFECTS

The following is a brief description of current "off-protocol" treatment regimens. It must be emphasized that many patients are treated according to research protocols, which vary considerably. Acute toxicities of radiation therapy typically result from direct tissue damage within the radiation path. Most radiation-alone acute effects can be managed on an outpatient basis. However, with concurrent chemoradiation, acute effects increase substantially and may require inpatient management. This is especially seen with head and neck, lung, and gastrointestinal cancers.

Palliative Therapy

Palliative treatment of brain and bone metastases is given at doses of 20 to 40 Gy over 1 to 3 weeks. This is a larger fraction size than used in most curative treatments, because there is less concern about late effects and a greater interest in minimizing treatment time for patient convenience.

Bone Metastases

Bone metastases can be treated with 6- to 8-Gy single doses, or with 30 Gy in fractions of 3 Gy/d, depending on the number and location of lesions and the patient's life expectancy. For patients with multiple bone metastases, an infusion of radioactive strontium, samarium, or yttrium can be used to decrease pain.

Lung Cancer

Stage III non-small-cell lung cancer is often treated with definitive radiotherapy, typically combined with chemotherapy and to a dose of 60 to 70 Gy. Recently, stereotactic radiation therapy has been shown to be promising for medically inoperable stage I and II lung cancer patients. In many patients, the mediastinum is irradiated, which can result in the acute toxicity of esophagitis. The resultant odynophagia can lead to dehydration or significant weight loss, which may require inpatient management. Shortly after the completion of radiotherapy, radiation pneumonitis or, very rarely, radiation pericarditis may occur. Anti-inflammatory steroid therapy is the mainstay of treatment for both of these conditions. Three-dimensional conformal radiation therapy, involving treatment planning based on CT scans, is being investigated as a method to increase dose to tumor while avoiding normal lung. Radiation therapy is used as

TABLE 17-1 NORMAL TISSUE TOLERANCE TO THERAPEUTIC IRRADIATION[a]

Critical Structure	Volume	Dose/Volume	Max Dose	Toxicity Rate	Toxicity Endpoint
Brain			<60 Gy	<3%	Symptomatic necrosis
Brain stem			<54 Gy	<5%	Neuropathy or necrosis
Optic nerve/chiasm			<55 Gy	<3%	Optic neuropathy
Spinal cord			50 Gy	0.2%	Myelopathy
Cochlea	Mean[b]	<=45 Gy		<30%	Sensory-neural hearing loss
Parotid, bilateral	Mean	<=25 Gy		<20%	Long-term salivary function <25%
Pharyngeal constrictors	Mean	<=50 Gy		<20%	Symptomatic dysphagia and aspiration
Larynx			<66 Gy	<20%	Vocal dysfunction
Larynx	Mean	<50 Gy		<30%	Aspiration
Lung	V20[c]	<=30%		<20%	Symptomatic pneumonitis
Lung	Mean	7 Gy		5%	Symptomatic pneumonitis
Esophagus	Mean	<34 Gy		5–20%	Esophagitis
Pericardium	Mean	<26 Gy		<15%	Pericarditis
Heart	V25	<10%		<1%	Long term cardiac events
Liver	Mean	<30–32 Gy		<5%	Radiation induced liver disease
Kidney, bilateral	Mean	<15–18 Gy		<5%	Clinical dysfunction
Rectum	V50	<50%		<10%	Proctitis
Bladder[d]			<65 Gy	<6%	Cystitis

[a]Based upon data from older 3D conformal radiation techniques.

[b]Mean <=45 Gy: The mean dose given to the whole organ should be <=45 Gy.

[c]V20 <=30%: The volume of tissue receiving >20 Gy should be <=30% of the total volume.

[d]Variations in bladder size/shape/location during RT hampers the ability to generate accurate data.

Data adapted from Bentzen SM, Constine LS, Deasy JO, et al. Quantitative analyses of normal tissue effects in the clinic (QUANTEC). *Int J Radiat Oncol Biol Phys.* 2010 Mar 1;76(3 Suppl):S10–S19.

adjuvant treatment in select cases of locally advanced non-small-cell lung cancer treated with definitive surgery. Both chemotherapy and radiation therapy play a central role in the definitive management of limited-stage small-cell lung cancer.

Esophageal Cancer

Radiation therapy with concurrent chemotherapy is used either as definitive treatment for esophageal/gastroesophageal junction tumors or as neoadjuvant treatment. Esophagitis is the major acute toxicity.

Central Nervous System Cancer

After maximal safe surgical resection, primary brain tumors may be treated to 50 to 60 Gy, depending on the area of the brain involved. Brain metastases are normally treated to 20 to 30 Gy. Stereotactic radiosurgery, either by linear accelerator or by gamma knife, can be used for patients with few metastatic lesions that are <4 cm in size. Radiosurgery involves a single day of treatment. Mild mental deterioration is seen in children and the elderly. Neurologic changes requiring hospitalization are generally due to tumor progression, not toxicity from radiosurgery.

Head and Neck Cancer

In general, early-stage head and neck cancers are treated equally well with surgery or radiation. Advanced head and neck cancers require surgery and postoperative radiation, radiotherapy alone, or chemoradiation. Doses are typically 60 to 70 Gy. Multiple treatments per day (hyperfractionation) are often used. Side effects include xerostomia, odynophagia, dysphagia, and hoarseness. Acute toxicity often results in dehydration, which may require administration of IV fluids or placement of a gastric tube for nutritional support. Chemotherapy has been shown to improve outcome in the definitive radiotherapy of advanced head and neck cancers at the cost of 1% to 3% treatment-associated mortality and 20% to 30% risk of hospitalization for esophagitis. Treatment-associated deaths are rare with radiotherapy alone, and the frequency of hospitalization for acute toxicity is generally ≤10%.

Breast Cancer

Radiation is used in breast conservation therapy as well as postmastectomy patients with large initial tumors, positive lymph nodes, or positive resection margins. The dose to the breast is normally 54 to 60 Gy. For early-stage breast conservation therapy, partial breast radiation therapy is being investigated as a shorter-course, lower-volume alternative to whole-breast radiation. Acute side effects are usually limited to skin reactions, but pneumonitis, lymphoedema, and carditis can occur as late reactions. Hospitalization is a distinctly rare event for any acute radiotherapy effect in the breast.

Prostate Cancer

Prostate cancer can be treated with either external-beam radiation therapy or prostate brachytherapy ("seeds"). External-beam radiation consists of 70 to 80 Gy. The most common side effects are urethritis and cystitis, which are managed on an outpatient basis in the vast majority of patients. Rates of impotence and cure are similar among external-beam radiation therapy, brachytherapy, and radical prostatectomy.

Colon/Rectal Cancer

Radiation is not often used in colon cancers, except in those that are locally advanced (often fixed or perforated) and require preoperative radiation therapy.

The confines of the pelvis make surgical resection of rectal cancer more challenging than that of colon cancer. Preoperative radiation therapy is used in most cases to facilitate surgical resection, for sphincter preservation, and to treat the poorly accessible presacral lymph nodes. Rectal cancer doses are 20 to 50 Gy, depending on the size of the lesion and whether radiation is given before or after surgery. Radiation therapy–induced proctitis is generally quite mild unless concurrent chemotherapy (generally 5-fluorouracil) is administered, in which case proctitis can be severe enough to cause dehydration leading to hospitalization. Patients may need nutritional support.

Anal Cancer

Most anal malignancies can be managed with definitive radiotherapy plus adjuvant chemotherapy, with surgery reserved for salvage. Although generally of squamous histology, anal cancers respond well to low doses of radiotherapy. Typical curative doses are 30 to 54 Gy, classically given with concurrent mitomycin-C and 5-fluorouracil. Acute toxicities are mainly myelosuppression caused by mitomycin-C, proctitis, cystitis, hemorrhoid exacerbation, and skin reaction in the perineum.

Pediatric Cancer

Radiation is used in many pediatric tumors. Total-body irradiation and irradiation of sanctuary sites are used in leukemia, and many lymphoma protocols involve local irradiation. Many sarcomas are treated with radiation after or instead of surgery. Most CNS tumors are treated in part with radiation. Treatment varies by site, and long-term effects on development limit dose.

Lymphoma

Lymphomas are very radioresponsive, and doses from 20 to 45 Gy are used, depending on the type of lymphoma and chemotherapy regimen. Treatment is normally very well tolerated, with some cytopenia and fatigue with larger fields and some nausea/vomiting when the abdomen is treated.

Total-Body Irradiation

Total-body irradiation is used as part of the preparative scheme for peripheral blood stem cell transplant protocols. Treatment with 550 cGy in a single fraction is very common, although fractionated total-body irradiation is also used in certain protocols. This is normally well tolerated, except for self-limiting parotitis and nausea and vomiting.

Gynecologic Cancer

Cervical and uterine corpus cancers are often treated with radiation therapy. Most advanced cervical cancers are treated with definitive radiotherapy, and numerous phase III trials have demonstrated equivalent survival outcome between radical hysterectomy and radiotherapy for early cervical cancer. Radiation is generally used as adjuvant therapy in uterine corpus tumors. Radiotherapy for most gynecologic malignancies uses brachytherapy, because it better delivers the dose to the at-risk tissues, while sparing the bladder and rectum. Doses are anywhere from 50 to 85 Gy. Patients can develop proctitis, enteritis, and urethritis/cystitis, depending on the dose and tumor location. As with other sites, the frequency of admission for acute toxicity increases with concurrent chemoradiation.

KEY POINTS TO REMEMBER

- Consult a radiation oncology specialist before starting therapeutic chemotherapy or surgery to allow for optimum multidisciplinary management of the malignancy. Evaluating patients in their presenting state is very valuable to the radiation oncologist.
- When radiation toxicity is in the differential diagnosis, consult a radiation oncologist, who can help with diagnosis and treatment.
- The only true radiation oncology emergency is spinal cord compression, although there are other "urgent" indications for radiation therapy.
- Consider urgent radiation oncology consults when faced with SVC syndrome, new brain metastases, or uncontrolled bleeding.

REFERENCES

1. Gunderson L, Tepper J, eds. *Clinical Radiation Oncology.* 2nd ed. Philadelphia: Churchill Livingstone; 2006.
2. Perez C, Brady L, eds. *Principles and Practices of Radiation Oncology.* 5th ed. Philadelphia: Lippincott-Raven; 2007.

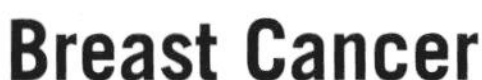

Breast Cancer

18

Yee Hong Chia, Gayathri Nagaraj, and Cesar Sanchez

GENERAL PRINCIPLES

- Other than skin cancer, breast cancer is the most common cancer diagnosed in women in North America. Breast cancer is second only to lung cancer as the leading cause of cancer deaths among American women.[1] Although the incidence of breast cancer has continued to rise in the United States over recent decades, the mortality appears to be declining, suggesting a benefit from screening, withdrawal of hormone replacement therapy (HRT), and improved therapy.

Definition

- Breast cancers are neoplasms that originate from breast tissue. Breast cancers, invasive and its precursor DCIS (ductal carcinoma in situ), most commonly arise from the inner lining of the milk ducts or the lobules.

Classification

- **Pathologic classification**
  - Most **invasive breast cancers** are adenocarcinomas that can be quite heterogeneous in histologic appearance. Infiltrating (invasive) ductal carcinoma accounts for ~80% of all breast cancers. Infiltrating ductal carcinomas metastasize predominantly to the bones, liver, lungs, and brain. Lobular carcinomas make up 10% of malignant breast cancers and are associated with bilateral tumors in up to 20% of cases. Lobular carcinomas also tend to be associated with multicentric disease within the same breast, and have a predilection to metastasize to the meninges, serosal surfaces, and mediastinal and retroperitoneal lymph nodes. The loss of E-cadherin, which plays a role in cell adhesion, is a key event in the development of invasive lobular breast cancers. Less common subtypes of ductal carcinomas include mucinous and tubular, which may carry a more favorable prognosis. Another variant, with aggressive histological appearance but relatively good prognostic, is medullary carcinoma. Metaplastic carcinoma of the breast, a neoplasm with both epithelial and mesenchymal elements, is a rare (<1% of all breast cancers) but aggressive breast tumor.
  - **Noninvasive carcinomas,** which are characterized pathologically by the lack of penetration through the basement membrane into the surrounding stroma, include DCIS and lobular carcinoma in situ (LCIS), which is not a true cancer but, instead, a marker for breast cancer risk. DCIS is most often identified with an abnormal mammogram showing clustered microcalcifications with or without a palpable mass. LCIS, on the other hand, is not detected on physical examination or mammography and is almost always an incidental finding in breast biopsies performed for another reason.

  - **Paget disease of the nipple** is a specialized form of ductal carcinoma that arises from the main excretory ducts in the breasts and involves the skin of the nipple and areola.
  - **Inflammatory carcinomas** involve the lymphatic structures in the dermis and infiltrate widely throughout the breast tissue. Inflammatory carcinomas are not a special morphologic pattern but are clinically diagnosed based on swelling, erythema, and tenderness in the involved breast and are associated with more aggressive disease.
- **Biomarker classification**
  Apart from histology, breast cancer can also be conceptualized on the basis of biomarkers, which bear implications for systemic treatment. Hormone receptor (HR)-positive breast cancers express the estrogen receptor (ER) and/or progesterone receptor (PgR), and are HER2 (human epidermal growth factor receptor 2) negative. HER2 positive breast cancers demonstrate overexpression or amplification of human epidermal growth factor Receptor 2/homologue of the oncogene neu (HER2/neu), a member of the epidermal growth factor receptor (EGFR) family. Triple negative breast cancers are negative for ER, PgR, and HER2/neu.
- **Intrinsic subtypes by molecular profiling**
  More recently, gene expression profiling techniques were used to separate breast cancer into distinctive molecular subtypes with prognostic significance.[2,3] Molecular subtypes include luminal A and luminal B, HER2 enriched, and basal. Luminal A breast cancers are typically HR positive with low proliferation indices. Like luminal A breast cancers, luminal B breast cancers are also HR positive. However, luminal B breast cancers have higher proliferation indices and are associated with poorer outcomes compared to luminal A breast cancers. The HER2-enriched breast cancers are usually, but not always, HER2 positive. Basal-like breast cancers are usually triple negative, although the two terms are not synonymous. More recently, a new subtype, the claudin-low, was identified. Claudin-low tumors tend to be ER-, PgR-, and HER2/neu-negative ("triple-negative") invasive ductal carcinoma with a high frequency of metaplastic differentiation. These tumors carry a poor prognosis.

Epidemiology

- 209,060 (1,970 men; 207,090 women) new cases of breast cancers will be diagnosed in 2010, and 40,230 deaths will occur. Although most breast cancers occur in women, ~1% of new cases annually occur in men. The lifetime risk of developing breast cancer in women (assuming a life expectancy of 85 years) is approximately one in eight women. The median age at diagnosis is in the seventh decade of life.[1]

Etiology

- The etiology of breast cancer is unknown and likely multifactorial. Several risk factors for developing breast cancer have been identified in the literature.[4]

Risk Factors

- Identifiable risk factors for breast cancer include a history of breast cancer, female gender, increasing age, early menarche, late menopause, nulliparity, older age at first live childbirth, family history of breast cancer, genetic mutations such as *BRCA1* and *BRCA2,* prolonged HRT, previous exposure to therapeutic chest wall irradiation, and benign proliferative breast disease such as atypical lobular or ductal hyperplasia.

- With regard to behavioral activities, such as weight and diet, controversy exists over whether there is a clear association of high-fat and low-fiber diets and obesity with increased breast cancer risk. It appears that regular physical activity has been shown to correlate with a reduced risk of breast cancer. More than minimal alcohol intake (such as one to two drinks per day) has been associated with an increased risk. Cigarette smoking is a controversial risk factor, with some studies showing a correlation with risk while other studies do not.
- While the majority of breast cancers are sporadic, inherited breast cancer is now well documented. *BRCA1* and *BRCA2* were identified as breast cancer susceptibility genes in the 1990s.[5,6] Mutations in *BRCA1* and *BRCA2,* which are inherited in an autosomal dominant fashion, are responsible for ~90% of hereditary breast cancer diagnoses. Approximately 5% to 10% of all women with breast cancer have a germline mutation of the gene *BRCA1* or *BRCA2. BRCA1* (chromosome 17q21) and *BRCA2* (chromosome 13q12–13) are associated with an autosomal dominant inheritance pattern, younger age at diagnosis, bilateral disease, multiple affected family members, and an association with other cancers, especially ovarian. Specific mutations of *BRCA1* and *BRCA2* are also more common in women of Ashkenazi Jewish descent. In a combined analysis of 22 studies, the average cumulative risk of developing breast cancer by age 70 years in *BRCA1* and *BRCA2* carriers were 65% (95% confidence interval of 44% to 78%) and 45% (31% to 56%), respectively. The corresponding risk of developing ovarian cancer was 39% (18% to 54%) and 11% (2.4% to 19%) for *BRCA1* and *BRCA2* carriers, respectively.[7] Other, less common but established hereditary causes for breast cancer include Li–Fraumeni syndrome (*p53* gene mutations), Cowden syndrome or multiple hamartoma syndrome (PTEN gene mutations), and Peutz–Jeghers syndrome (*STK11* gene mutations).

Prevention

- The Gail model is a statistical tool that calculates a woman's risk of developing breast cancer.[8] Variables in the model include age, age at menarche, age at first live birth, number of previous breast biopsies, history of atypical ductal hyperplasia, and number of first-degree relatives with breast cancer.
- **Primary prevention** of breast cancer with selective estrogen receptor modulators (SERMs) has been evaluated in a number of studies including the National Surgical Adjuvant Breast and Bowel Project (NSABP) P-1 trial and the Study of Tamoxifen and Raloxifene (STAR) trial. The NSABP P-1 trial included women who were 35 years of age and older and had either an absolute risk of at least 1.66% over a 5-year period on the basis of the Gail model or a history of LCIS. In this trial, tamoxifen at a dose of 20 mg daily for 5 years demonstrated a 49% reduction in the incidence of invasive breast cancer.[9] In the STAR trial, raloxifene was compared to tamoxifen in high-risk postmenopausal women. Raloxifene was equivalent to tamoxifen, but had a better side-effect profile, including a lower incidence of thromboembolic events and uterine hyperplasia.[10]
- **Secondary prevention** (screening) measures include monthly breast self-examination and radiographic imaging to detect early cancers.

- **Monthly breast self-exam** (BSE) is frequently advocated as a screening tool for breast cancer, but there is little evidence showing its effectiveness in reducing mortality rates in breast cancer.[11] The United States Preventive Services Task Force (USPSTF) recommends against clinicians teaching women how to perform BSE.[12]
- **Regular mammographic screening** has a sensitivity and specificity of 77% to 95% and 94% to 97%, respectively.[11] Younger women have more false-positive mammograms and require additional imaging, but fewer biopsies than older women. The USPTF modified its recommendations on screening mammography. The revised version recommended against routine screening mammography for women between the ages of 40 and 49 years (in the absence of known genetic predisposition), while recommending biennial mammography for women aged 50 to 74 years.[12] Although the relative risk reduction of screening mammography on breast cancer mortality is similar between the two groups (around 15%), the absolute risk reduction is higher in the older women (ages 50 to 74 years) than in the younger women (ages 40 to 49 years).
- **Magnetic resonance imaging** (MRI) has also been found to be superior to mammogram and ultrasound in young women and in women with *BRCA1* and *BRCA2* mutations, where mammography is less sensitive and multicentric disease is more common.[13]

DIAGNOSIS

Clinical Presentation

- A majority of breast cancers these days are diagnosed as the result of an abnormal mammogram; however, any woman who presents with a new breast mass should be evaluated with a complete history and physical examination.

History

- For patients presenting with a new breast mass, symptoms related to the new mass, including duration, tenderness, relationship to menstrual cycle, presence of nipple changes, and discharge, should be elicited. A heightened concern for malignancy arises if nipple discharge is unilateral, spontaneous, or bloody, especially in a postmenopausal woman. A negative family history does not exclude malignancy, given that most women who develop breast cancer do not have a family history. Patients should be asked a detailed history concerning any prior breast biopsies and personal and family history of breast, ovarian, and other malignancies, as well as any personal history of breast cancer or other malignancies. A full gynecologic history should be taken, including age at menarche, age at menopause, use of oral contraceptives or exogenous HRT (type and duration), age at first live birth, and number of pregnancies.

Physical Examination

- The physical characteristics of a breast mass can be helpful in determining a diagnosis. One should begin with a careful inspection for breast symmetry, contours, and retraction of the skin. Other changes in the skin can include erythema, thickening, skin nodules, and peau d'orange appearance. Close inspection of the nipple can reveal rashes, ulceration, thickening, or discharge that may help identify an underlying malignancy or Paget disease of the breast.

The characteristics of any palpable lumps in the breast should be noted, including the location, size, shape, consistency, demarcation, tenderness, and mobility. A complete examination for lymphadenopathy includes evaluation for axillary, supraclavicular, and infraclavicular lymph nodes. The final element of the breast examination is compression of the areola to try to elicit any nipple discharge. A nonmilky or bloody unilateral nipple discharge suggests underlying breast pathology and should be evaluated further. The most common source of nipple discharge is an intraductal papilloma, which is a benign lesion.

Differential Diagnosis

- The individual risk of a primary breast cancer can be characterized as high or low based on the patient's age, presenting symptoms, history of breast pathology, and family history. For example, a new breast mass in a woman >40 years old should be considered malignant until proven otherwise, whereas in women <35 years old with a similar lesion, cancer is a possibility, which needs to be investigated further. The differential diagnosis of a breast mass can be broad, including malignancies, such as primary breast cancer, lymphoma, and sarcoma, and benign breast lesions, such as cysts, fibroadenomas, and fat necrosis. Skin conditions, such as sebaceous cysts, abscesses, or thrombophlebitis, may present with a palpable mass. The history and physical exam will help aid in the differential diagnosis, but ultimately a biopsy is required for confirmation.

Diagnostic Testing

- Patients suspected of having breast cancer should undergo a biopsy to obtain tissue for diagnosis and for biomarker evaluation. Imaging studies are useful in the staging of the cancer.

Laboratories

- Laboratory tests do not directly aid in the diagnosis or staging of breast cancer, but can allow the clinician to focus on possible metastatic sites of disease. Routine laboratory studies obtained are complete blood count (bone marrow infiltration), liver function tests (liver metastasis), and alkaline phosphatase (bone metastasis). Abnormal blood tests can also give the physician an objective marker to assess for clinical response after therapy in patients without identifiable measurable disease.
- Tumor markers (CA15–3, CA27–29, CEA), although not specific, may be elevated in patients with breast cancer. Tumor markers are not accurate for screening or diagnostic purposes; thus they are not indicated in the initial assessment of breast cancer. In the metastatic setting, however, tumor markers may be elevated and the trend of elevation can assist in monitoring for response to therapy.

Imaging

- A solid mass is best evaluated with **diagnostic mammography.** Mammography allows the physician to assess the radiographic characteristics of the mass and the remainder of breast tissue in the ipsilateral and contralateral breast. **Ultrasound** (US) can be useful to determine whether a lesion is cystic or solid. In the evaluation of a patient with breast cancer, especially in the setting where neoadjuvant systemic therapy is contemplated, evaluation of the axillary lymph nodes with US is indicated. In select situations, **breast MRI** may be useful in identifying additional lesions or bilateral disease.

- In patients with locally advanced disease or suspected metastatic disease, computed tomography (CT) examination of the chest, abdomen, and pelvis can be performed as clinically indicated, and may be useful in identifying sites of metastatic disease. In patients with neurological findings suggestive of brain metastases, a contrast-enhanced MRI of the brain will be helpful.

Diagnostic Procedures

- Any distinct breast mass should be considered for biopsy, even if the mammogram is negative. Aspiration of a cystic mass may be helpful. Cytology may reveal malignant cells, but the absence of malignant cells does not rule out a malignant lesion.
- After radiographic evaluation to determine the location and characteristics of the mass, a biopsy can be obtained using several different methods. Fine-needle aspiration (FNA) is a simple method for obtaining material for cytologic exam that can be performed in the clinician's office. False-negative rates for FNA can be as high as 10%, even among the most experienced technicians. FNA also cannot distinguish in situ disease from invasive carcinoma. If a negative result is obtained from FNA, a core-needle or excisional biopsy should be done to obtain appropriate tissue for pathologic review. The majority of these biopsies can also be performed in the outpatient setting. If the biopsy reveals only normal breast tissue, then further surgical biopsy is recommended if the lesion is suspicious for cancer. Needle localization or stereotactic biopsies may be helpful in this situation. **Excisional biopsy is the gold standard,** allowing complete histologic characterization with regard to biomarkers as well as tumor grade. Excisional biopsy also may serve as the definitive lumpectomy in certain clinical situations. In patients who are slated to undergo neoadjuvant systemic therapy, a biopsy of an abnormal-appearing axillary lymph node may be warranted as well for accurate staging.

TREATMENT

- The treatment of breast cancer utilizes a multidisciplinary approach, including local-regional treatment with surgery ± radiation therapy and treatment of systemic disease with cytotoxic chemotherapy, hormonal therapy, biologic therapy, or a combination of these agents. The treatment plan for each patient is individualized based on the stage of disease, patient's age, comorbidities, menopausal status, and biomarker profile. A simplified version of the American Joint Committee on Cancer staging system is provided in Table 18-1.[14] In addition to the various prognostic and predictive factors, a patient's preference is also a major component of the decision-making process, especially when more than one option may provide similar benefits.
- In terms of treatment, breast cancer can be divided into four general categories:
  - Noninvasive carcinoma, DCIS, and LCIS (stage 0)
  - Early-stage breast cancer that is operable (clinical stage I, stage II, and some stage IIIA tumors)
  - Locally advanced or inoperable local-regional invasive carcinoma (clinical stage IIIB, stage IIIC, and some stage IIIA)
  - Metastatic carcinoma (stage IV)

TABLE 18-1 TNM CLASSIFICATION AND AMERICAN JOINT COMMITTEE ON CANCER (AJCC) STAGING FOR BREAST CANCER

Primary tumor (T)

Tis:	**Carcinoma in situ**
T1:	Tumor ≤2 cm in greatest dimension
T2:	Tumor >2 cm but not >5 cm in greatest dimension
T3:	Tumor >5 cm in greatest dimension
T4:	Tumor of any size with direct extension to (1) chest wall, not including pectoralis muscle, or (2) skin including peau d'orange, skin ulceration, satellite skin nodules in the same breast. T4c applies when both T4a and T4b present. T4d indicates inflammatory carcinoma

Axillary nodal status (N)

Clinical

N0:	No axillary nodal involvement
N1:	Ipsilateral movable axillary nodal involvement
N2:	Ipsilateral, fixed, or matted axillary nodal involvement; or clinically apparent ipsilateral internal mammary nodal involvement in the absence of clinically evident axillary nodal involvement
N3:	Ipsilateral infraclavicular nodal involvement with or without axillary nodal involvement; or clinically apparent ipsilateral internal mammary nodal involvement in the presence of clinically evident axillary nodal involvement; or ipsilateral supraclavicular nodal involvement with or without axillary or internal mammary involvement

Distant metastatic disease (M)

M0:	No distant sites of disease detected
M1:	Distant metastasis

AJCC stage

Stage I:	T1	N0	M0
Stage IIA:	T0	N1	M0
	T1	N1	M0
	T2	N0	M0
Stage IIB:	T2	N1	M0
	T3	N0	M0
Stage IIIA:	T0	N2	M0
	T1 or T2	N2	M0
	T3	N1 or N2	M0
Stage IIIB:	T4	N0, N1 or N2	M0
Stage IIIC:	Any T	N3	M0
Stage IV:	Any T	Any N	M1

Adapted from American Joint Committee on Cancer. *AJCC Cancer Staging Manual.* 7th ed. New York: Springer; 2010.

- **Noninvasive carcinoma/carcinoma in situ**
  - **Lobular carcinoma in situ** (LCIS) is a misleading term, as it is not a premalignant lesion. It is noted as an incidental finding on breast biopsies performed for another reason. It is a marker that identifies women at an increased risk (21% over 15 years) for the development of invasive breast cancer that may occur equally in either breast. Of note, the majority of subsequent cancers are infiltrating ductal rather than lobular carcinomas. LCIS can be managed by observation alone after biopsy. There is no evidence that re-excision after the initial biopsy to obtain histologically negative surgical margins is required. The increased risk of breast cancer persists beyond 20 years, so careful observation and diagnostic mammography should be performed indefinitely in these women. Bilateral prophylactic mastectomies are an alternate option for women who are uncomfortable with the increased risk of developing breast cancer, for patients with a strong family history of breast cancer, or for patients with known *BRCA1/BRCA2* mutations. Radiation therapy has no role in the management of LCIS. According to results from the NSABP-P1 study, tamoxifen, when taken for 5 years, is associated with a 56% decrease in the risk of all breast cancer events in women with LCIS. Results from the NSABP Study of Tamoxifen and Raloxifene (STAR) trial has also shown raloxifene to be as effective as tamoxifen in reducing the risk of invasive cancer in postmenopausal patients with LCIS.[9,10]
  - **Ductal carcinoma in situ** (DCIS), also known as intraductal carcinoma, is being encountered more frequently with the increased use of screening mammography. Surgical treatments for DCIS range from local excision to total mastectomy. Total mastectomy results in a 98% long-term disease-free survival (DFS) rate for noninvasive cancer; however, it is now generally accepted that a lumpectomy followed by radiation therapy to the breast represents the optimal treatment option, as no difference in mortality has been found between lumpectomy and mastectomy.[15] Local chest wall irradiation reduces the rate of ipsilateral breast tumor recurrences by >50% compared to lumpectomy alone. Contraindications for breast-conserving surgery followed by radiation include (1) inability to completely excise the underlying disease to negative surgical margins, (2) multifocal disease, and (3) patient contraindication to receive radiation. Routine axillary nodal dissection is not recommended, given a low (<5%) incidence of axillary nodal metastases in patients with DCIS. According to the NSABP-B24 trial, tamoxifen given after surgery and radiation has been demonstrated to reduce the rate of all breast cancer events (noninvasive or invasive), ipsilateral tumors and new contralateral tumors.[16]
- **Early breast cancer**
  - **Surgery.** The surgical options for the management of early breast cancer include breast-conserving therapy (BCT) followed by radiation therapy or total mastectomy. Randomized clinical trials have proven that overall survival (OS) is equivalent between BCT followed by radiation therapy and mastectomy in women with early breast cancer. The selection of a surgical approach depends on the location and size of the tumor, other abnormalities present on the mammogram, the breast size, and the patient's attitude toward breast preservation. Multicentric disease (two or more primary tumors in separate quadrants), extensive malignant-appearing microcalcifications on

imaging, pregnancy, and previous breast or mantle irradiation are absolute contraindications for BCT. Relative contraindications for BCT include tumors >5 cm and active connective tissue disease involving the skin, such as scleroderma.

- **Axillary lymph node dissection:** This remains an important part of the surgical approach, given the prognostic importance of lymph node involvement. In an effort to decrease the morbidity associated with axillary lymph node dissection (especially lymphedema and pain), while maintaining accurate staging, a sentinel lymph node (SLN) biopsy can be obtained. The SLN (the first node in the lymphatic chain that receives lymphatic flow from the entire breast) is at the highest risk for harboring occult metastatic disease in breast cancer patients. Vital blue dye and/or technetium-labeled sulfur are injected in and around the tumor or biopsy site. The surgeon maps the dye or radioactive compound drainage to the axilla and identifies the SLN, which is then biopsied. The SLN can be identified in >90% of patients with breast cancer, with false-negative rates ranging from 0% to 10%. No further axillary node dissection is needed if the SLN biopsy is negative. If the SLN is positive for malignancy, further treatment options include a full axillary lymph node dissection (ALND), axillary radiation with no further surgery, and adjuvant chemotherapy. One recent randomized clinical trial suggested that complete ALND can be avoided in patients with small tumors (T1,T2), with fewer than 3 SLN involvement.[17] SLN biopsies are only performed on women without palpable, clinically suspicious, axillary lymph nodes on physical examination.
- **Adjuvant radiation therapy:** Radiation therapy to the intact breast after BCT is the standard treatment based on several randomized trials that have shown higher local recurrence rates with BCT alone compared to BCT with radiation therapy. Radiation treatments are administered daily to the intact breast over a 5- to 6-week period to a total dose of 45 to 50 Gy. A radiation boost to the tumor bed is often administered. Patients with positive axillary nodes may benefit from regional nodal irradiation in addition to irradiation of the intact breast. Postmastectomy adjuvant chest wall and axillary radiation is considered for the following: positive surgical margins, primary tumors >5 cm, and involvement of four or more lymph nodes. Radiation therapy can decrease the rates of local recurrence even among patients who receive adjuvant chemotherapy. Certain chemotherapy agents such as anthracyclines have radiation-sensitizing effects and should not be given concurrently with radiation. Typically, adjuvant radiation is given following the completion of adjuvant chemotherapy.
- **Adjuvant systemic therapy.** Systemic treatment has the greatest impact when used in the adjuvant setting rather than metastatic setting. Adjuvant systemic therapy with cytotoxic chemotherapy, hormonal therapy, and HER2-targeted agents has demonstrated significant improvement in DFS and OS in both premenopausal and postmenopausal women in general. Given that not all patients with early state breast cancers recur, it is important to identify high-risk patients who will benefit the most and spare cytotoxic chemotherapy for the subset of patients with low-risk features. Selecting candidates for adjuvant systemic therapy of early breast cancers is thus based on clinicopathologic factors and more recently based on gene expression analysis.

- **Predicting benefits of systemic therapy.** The development and validation of prognostic and predictive models is an area of active research and can be useful in the right clinical scenario for decision making. The clinical and pathologic prognostic determinants of adjuvant therapy are patient age, comorbidities, tumor size, histologic grade or differentiation, histologic type, number of involved axillary lymph nodes, dermal lymphatic invasion, markers of proliferation, HR status, and HER2 status. Several clinically useful prognostic indices that incorporate some of these clinical variables have been developed. Adjuvantonline, is one such validated Web-based tool that includes patient age, comorbidities, HR status, tumor grade, tumor size, and lymph node status to estimate risk of death and relapse from breast cancer and can estimate benefits of adjuvant chemotherapy and hormonal therapy (**www.adjuvantonline.com**). Several gene expression–based prognostic assays, such as Oncotype Dx and Mammaprint, are also commercially available. These multigene assays are mostly independent of clinicopathologic prognostic factors, and hence the treating oncologist has to familiarize the clinical contexts when these tests are applicable.
- **Adjuvant chemotherapy.** Polychemotherapy in the adjuvant setting in early breast cancer reduces the annual breast cancer death rate by ~38% for women <50 years of age and by ~20% for those aged 50 to 69 years, largely irrespective of use of tamoxifen, nodal status, tumor characteristics, and HR status.[18] Chemotherapy is recommended for most patients with node-positive disease, and adjuvant chemotherapy in node-negative patients is usually recommended if the tumor is >1 cm. The benefit of adding adjuvant chemotherapy to hormonal therapy in ER+ stage 1 or node-negative stage 2 is very small when compared to the benefits of hormonal therapy alone. The risk and benefits of adding chemotherapy in such situations have to be based on available clinicopathologic prognostic factors, existing comorbid conditions, and further evaluation with the aid of modern Web-based and genome-based prognostic tools. If chemotherapy is considered, less aggressive regimens should be considered in this patient population. The current standard of practice is to initiate adjuvant chemotherapy 4 to 5 weeks after surgery, before the initiation of radiation. Some of the adjuvant chemotherapy regimens are outlined in Table 18-2. Most modern and widely used chemotherapy regimens are taxanes and anthracycline-based regimens. Current literature supports that four to six courses of treatment provide optimal benefit. Available data also suggest a possible improved response with anthracycline-containing regimens for HER2-positive patients. For node-positive breast cancer, the addition of a taxane to anthracycline-containing chemotherapy improves DFS and OS. Dose-dense chemotherapy for node-positive patients with Adriamycin and cyclophosphamide followed by paclitaxel with growth factor support is a more intensive regimen that has also shown to improve DFS and OS.
- **Adjuvant hormonal therapy.** Patients with invasive breast cancer that is ER or PR positive should be considered for adjuvant hormonal therapy, regardless of the patient's age, menopausal status, or lymph node status or whether or not adjuvant chemotherapy is to be administered. Adjuvant hormonal therapy should not be recommended in patients whose breast cancers are ER or PR negative because clinical trials have not shown any benefit in DFS or OS.

TABLE 18-2 **OVERVIEW OF COMMON NON-TRASTUZUMAB-CONTAINING AND TRASTUZUMAB-CONTAINING ADJUVANT CHEMOTHERAPY REGIMENS FOR BREAST CANCER**

Non-trastuzumab-containing regimens

Fluorouracil/Adriamycin/cyclophosphamide (FAC) × 6 cycles
Fluorouracil/epirubicin/cyclophosphamide (FEC) × 6 cycles
Fluorouracil/epirubicin/cyclophosphamide (FEC) × 3 cycles followed by docetaxel q3wk × 3 cycles or paclitaxel q1wk.
Adriamycin/cyclophosphamide (AC) × 4 cycles
Docetaxel/cyclophosphamide (TC) × 4 cycles
Docetaxel/doxorubicin/cyclophosphamide (TAC) × 6 cycles (with growth factor support)
Cyclophosphamide/methotrexate/fluorouracil (CMF) × 6 cycles
Adriamycin (A) × 4 cycles → paclitaxel (T) × 4 cycles → cyclophosphamide (C) × 4 cycles
Adriamycin/cyclophosphamide (AC) × 4 cycles → paclitaxel (T) × 4 cycles (q21d or dose-dense q14d with growth factor support

Trastuzumab-containing regimens

AC × 4 cycles → paclitaxel/trastuzumab (TH) (paclitaxel × 4 cycles; trastuzumab for 52 wk)
Docetaxel/carboplatin/trastuzumab (TCH) (docetaxel and carboplatin × 6 cycles; trastuzumab for 52 wk)
AC × 4 cycles → docetaxel/trastuzumab (docetaxel × 4 cycles; trastuzumab for 52 wk)

- **Tamoxifen.** It belongs to the group of drugs called SERM, inhibits the growth of breast cancer cells by competitive antagonism of estrogen at the ER. Tamoxifen is a well-established form of hormonal therapy for both premenopausal and postmenopausal women. In women with ER-positive early breast cancer, adjuvant tamoxifen decreased the risk of recurrence by 40% to 50% and the risk of death by 30% to 40% irrespective of the use of chemotherapy, age, menopausal status, or axillary lymph node status.[18] Tamoxifen also decreased the incidence of breast cancer in the contralateral breast by ~50%. Prospective randomized trials have demonstrated that the optimal duration of tamoxifen is 5 years and that longer treatment may trend toward a detrimental effect. In patients receiving both tamoxifen and chemotherapy, chemotherapy should be given first.
- **Aromatase inhibitors (AIs).** In postmenopausal women the primary source of estrogen is the peripheral conversion of androgens to estrogen by the enzyme aromatase. Several studies have utilized AIs in the treatment of postmenopausal women with early-stage breast cancer. These studies have utilized AI as upfront initial therapy, as sequential therapy following 2 to 3 years of tamoxifen, or as extended therapy following 5 years of tamoxifen. Two upfront studies, BIG I-98 and ATAC, have compared letrozole versus tamoxifen and anastrozole versus tamoxifen, respectively. Both studies have shown an improved DFS with the AI compared to tamoxifen when used in the upfront setting.[19,20] Several trials have also studied the

use of sequential AI following either 2 to 3 years of tamoxifen or 5 years of tamoxifen. The NCIC MA 17 trial showed an improved DFS with continuation of letrozole versus placebo following 5 years of tamoxifen. The Intergroup Exemestane Study showed an improved DFS as well as a trend toward improved OS with switching to exemestane following 2 to 3 years of tamoxifen versus continuation of tamoxifen. Given the available data, aromatase inhibitors are now largely used as the treatment of choice for postmenopausal women with HR-positive early breast cancer.

- **Tamoxifen versus aromatase inhibitors.** The two classes of drugs have slightly different side-effect profiles. While both the agents can cause hot flashes, night sweats, and vaginal dryness, AIs are more commonly associated with musculoskeletal symptoms, osteoporosis, and an increased rate of bone fracture, whereas tamoxifen is associated with an increased risk of uterine cancer and deep vein thromboses.

- **Adjuvant HER2 targeted therapy.** Trastuzumab is a humanized, monoclonal antibody with specificity for the extracellular domain of HER2/neu. A meta-analysis from five randomized trials of adjuvant trastuzumab in HER2-positive breast cancer has shown significant reduction in the mortality, recurrence, and metastases rate in patients receiving trastuzumab with or following chemotherapy.[21] A 33% to 52% reduction in the risk of recurrence was seen across these four important initial trials (NSABP B-31, NCCTG 9831, BCIRG 006, and HERA), with a 34% to 41% reduction in the risk of death.[22] These data are compelling to consider use of 1 year of adjuvant trastuzumab in combination with anthracycline- and/or taxane-containing adjuvant chemotherapy regimens and should be offered to all patients with HER2-positive early breast cancer. The likelihood of cardiac toxicity was 2.4-fold higher in trastuzumab arms in the clinical trials. A non-anthracycline-containing regimen is the TCH (taxotere, carboplatin, trastuzumab), which offers less cumulative cardiac toxicity.

- **Neoadjuvant therapy.** Preoperative or neoadjuvant therapy with the use of hormonal or chemotherapeutic agents has been shown to be effective in downsizing the dimensions of the primary tumor, thus allowing for BCT. Results of randomized trials suggest that this strategy is safe and is equivalent to postoperative adjuvant chemotherapy with the same regimen for operable stage I and II breast cancers. Between 10% and 15% of patients are noted to have a complete pathologic response in the primary tumor after three or four cycles of an anthracycline-containing regimen, and 20% to 30% of patients with biopsy-proven lymph node metastases before neoadjuvant chemotherapy have pathologically negative lymph nodes after neoadjuvant chemotherapy. In postmenopausal women with HR-positive cancer, a hormonal agent, such as an aromatase inhibitor, can be used to shrink the primary tumor. While pathologic response rates following neoadjuvant systemic therapy are prognostic, this modality of treatment also has the advantage of testing in vivo sensitivity of the tumor to systemic therapy and is an ideal setup to evaluate newer therapies and develop predictive biomarkers of response.

- **Locally advanced breast cancer.** Locally advanced breast cancer is associated with a poor prognosis and a high rate of local and distant recurrences. This group includes subsets of patients with tumors >5 cm, inflammatory breast tumors, and any tumor with fixed or matted axillary lymphadenopathy or internal mammary lymph node involvement. Patients with locally advanced breast cancer need to be evaluated in order to determine whether or not an initial surgical approach is likely to achieve pathological negative margins and provide long-term local control. Patients who present with clinical stage IIIA (except T3N1M0), IIIB, or IIIC considered to have inoperable breast cancer at presentation should receive more aggressive third-generation chemotherapy regimens, such as dose-dense AC-T or TAC as the initial therapeutic strategy. Neoadjuvant chemotherapy is an effective treatment approach in this setting and may allow for tumor shrinkage to perform adequate surgical resection with clear margins. Total mastectomy with lymph node dissection with or without reconstruction or lumpectomy with axillary dissection is recommended for local control. Given the high risk of recurrence, all patients need radiation therapy after surgery. Adjuvant systemic therapy with cytotoxic chemotherapy, hormonal therapy (ER positive), and trastuzumab therapy (in HER2 positive) is considered standard. Table 18-2 lists a few of the commonly used chemotherapy regimens.

- ○ **Inflammatory breast cancer.** This subset of stage III breast cancer is one of the most aggressive forms of breast cancer. It is characterized by a triad of clinical findings, namely, erythema, warmth, and edema of the skin (peau d'orange) secondary to involvement of dermal lymphatics. While an underlying mass may or may not be palpable, the condition can be misdiagnosed for inflammatory or infectious condition. The biomarker profile is most often (not always) HR and HER2 negative, and they are characterized by rapid growth potential. Inflammatory breast cancers should be treated aggressively with multiagent chemotherapy followed by mastectomy and radiation. The overall prognosis is improving in the recent years with more aggressive multimodality approach compared to their historical dismal outcome.

- **Metastatic breast cancer (MBC).** Patients with MBC are a heterogeneous group of patients with varied presentations and clinical course. The disease can vary from clinically indolent disease to rapidly progressing disease with visceral involvement and resistance to therapy. The primary goals of treatment for patients with metastatic disease are to control the disease, palliate symptoms, and prolong survival. The management of MBC depends on the site and extent of metastases, comorbid conditions, HR status, and HER2/neu overexpression. Patients with MBC can be divided into two groups for the sake of making treatment decisions: patients with locoregional relapse and those with systemic metastatic disease. Patients who have had BCT or mastectomy and present with local recurrence are generally treated with mastectomy and local resection respectively (if obtaining clear surgical margins seems plausible) and radiation therapy if not received in the adjuvant setting. Unresectable chest wall recurrences should be treated with radiation therapy if the patient has not previously received this modality of treatment. After local control, patients should be considered for systemic chemotherapy or hormonal therapy given adjuvantly. Regional lymph node recurrence is managed with surgical resection (or axillary lymph node dissection, if not done before) and radiation therapy. Systemic therapy is again considered for these patients as in the adjuvant setting.
- With regard to systemic metastatic disease, some of the important decisions regarding treatment are made based on risk categories. Patients in the low-risk group include those with a long disease-free interval; HR-positive tumors; and bone, soft tissue, or limited visceral organ involvement. High-risk groups

include patients with rapidly progressing disease or extensive visceral involvement, as well as patients whose disease becomes refractory to hormonal therapy.

- MBC treatment should be multidisciplinary, and support groups tend to be very helpful. At some point in the clinical course, the disease burden from MBC may interfere with the patient's ability to tolerate further treatment options, and supportive or palliative care should be offered to the patient and family. Failure to achieve response to three sequential chemotherapy regimens or an Eastern Cooperative Oncology Group (ECOG) performance status of ≥3 is believed to be an indication for supportive therapy only.
  - **Hormonal therapy.** In low-risk patients with advanced or MBC and ER-positive disease, hormonal therapy can achieve high initial response rates. ER-negative tumors exhibit no clinical benefit from first-line hormonal therapy. The modern hormonal interventions are more selective and are well tolerated. The list of the commonly used hormonal agents in clinical practice is shown in Table 18-3. In postmenopausal women with ER-positive tumors, a selective aromatase inhibitor is the preferred first-line therapy. Hormonal therapy options such as antiestrogen, fulvestrant, SERMs, and tamoxifen can be used in both premenopausal and postmenopausal women. In premenopausal women, although surgical or radiotherapeutic oophorectomy remains an option, this has largely been replaced by luteinizing hormone–releasing hormone (LHRH) analogs for effective hormonal ablation. The current options for first-line treatment in premenopausal ER-positive women with locally advanced or MBC include tamoxifen, some form of ovarian ablation, or the combination of an LHRH agonist and tamoxifen. The combination of LHRH agonist with tamoxifen in recent trials has resulted in better outcomes when compared to LHRH alone with regard to improvement in time to disease progression and survival.[23] Single-agent, sequential hormonal therapy is the preferred management in both premenopausal and postmenopausal ER-positive breast cancer patients. With each subsequent hormonal therapy, the duration of a clinical response becomes shorter, and ultimately, the disease will become refractory to

TABLE 18-3 HORMONAL AGENTS COMMONLY USED IN BREAST CANCER

Nonsteroidal aromatase inhibitor
- Anastrozole (Arimidex) 1 mg PO daily
- Letrozole (Femara) 2.5 mg PO daily

Steroidal Aromatase inhibitor
- Exemestane (Aromasin) 25 mg PO daily

Selective estrogen receptor modulator (SERM)
- Tamoxifen 20 mg PO daily

Antiestrogen
- Fulvestrant (Faslodex) 250 mg IM × 2 on day 1, 15, and 29, then monthly

LHRH analogs
- Goserelin (Zoladex) 3.6 mg subcutaneous monthly

LHRH, luteinizing hormone–releasing hormone.

hormone treatment. Second- and third-line hormonal therapy should be chosen based on the adverse side-effect profile of each drug. Interestingly, estradiol therapy can resensitize a patient to antiestrogen therapies.[24] Systemic chemotherapy can be recommended in patients whose disease becomes refractory to multiple lines of hormonal therapy.

- **Chemotherapy.** High-risk patients with rapidly progressive disease, extensive visceral involvement, or disease that becomes refractory to hormonal therapy may benefit from chemotherapy. Combination chemotherapy generally provides higher rates of objective responses and longer time to progression; however, these regimens are associated with increased toxicity without adding survival benefit. Several chemotherapy agents produce objective responses in MBC; while there are overlapping toxicities of these agents, their specific toxicity profile and metabolism should be kept in mind, especially given the relatively higher frequency of renal and hepatic impairment in this patient population. Single-agent sequential therapies are preferred in patients who are candidates for chemotherapy, but are relatively asymptomatic with no impending visceral crises. There is no convincing data if combination chemotherapy provides better long-term outcomes than single-agent sequential therapy. There is no consensus with regard to duration of therapy or "chemotherapy holidays." If the patient is tolerating chemotherapy well, it is reasonable to continue therapy, and the basic management plan would be to switch to a different regimen when patient develops progressive disease if the patient desires further treatment. The list of preferred chemotherapy options including sequential single agents and combination chemotherapy as listed by the National Cancer Institute (NCI) based on available data is shown in Table 18-4.[25]

TABLE 18-4 CHEMOTHERAPY AGENTS USED IN METASTATIC BREAST CANCER

Single agents that have shown activity in MBC
Anthracyclines: doxorubicin, epirubicin, liposomal doxorubicin, mitoxantrone
Taxanes: paclitaxel, docetaxel, albumin-bound nanoparticle paclitaxel
Alkylating agents: cyclophosphamide
Fluoropyrimidines: capecitabine, 5-fluorouracil
Antimetabolites: methotrexate
Vinca alkaloids: vinorelbine, vinblastine, vincristine
Platinum: carboplatin, cisplatin
Other: Gemcitabine, Mitomycin C, ixabepilone, eribulin

Combination regimens that have shown activity in MBC
AC: cyclophosphamide and doxorubicin

Docetaxel and doxorubicin
CAF: cyclophosphamide, doxorubicin, 5-fluorouracil
CMF: cyclophosphamide, methotrexate, 5-fluorouracil
Doxorubicin and paclitaxel
Docetaxel and capecitabine
Vinorelbine and epirubicin
Capecitabine and ixabepilone

- **Immunotherapies.**
  - **Trastuzumab.** Among patients with MBC, HER2/neu overexpression occurs in 25% to 30% of cases. Trastuzumab is approved for use in combination chemotherapy or as a single agent in MBC. In the original trials, the response rates using trastuzumab as a single agent in first-line therapy were 20% to 25%. There are data suggesting benefit from adding trastuzumab to anastrozole (in HR positive) and chemotherapy agents such as taxanes, capecitabine, anthracyclines, vinorelbine, and platinum compounds. It is also considered safe and effective to incorporate trastuzumab in subsequent lines of therapy after progression on trastuzumab.[26,27] The use of trastuzumab in combination with anthracyclines was associated with severe cardiac toxicity in up to 27% of patients in the registration trial. Trastuzumab is not advised to be used in combination with this drug class outside of a clinical trial.[28]
  - **Bevacizumab** is a humanized monoclonal antibody against vascular endothelial growth factor (VEGF). The FDA granted accelerated approval for bevacizumab in February 2008 to be used in combination with paclitaxel for treatment of patients with MBC, based on clinical trial that showed an improvement in PFS with no impact on overall survival. In December 2010, the FDA announced its recommendation to remove this indication from the label because of lack of demonstration of overall survival benefit with added adverse effects in subsequent studies. The treating oncologists are advised to use their clinical judgment when deciding whether to use this agent in treating MBC patients.
- **Other targeted therapies**
  - **Lapatinib** is an epidermal growth factor receptor (EGFR) and ErbB-2 (HER2/neu) dual tyrosine kinase inhibitor. Lapatinib is approved for use in the United States in HER2-overexpressing metastatic breast cancer in combination with capecitabine and in combination with letrozole, if the tumor is also HR positive.[29,30]
  - **PARP inhibitors.** The poly(ADP-ribose) polymerase is an enzyme used by cancer cells to repair DNA damage. Tumors with *BRCA1/BRCA2* mutations lose a form of DNA repair and thus rely heavily on the PARP pathway. By blocking PARP in the already-compromised tumor cells, the PARP inhibitors can cause cell death through a synthetic lethality mechanism. Very promising data are emerging of its use in patients with BRCA-mutated and triple-negative metastatic breast cancer, as a single agent, and in combination with chemotherapy.[31,32]
- **Treatment of bone metastases.** Although patients with bone-only metastatic disease have a better prognosis than those with visceral metastases, bone metastases can lead to serious complications such as pain, fractures, spinal cord compression, and hypercalcemia. Traditionally, treatment of symptomatic bone metastases has been with analgesics, localized radiation, or surgery. Although improvements in pain and quality of life have been achieved with the use of these therapeutic options, their use for the prevention of progression of bone lytic metastases has been ineffective.
  - **Bisphosphonates.** These agents improve bone health by inhibiting osteoclast-mediated bone resorption. Their use, alone or in combination with chemotherapy or hormonal therapy, has shown to reduce bone pain, improves quality of life, reduces the risk of developing a skeletal event, as

well as increases the time to skeletal event. Intravenous bisphosphonates commonly used are pamidronate (Aredia), as an IV infusion of 90 mg over 2 hours and zoledronate (Zometa) with a much shorter infusion time of 4 mg IV over 15 minutes. The optimal timing of initiation and the duration of treatment remains uncertain.[33]

- **Denosumab.** Denosumab is a fully humanized antibody against receptor activator of nuclear factor κ B (RANK) ligand. Recently reported randomized clinical trial comparing denosumab against zoledronic acid showed superiority of denosumab with regard to delaying or preventing skeletal-related events and equivalency with regard to overall survival. With the convenience of a subcutaneous injection and no requirement for renal monitoring, denosumab represents a potential treatment option for patients with bone metastases.[34]

- **CNS metastases.** Metastatic involvement of the CNS is commonly seen in ER-negative, HER2-positive breast cancers that are poorly differentiated. Solitary metastatic lesions are treated by either surgery or radiosurgery, while whole-brain radiation should be considered for patients with multiple metastatic lesions. Given the frequency of occurrence in HER2-overexpressing breast cancers, it is important to remember that trastuzumab, being a large molecule, **does not cross** the blood–brain barrier while lapatinib, being a small molecule, is more effective in CNS penetration. There is no standard treatment approach at this time with regard to the use of other systemic therapy, and this is an area of active research.

SPECIAL CONSIDERATIONS

- **Genetic testing.** Several indications for genetic testing for breast and ovarian cancer exist: two or more family members with breast and/or ovarian cancer at <50 years of age, breast or ovarian cancer at a very young age, known *BRCA1* and *BRCA2* mutations in a family member, personal history of both breast and ovarian cancers, Ashkenazi Jewish ancestry plus a family member younger than 50 years with breast cancer, and a personal history of ovarian cancer. All patients should undergo genetic counseling before undergoing genetic testing.
- **Breast cancer in pregnancy** is an uncommon phenomenon, but one that poses dilemmas for patients and their physicians. A multidisciplinary approach, in consultation with a maternal-fetal medicine specialist, is recommended for optimal clinical decision making. It has been estimated that there are approximately 13 cases of breast cancer diagnosed per 100,000 live births.[35,36] Breast cancer during pregnancy tends to present at advanced stages with lymph node involvement, sometimes because there is a delay in the diagnosis. Tumors tend to be poorly differentiated, HR negative, and HER2 positive in 30% of cases. The initial workup should evaluate for the presence of metastatic disease, as this may influence the patient's decision regarding maintenance of the pregnancy. Estimation of delivery time will help in establishing the best treatment options. Fetal growth needs to be monitored during treatment. Much of the data regarding the management of pregnant breast cancer patients with modalities such as surgery, chemotherapy, etc., are retrospective in nature.[36] Surgery remains the mainstay of treatment of breast cancer during pregnancy, and in some circumstances breast-conserving surgery is an acceptable option. SLN biopsy with

technetium 99m is considered safe; however, isosulfan blue dye should be avoided because of unknown fetal effects and risk for anaphylaxis for the patient. Indications for chemotherapy are the same as for nonpregnant patients, but it should ideally not be given during the first trimester (may be teratogenic) or after week 35, to avoid complications at the time of delivery. Reports of fetal malformations fall in the range of 14% to 19% when chemotherapy has been given in the first trimester. Chemotherapy regimens containing anthracyclines or alkylating agents are most commonly used; if taxanes are indicated, they should be used after delivery. Concern of the effectiveness of taxanes during pregnancy has been raised secondary to the upregulation of the cytochrome P-450 system during the third trimester, thus potentially increasing drug metabolism. Trastuzumab, hormonal therapy, and radiation therapy should be initiated only in the postpartum period. Trastuzumab administration during pregnancy was associated with oligo- and anhydramnios. Decisions regarding lactation and future fertility should be addressed on a per-patient basis.

- **Male breast cancer** is a rare disease. Less than 1% of breast cancer patients are males. In contrast to female breast cancer, an estimated 4% to 40% of cases are thought to result from autosomal dominant inheritance. Familial cases tend to be associated with *BRCA2,* and 20% of patients with male breast cancer have a first-degree relative with the disease.[37] Known risk factors are those associated with hormonal imbalance in estrogen and androgen levels. Patients with Klinefelter syndrome, testicular pathology (e.g., cryptorchidism, testicular injury, orchitis, or any other form of gonadal dysfunction), and infertility have an increased risk. Obesity, increased alcohol intake, exposure to radiation, high temperatures, and exhaust fumes are also considered risk factors. Gynecomastia does not increase the risk of male breast cancer. Ninety percent of the tumors are ER positive, and therefore, hormonal therapy is a mainstay of treatment. At presentation, patients usually have stage III or IV disease, but survival is comparable to that for female breast cancer when matched for stage and grade. As male breast cancer is rare, the principles of treatment are derived from randomized studies in women with breast cancer. Mastectomy is the type of surgery usually performed, followed usually by radiation therapy. Tamoxifen is the first-line therapy in ER-positive tumors. Chemotherapy can be used in cases of hormone-refractory disease.

COMPLICATIONS

- **Lymphadema** is a complication of breast cancer treatment. Impaired lymphatic drainage in the ipsilateral arm may result from removal or injury to axillary lymph nodes from lymph dissection and/or radiation. Treatment of lymphadema depends on its severity and is usually handled with the assistance of specially trained lymphadema specialists. The most common treatments for lymphedema involve a combination of compression garments or wraps, intermittent sequential multichambered overlapping gradient pumps, and manual compression lymphatic massage. Any of the treatments can be done individually.

MONITORING/FOLLOW-UP

- Follow-up exams should be individualized either to reflect the patient's risk of recurrence or to monitor treatment or disease progression. Posttreatment follow-up includes regular physical exam and mammography. The first mammogram in patients undergoing BCT should be after 6 months, and then yearly. No randomized trials have demonstrated a benefit from routine laboratory or radiology testing compared to a careful history and physical exam. The clinical role of tumor markers (CEA, CA 15–3, CA 27–29) is also unproven. According to the most recent **NCCN guidelines,** routine liver function tests, bone scans, chest x-rays, CT scans, PET scans, or US is not recommended unless clinical suspicion for recurrent/metastatic disease is suggested by the history and/or physical exam. MRI can be considered as an option for surveillance in women at high risk for bilateral disease, such as *BRCA1/BRCA2* mutation carriers, or in young women with dense breasts. Female patients who are taking tamoxifen should undergo yearly gynecologic evaluation if they have a uterus. Patients taking aromatase inhibitors should have bone health monitoring, given the associated increased risk of osteopenia and osteoporosis.

OUTCOME/PROGNOSIS

- The most reliable and reproducible prognostic factor is the involvement of axillary lymph nodes. Tumors <1 cm without nodal involvement have a good prognosis. Tumors with a poorly differentiated histology and a high nuclear grade have a worse prognosis. Estrogen receptor (ER) and progesterone receptor (PgR) statuses are prognostic and also predictive factors for the likelihood of benefit from hormonal therapy. The HER2 overexpression has been associated with a poor prognosis, but is a strong predictive factor for response to anti-HER2 therapy, which has altered its previously aggressive evolution.

REFERENCES

1. Jemal A, Siegel R, Xu J, et al. Cancer statistics, 2010. *CA Cancer J Clin.* 2010;60:277–300.
2. Perou CM, Sorlie T, Eisen MB, et al. Molecular portraits of human breast tumours. *Nature.* 2000;406:747–752.
3. Prat A, Perou CM. Deconstructing the molecular portraits of breast cancer. *Mol Oncol.* 2011:5:5–23.
4. Amir E, Freedman OC, Seruga B, et al. Assessing women at high risk of breast cancer: a review of risk assessment models. *J Natl Cancer Inst.* 2010;102:680–691.
5. Miki Y, Swensen J, Shattuck-Eidens D, et al. A strong candidate for the breast and ovarian cancer susceptibility gene BRCA1. *Science.* 1994;266:66–71.
6. Wooster R, Bignell G, Lancaster J, et al. Identification of the breast cancer susceptibility gene BRCA2. *Nature.* 1995;378:789–792.
7. Antoniou A, Pharoah PD, Narod S, et al. Average risks of breast and ovarian cancer associated with BRCA1 or BRCA2 mutations detected in case series unselected for family history: a combined analysis of 22 studies. *Am J Hum Genet.* 2003;72:1117–1130.
8. Gail MH, Brinton LA, Byar DP, et al. Projecting individualized probabilities of developing breast cancer for white females who are being examined annually. *J Natl Cancer Inst.* 1989; 81:1879–1886.
9. Fisher B, Costantino JP, Wickerham DL, et al. Tamoxifen for prevention of breast cancer: Report of the National Surgical Adjuvant Breast and Bowel Project P-1 Study. *J Natl Cancer Inst.* 1998;90:1371–1388.
10. Vogel VG, Costantino JP, Wickerham DL, et al. Effects of tamoxifen vs raloxifene on the risk of developing invasive breast cancer and other disease outcomes: the NSABP Study of Tamoxifen and Raloxifene (STAR) P-2 trial. *JAMA.* 2006;295:2727–2741.

11. Nelson HD, Tyne K, Naik A, et al. Screening for breast cancer: an update for the U.S. Preventive Services Task Force. *Ann Intern Med.* 2009;151:727–737, W237–42.
12. Calonge N, Petitti DB, DeWitt TG, et al. Screening for breast cancer: U.S. Preventive Services Task Force recommendation statement. *Ann Intern Med.* 2009;151:716–726, W-236.
13. Warner E, Plewes DB, Hill KA, et al. Surveillance of BRCA1 and BRCA2 mutation carriers with magnetic resonance imaging, ultrasound, mammography, and clinical breast examination. *JAMA.* 2004;292:1317–1325.
14. Edge S, Byrd DR, Compton CC, et al. *AJCC Cancer Staging Manual.* 7th ed. New York: Springer; 2010:417–460.
15. Schwartz GF, Solin LJ, Olivotto IA, et al. Consensus conference on the treatment of in situ ductal carcinoma of the breast. April 22–25, 1999. *Cancer.* 2000;88:946–954.
16. Fisher B, Dignam J, Wolmark N, et al. Tamoxifen in treatment of intraductal breast cancer: National Surgical Adjuvant Breast and Bowel Project B-24 randomised controlled trial. *Lancet.* 1999;353:1993–2000.
17. Giuliano AE, McCall LM, Beitsch PD, et al. A randomized trial of axillary node dissection in women with clinical T1–2 N0 M0 breast cancer who have a positive sentinel node. *J Clin Oncol.* 2010;28(Suppl; Abstract CRA506).
18. Early Breast Cancer Trialists' Collaborative Group (EBCTCG). Effects of chemotherapy and hormonal therapy for early breast cancer on recurrence and 15-year survival: an overview of the randomized trials. *Lancet.* 2005;365:1687–1717.
19. Mouridsen H, Giobbie-Hurder A, Goldhirsch A, et al. Letrozole therapy alone or in sequence with tamoxifen in women with breast cancer. *N Engl J Med.* 2009;361:766–776.
20. Howell A, Cuzick J, Baum M, et al. Results of the ATAC (Arimidex, Tamoxifen, alone or in combination) trial after completion of 5 years adjuvant treatment for breast cancer. *Lancet.* 2005;365:60–62.
21. Viani GA, Afonso SL, Stefano EJ, et al. Adjuvant trastuzumab in the treatment of HER-2-positive early breast cancer: a meta-analysis of published randomized trials. *BMC Cancer.* 2007;7:153.
22. Jahanzeb M. Adjuvant trastuzumab therapy for HER2-positive breast cancer. *Clin Breast Cancer.* 2008;8:324–333.
23. Klijn JG, Blamey RW, Boccardo F, et al. Combined tamoxifen and luteinizing hormone-releasing hormone (LHRH) agonist versus LHRH agonist alone in premenopausal advanced breast cancer: a meta-analysis of four randomized trials. *J Clin Oncol.* 2001;19:343–353.
24. Ellis MJ, Gao F, Dehdashti F, et al. Lower-dose vs high-dose oral estradiol therapy of hormone receptor-positive, aromatase inhibitor-resistant advanced breast cancer: a phase 2 randomized study. *JAMA.* 2009;302:774–780.
25. Breast cancer Treatment -National Cancer Institute. NCI. http://www.cancer.gov/cancertopics/pdq/treatment/breast/HealthProfessional/page7#Section_211. 2010.
26. Goel S, Chirgwin J, Francis P, et al. Rational use of trastuzumab in metastatic and locally advanced breast cancer: implications of recent research. *Breast.* 2010;20:101–110.
27. Harris CA, Ward RL, Dobbins TA, et al. The efficacy of HER2-targeted agents in metastatic breast cancer: a meta-analysis. *Ann Oncol.* 2010;22:1308–1317.
28. Slamon DJ, Leyland-Jones B, Shak S, et al. Use of chemotherapy plus a monoclonal antibody against HER2 for metastatic breast cancer that overexpresses HER2. *N Engl J Med.* 2001;344:783–792.
29. Geyer CE, Forster J, Lindquist D, et al. Lapatinib plus capecitabine for HER2-positive advanced breast cancer. *N Engl J Med.* 2006;355:2733–2743.
30. Johnston S, Pippen J Jr, Pivot X, et al. Lapatinib combined with letrozole versus letrozole and placebo as first-line therapy for postmenopausal hormone receptor-positive metastatic breast cancer. *J Clin Oncol.* 2009;27:5538–5546.
31. O'Shaughnessy J, Osborne C, Pippen JE, et al. Iniparib plus chemotherapy in metastatic triple-negative breast cancer. *N Engl J Med.* 2011;364:205–214.

32. Annunziata CM, O'Shaughnessy J. Poly (ADP-ribose) polymerase as a novel therapeutic target in cancer. *Clin Cancer Res.* 2010;16:4517–4526.
33. Pavlakis N, Schmidt R, Stockler M. Bisphosphonates for breast cancer. *Cochrane Database Syst Rev.* 2005:CD003474.
34. Stopeck AT, Lipton A, Body JJ, et al. Denosumab compared with zoledronic acid for the treatment of bone metastases in patients with advanced breast cancer: a randomized, double-blind study. *J Clin Oncol.* 2010;28:5132–5139.
35. Smith LH, Dalrymple JL, Leiserowitz GS, et al. Obstetrical deliveries associated with maternal malignancy in California, 1992 through 1997. *Am J Obstet Gynecol.* 2001;184:1504–1512; discussion 12-3.
36. Litton JK, Theriault RL. Breast cancer and pregnancy: current concepts in diagnosis and treatment. *Oncologist.* 2010;15:1238–1247.
37. Fentiman IS, Fourquet A, Hortobagyi GN. Male breast cancer. *Lancet.* 2006;367:595–604.

19 Lung Cancer

Saiama Waqar

GENERAL PRINCIPLES

Lung cancer is first divided into two broad groups: small-cell lung cancer (SCLC) and non-small-cell lung cancer (NSCLC), based on histology. Their clinical behavior and management are different and, therefore, discussed separately.

Epidemiology

Lung cancer is the leading cause of cancer-related mortality in the United States with an estimated 222,520 new cases and 157,300 deaths attributable to lung cancer in 2010.[1] The incidence of lung cancer is continuing to decline in men. However, in women the rates appear to be plateauing after several years of rising incidence.[2]

Risk Factors

- **Tobacco smoke** is the major risk factor for lung cancer. There is a clear, dose-dependent relationship between tobacco use and lung cancer. A major public health goal in reducing total mortality from lung cancer remains reducing the prevalence of smoking. Smoking reduction by 50% in heavy smokers significantly reduces the risk of lung cancer.[3] Squamous cell lung cancers and SCLCs, in particular, are associated with tobacco smoking.
- Other exposures have also been associated with lung cancer, including asbestos, radon, chromium, nickel, and arsenic compounds.[4] Genetic predisposition is an important risk factor, and there are well-identified familial clusters of lung cancers. A major inheritable lung cancer susceptibility locus has been reported to be within 6q23–25.[5] Genetic polymorphisms of enzymes regulating tobacco carcinogen metabolism, such as an exon 7 cytochrome p450 (CYP1A1) polymorphism, and GSTM1 null genotype are associated with increased risk of lung cancer.[6–8] In addition, polymorphisms of genes regulating DNA repair (ERCC2 and XRCC1) and inflammation (COX-2, IL-6, and IL-8) have also been reported to be associated with increased risk of lung cancer.[9]

Prevention and Screening

Current and former smokers have a significant risk of lung cancer, and **smoking cessation** should be encouraged. Chemoprevention agents for lung cancer have not been established. The National Lung Screening Trial (NLST) is a randomized National Cancer Institute–sponsored trial comparing the effect of low-dose helical computed tomography (CT) and standard chest x-ray on lung cancer mortality in former and current smokers. According to the press release, 20% fewer lung cancer deaths were seen among trial participants screened with low-dose helical CT.[10] The National Comprehensive Cancer Network (NCCN) does not currently recommend screening CT use.[11]

NON-SMALL-CELL LUNG CANCER

GENERAL PRINCIPLES

Non-small-cell lung cancer accounts for ~87% of lung cancers in the United States. NSCLC encompasses four pathologic subtypes:

- **Squamous cell lung cancer** usually arises in proximal bronchi and can cause obstruction of the larger airways.
- **Adenocarcinoma** is the most common subtype, representing 40% of lung cancers in North America. It usually arises in the lung periphery.
- **Bronchoalveolar carcinoma** is a subtype of adenocarcinoma that grows along alveolar septa. It can present as a single nodule, as multiple nodules, or as a rapidly progressive multilobar disease that radiographically resembles pneumonia. It is not associated with tobacco smoking.
- **Large-cell carcinoma** is the least common subtype.

DIAGNOSIS

Clinical Presentation

- Presenting signs and symptoms of lung cancer depend on the size, location, and degree of spread of the tumor. Lung cancer can present as an asymptomatic lung nodule found incidentally on chest x-ray (CXR). Local symptoms can include cough, wheeze, hemoptysis, dyspnea, postobstructive pneumonia (due to tumors that occlude major bronchi), pain (particularly with pleural or chest wall involvement), dysphagia (due to esophageal compression by tumor or lymphadenopathy), and hoarseness (caused by laryngeal nerve involvement). Apical tumors that invade the lower brachial plexus can present with **Pancoast syndrome,** which is a brachial plexopathy, Horner syndrome, and shoulder pain. Mediastinal lymphadenopathy that compresses the superior vena cava (SVC) can cause **SVC syndrome,** which most commonly presents with dyspnea and facial swelling. Systemic symptoms usually accompany disease that is more advanced and can include weight loss, fatigue, and loss of appetite. Metastatic disease may cause symptoms specific to the involved organs. For example, patients may have pain from bony metastases, dyspnea from pericardial or pleural effusions, or headache and neurologic deficits from brain metastases. Although adrenal and liver metastases are common, they are usually asymptomatic.
- NSCLC has been associated with numerous paraneoplastic syndromes. Clubbing results from proliferation of connective tissue at the ends of the digits and usually improves with treatment of the tumor. Hypercalcemia may be due to ectopic parathyroid hormone production by the tumor. **Pulmonary hypertrophic osteoarthropathy** is a syndrome consisting of bone and joint pain, clubbing, and increased alkaline phosphatase. It can be diagnosed by plain films (which show periosteal inflammation) or bone scan (which shows increased uptake symmetrically in long bones).

Diagnostic Testing

The goal of the initial workup is to establish the diagnosis of malignancy and to determine accurately the clinical stage of the cancer so that candidates for potentially curable surgical resection are identified. Strategies for obtaining a pathologic diagnosis of a lung mass include sputum cytology (optimally from three early morning sputum collections), biopsy by percutaneous fine-needle aspiration, and bronchoscopy with biopsy.

Imaging

Once the diagnosis of NSCLC has been confirmed, recommended imaging studies include a **chest x-ray** and a **chest CT scan,** which can reveal the size of the tumor, extent of invasion of local structures, and presence of regional lymph node metastases. **PET scan** is also useful, as it has high accuracy in detecting disease metastatic to lymph nodes and distant sites, and it can aid in the differentiation of benign and malignant lung nodules.

Diagnostic Procedures

Potential lymph node metastases identified on imaging studies should be confirmed with direct biopsy. **Mediastinoscopy** is the most accurate means of staging mediastinal lymph nodes and should be performed when nodal involvement cannot be defined with chest CT. Pleural effusions should always be examined by **thoracentesis,** as a tumor associated with a malignant effusion is inoperable. The best way to identify the presence of distant metastases is with a thorough history and physical exam. Further imaging exams (i.e., head CT, abdominal CT, bone scan) should be directed by the patient's symptoms and are not required in asymptomatic patients who have early-stage tumors.

Staging

If tissue sampling confirms the diagnosis of NSCLC, the stage of disease should be determined using the tumor, node, metastasis (TNM) staging. The 7th edition of TNM staging was developed by the International Association for the Study of Lung Cancer (IASLC), based on retrospective analysis of survival data from patients with NSCLC. It was approved by the American Joint Committee on Cancer (AJCC) for use starting January 1, 2010. See Table 19-1 for details regarding TNM staging. The major changes in this edition include reclassification of malignant pleural effusions as M1a rather than T4, downstaging of additional tumor nodules in a different lobe of the same lung to T4 rather than M1. T4 tumors with separate tumor nodules in the same lobe have been reclassified as T3. In addition, T1 and T2 tumors are divided into additional categories (a and b) based on size cutoffs. Finally, T2 tumors larger than 7 cm were reclassified as T3.[12,13]

TREATMENT

Stages I and II

- Stage I and II tumors are considered **resectable,** as they have extended no further than adjacent resectable structures or first-level lymph nodes. The optimal treatment is surgical resection with lobectomy or pneumonectomy. Preoperative workup includes spirometry, arterial blood gases, and V/Q scan to establish both that the FEV1 will be >1.2 L post-resection and that the patient does not have hypercapnia or cor pulmonale.
- Patients who are not candidates for surgery because of poor lung function or comorbid conditions should be considered for **radiation therapy** (RT) administered with curative intent. Toxicities of RT include pneumonitis (shortness of breath, tachypnea, tachycardia, fever, nonproductive cough, and infiltrate on

TABLE 19-1 TNM STAGING SYSTEM FOR NON-SMALL-CELL LUNG CANCER (7TH EDITION)

Primary tumor (T)	
TX:	Primary tumor cannot be assessed
T1:	Tumor ≤3 cm in greatest dimension, surrounded by lung or visceral pleura, without bronchoscopic evidence of invasion more proximal than the lobar bronchus a (i.e., not in the main bronchus)
T1a:	Tumor ≤2 cm
T1b:	Tumor >2 cm but ≤3 cm
T2:	Tumor size >3 cm in greatest dimension but ≤7cm; or tumor with any of the following features: involves main bronchus, ≥2 cm distal to the carina; invades the visceral pleura; associated with atelectasis or obstructive pneumonitis that extends to the hilar region but does not involve the entire lung
T2a:	Tumor >3 cm but ≤5 cm
T2b:	Tumor >5 cm but ≤7 cm
T3:	Tumor >7 cm or any of the following: tumor of any size that directly invades any of the following: chest wall, diaphragm, phrenic nerve, mediastinal pleura, or parietal pericardium; or tumor in the main bronchus <2 cm distal to the carina, but without involvement of the carina; associated atelectasis or obstructive pneumonitis of the entire lung, separate tumor nodules in the same lobe
T4:	Tumor of any size that invades any of the following: mediastinum, heart, great vessels, trachea, esophagus, recurrent laryngeal nerve, vertebral body, or carina; or separate tumor nodules in a different ipsilateral lobe of the lung
Regional lymph nodes (N)	
NX:	Regional lymph nodes cannot be assessed
N0:	No regional lymph node metastasis
N1:	Metastasis to ipsilateral peribronchial and/or ipsilateral hilar lymph nodes, and intrapulmonary nodes involved by direct extension of the primary tumor
N2:	Metastasis to ipsilateral mediastinal and/or subcarinal lymph node(s)
N3:	Metastasis to contralateral mediastinal, contralateral hilar, ipsilateral or contralateral scalene, or supra clavicular lymph node(s)
Distant metastasis (M)	
MX:	Presence of distant metastasis cannot be assessed
M0:	No distant metastasis
M1:	Distant metastasis
M1a:	Separate tumor nodule(s) in a contralateral lobe, tumor with pleural nodules or malignant pleural or pericardial effusion
M1b:	Distant metastasis

(*continued*)

TABLE 19-1 TNM STAGING SYSTEM FOR NON-SMALL-CELL LUNG CANCER (7TH EDITION) (*Continued*)

Stage grouping:	**TNM subsets**
Stage IA:	T1a-T1b N0 M0
Stage IB:	T2a N0 M0
Stage IIA:	T1a,T1b,T2a N1 M0
	T2b N0 M0
Stage IIB:	T2b N1 M0
	T3 N0 M0
Stage IIIA:	T1a,T1b,T2a,T2b N2 M0
	T3 N1,N2 M0
	T4 N0,N1 M0
Stage IIIB:	T4 N2 M0
	Any T N3 M0
Stage IV:	Any T Any N M1a or M1b

Adapted from American Joint Committee on Cancer. *AJCC Cancer Staging Manual.* 7th ed. New York: Springer; 2010.

CXR 1 to 3 months after RT), pulmonary fibrosis, acute esophagitis, pericarditis, and Lhermitte's phenomenon or radiation myelitis (transient electric sensation radiating down the spine or into the limbs with neck flexion). Adjuvant RT is indicated if the surgical margins are positive for tumor.

- Several prospective studies have reported that the addition of adjuvant platinum-based chemotherapy to resected stage II patients with good performance status significantly improves survival.[14–16] In patients with stage I patients, there is currently not enough evidence to recommend adjuvant chemotherapy, although there is a suggestion that stage IB tumors >4 cm in size may benefit.[17,18]

Stage III

Treatment of patients with stage III disease requires a multidisciplinary approach, involving input from surgeons, medical oncologists, and radiation oncologists. In patients with surgically resectable stage IIIA disease (T3N1), the addition of adjuvant chemotherapy following surgical resection significantly improves survival.[19] Patients with N2 disease are generally considered to be unresectable. Concurrent chemotherapy and radiation has been shown to improve long-term survival compared with sequential chemotherapy followed by radiation in patients with unresectable IIIA and IIIB NSCLC.[20] However, survival benefit was seen only in patients with good performance status. The addition of surgery after receiving chemoradiation in patients with stage IIIA disease (N2) has not shown a significant survival advantage; however, a subset analysis suggested a survival advantage in a subset of patients who underwent lobectomy, but not pneumonectomy.[21] In patients with poor performance status, a palliative treatment approach is preferred.

Stage IV

- Patients with stage IV disease are considered to be **incurable.** Recent advances in the treatment of stage IV NSCLC include the use of targeted agents, such as bevacizumab and erlotinib, factoring histology and genetic mutations into treatment decisions. Front-line platinum-based doublet chemotherapy provides modest improvement in survival.[22] In patients with non-squamous histology, treatment options include front-line platinum and pemetrexed (a folate antagonist) doublet therapy or addition of bevacizumab, a vascular endothelial growth factor (VEGF) inhibitor, to platinum-based doublet chemotherapy.[23,24] Epidermal growth factor receptor tyrosine kinase inhibitors (EGFR-TKIs) have been studied in the front-line setting. Single-agent gefitinib, an oral EGFR-TKI, has been shown to improve progression-free survival over combination chemotherapy in patients with EGFR mutations, but not in patients with EGFR wild-type tumors.[25] However, neither gefitinib nor erlotinib improved outcome when combined with cytotoxic chemotherapy.[26,27]

- Front-line **platinum-based chemotherapy** is generally given for 4 to 6 cycles. Maintenance chemotherapy is an option for patients with good performance status who do not have disease progression after 4 cycles of front-line platinum-based doublet therapy. Agents approved for this indication include pemetrexed and erlotinib.[28,29] Selection of agent is based on histology (pemetrexed for non-squamous histology) and presence of EGFR mutation (erlotinib in patients with EGFR mutations). In patients who have had significant toxicities with first-line therapy, or those who desire a treatment break, waiting until disease progression to start second-line therapy is appropriate.
- Single-agent **docetaxel** in the second-line setting has been shown to improve survival compared to best supportive care.[30] In addition, pemetrexed is approved as a second-line agent for patients with non-squamous histology.[31] Second-line erlotinib is also approved for NSCLC.[30]
- For patients with poor performance status, who may not benefit from chemotherapy, treatment should focus on palliation of symptoms. A brief palliative course of RT may reduce disease bulk, relieving dyspnea, pain, or other symptoms. Targeted RT may also treat pain and complications from bony or brain metastases. Early palliative care in patients with metastatic NSCLC integrated with standard oncologic care improves quality of life.[32]

SPECIAL CONSIDERATIONS

- Somatic activating mutations in EGFR are present in 10% of unselected NSCLC tumors. These mutations are further enriched in never smokers, with a frequency of ~50%. Exon 19 deletions and exon 21 L858R mutations account for 85% of EGFR mutations and are predictive for response to EGFR-TKIs, such as erlotinib and gefitinib. The most common mutations are exon 19 deletions and L858R mutations. Resistance to EGFR-TKI therapy in previously responsive patients is mediated by EGFRT90M mutations or MET amplification.
- Crizotinib is an anaplastic lymphoma kinase (ALK) inhibitor under study in patients with advanced NSCLC carrying the EML4-ALK fusion gene.[33] Patients carrying this fusion gene are typically nonsmokers and do not have the EGFR mutation. EML4-ALK fusion gene is seen in 3% to 5% of patients with NSCLC. There is currently no standard test for detecting the EML4-ALK fusion gene.

MONITORING/FOLLOW-UP

According to the NCCN guidelines, in patients with no evidence of disease, a careful history and physical exam and CT of the chest with contrast should be performed every 4 to 6 months for 2 years. After 2 years, history, physical exam and non-contrast

CT of the chest should be performed annually.[11] Patients should be counseled regarding smoking cessation. Further tests such as PET scan, abdominal CT, bone scan, and MRI of the brain are not part of routine surveillance and should be obtained only if signs or symptoms suggest recurrent disease. Blood tests and sputum cytology do not have a role in routine follow-up. Unfortunately, even with close follow-up, it is unlikely that recurrent disease will be resectable and curable.

OUTCOME/PROGNOSIS

Prognosis varies by stage. Recurrences may be local or distant and will occur in up to 30% of patients with stage I disease and 50% of patients with stage II disease over the subsequent 5 years. The 3-year survival in patients with stage III disease treated with chemoradiation is 25%.[34] Patients with advanced stage disease treated with platinum-based doublets have a median survival of 8 to 10 months, with a 1-year survival of 30% to 40% and 2-year survival of 10% to 15%.[22]

SMALL-CELL LUNG CANCER

GENERAL PRINCIPLES

SCLC accounts for ~13% of lung cancers in the United States. As opposed to NSCLC, SCLC grows more rapidly, is more often associated with diverse paraneoplastic syndromes, and is initially more chemosensitive.[35]

DIAGNOSIS

Clinical Presentation

The presenting signs and symptoms of SCLC are similar to those of NSCLC. SCLCs are often centrally located and symptoms result from obstruction of the airway lumen. Common symptoms are cough, dyspnea, hemoptysis, wheezing, and post-obstructive pneumonia. Ten percent of patients have SVC syndrome at presentation. Occasionally, SCLCs can present as asymptomatic lung nodules found on imaging studies.

- **Paraneoplastic syndromes** associated with SCLC include syndrome of inappropriate secretion of antidiuretic hormone (SIADH), Cushing syndrome from ectopic adrenocorticotropic hormone production, and neurologic paraneoplastic syndromes, including peripheral neuropathy and encephalomyelitis, are thought to be due to the production of autoantibodies. Lambert–Eaton syndrome is caused by an autoantibody that impairs acetylcholine release at the neuromuscular junction, leading to proximal muscle weakness and hyporeflexia.

Diagnostic Testing

Initial workup should include a comprehensive history and physical exam. Initial studies include **CBC** and **CMP**. Tumor lysis syndrome may occur with bulky disease, so **lactate dehydrogenase** and **uric acid** should also be checked. In addition to a baseline **chest x-ray, CT scan of the chest and abdomen** should be performed to define the extent of intrathoracic disease and to detect abdominal metastases. Further workup may include a head CT and bone scan. Once disease has been found outside of the thorax, workup for additional sites of metastasis is not necessary unless a metastasis requiring immediate intervention (e.g., to weight-bearing bone or CNS) is suspected.

Staging

The TNM (tumor, node, metastases) staging system is not widely used to classify SCLC, although the IASLC has proposed the use of TNM staging.[36] Currently, SCLC is described either as **limited stage,** with disease confined to one hemithorax that is encompassed in a single radiation field, or as **extensive stage,** which describes all other patterns of disease.

TREATMENT

- **Chemotherapy** is the primary modality used for the treatment of SCLC, as inferior results are obtained when RT is used alone. For patients with **limited-stage disease,** combined modality treatment with chemotherapy and RT to the chest is standard of care.[37] **Extensive stage disease** is treated with chemotherapy alone. The commonly used standard chemotherapy regimens for SCLC include combinations of carboplatin or cisplatin with etoposide. Irinotecan, topotecan, and epirubicin are acceptable alternatives to etoposide and have a lower incidence of myelosuppression. Overall response rate to chemotherapy is ~60%, but nearly all patients eventually have disease relapse.
- **Prophylactic cranial radiation** (PCI) is recommended for patients with limited-stage SCLC who achieve complete response after initial chemoradiation to prevent intracranial metastases.[38] It can also be considered in patients with extensive-stage SCLC with a complete response to treatment.[39] However, it should not be administered to patients with poor performance status or impaired mental function.
- Patients with poor performance status or significant comorbidities may not be able to tolerate aggressive chemotherapy. These patients may receive only RT or attenuated schedules of chemotherapy, with the goal of relieving symptoms.

MONITORING/FOLLOW-UP

Most patients treated for SCLC will relapse, usually in the first 2 years after diagnosis. Therefore, they should have close follow-up with a medical oncologist for the identification of symptoms, physical exam findings, or lab and CXR abnormalities that suggest recurrent disease. According to the NCCN guidelines, patients with no evidence of disease should have a follow-up visit every 2 to 3 months during year 1, every 3 to 4 months during years 2 to 3, and then every 4 to 6 months during years 4 to 5.[40] After this, follow-up visits should be scheduled annually. At every visit, a careful history and physical exam, labs, and CXR should be performed. Patients should be counseled regarding smoking cessation.

OUTCOME/PROGNOSIS

Stage (limited vs. extensive), performance status, and markers of disease burden, such as serum lactate dehydrogenase, are the factors that most reliably correlate with outcome. The median survival of limited-stage disease treated with chemotherapy and

RT is 15 to 26 months. However, long-term survival can be achieved in 20% to 40% of patients with limited-stage SCLC with chemoradiation. The median survival of extensive-stage disease treated with chemotherapy is 7 to 12 months. Only 5% of patients with extensive disease survive to 2 years.

OTHER MALIGNANT TUMORS OF THE LUNG

Malignant tumors of the lung, other than NSCLC and SCLC, are uncommon and include carcinoid tumors, mucoepidermoid carcinoma, and sarcomas. Carcinoid tumors account for 1% of lung malignancies and are derived from neuroendocrine cells. They arise in the bronchi and may cause bronchial obstruction and can produce a variety of systemically active substances that cause the **carcinoid syndrome:** flushing, diarrhea, and wheezing. Carcinoid tumors of the lung tend to grow slowly and are associated with a 5-year survival of 77% to 87%.

REFERENCES

1. Jemal A, Siegel R, Xu J, et al. Cancer statistics, 2010. *CA Cancer J Clin.* 2010;60:277–300.
2. Jemal A, Thun MJ, Ries LA, et al. Annual report to the nation on the status of cancer, 1975–2005, featuring trends in lung cancer, tobacco use, and tobacco control. *J Natl Cancer Inst.* 2008;100:1672–1694.
3. Godtfredsen NS, Prescott E, Osler M. Effect of smoking reduction on lung cancer risk. *JAMA.* 2005;294:1505–1510.
4. Neuberger JS, Field RW. Occupation and lung cancer in nonsmokers. *Rev Environ Health.* 2003;18:251–267.
5. Bailey-Wilson JE, Amos CI, Pinney SM, et al. A major lung cancer susceptibility locus maps to chromosome 6q23–25. *Am J Hum Genet.* 2004;75:460–474.
6. Hirvonen A, Husgafvel-Pursiainen K, Anttila S, et al. Polymorphism in CYP1A1 and CYP2D6 genes: possible association with susceptibility to lung cancer. *Environ Health Perspect.* 1993;101(Suppl 3):109–112.
7. Sobti RC, Sharma S, Joshi A, et al. Genetic polymorphism of the CYP1A1, CYP2E1, GSTM1 and GSTT1 genes and lung cancer susceptibility in a north Indian population. *Mol Cell Biochem.* 2004;266:1–9.
8. Shi X, Zhou S, Wang Z, et al. CYP1A1 and GSTM1 polymorphisms and lung cancer risk in Chinese populations: a meta-analysis. *Lung Cancer.* 2008;59:155–163.
9. Schwartz AG, Prysak GM, Bock CH, et al. The molecular epidemiology of lung cancer. *Carcinogenesis.* 2007;28:507–518.
10. http://www.cancer.gov/newscenter/pressreleases/NLSTresultsRelease. Accessed on 12/02/10.
11. http://www.nccn.org/professionals/physician_gls/PDF/nscl.pdf. Accessed on 12/01/10.
12. Goldstraw P, Crowley J, Chansky K, et al. The IASLC Lung Cancer Staging Project: proposals for the revision of the TNM stage groupings in the forthcoming (seventh) edition of the TNM classification of malignant tumours. *J Thorac Oncol.* 2007;2:706–714.
13. Groome PA, Bolejack V, Crowley JJ, et al. The IASLC Lung Cancer Staging Project: validation of the proposals for revision of the T, N, and M descriptors and consequent stage groupings in the forthcoming (seventh) edition of the TNM classification of malignant tumours. *J Thorac Oncol.* 2007;2:694–705.
14. Arriagada R, Dunant A, Pignon JP, et al. Long-term results of the international adjuvant lung cancer trial evaluating adjuvant Cisplatin-based chemotherapy in resected lung cancer. *J Clin Oncol.* 2010;28:35–42.
15. Douillard JY, Tribodet H, Aubert D, et al. Adjuvant cisplatin and vinorelbine for completely resected non-small cell lung cancer: subgroup analysis of the Lung Adjuvant Cisplatin Evaluation. *J Thorac Oncol.* 2010;5:220–228.

16. Douillard JY, Rosell R, De Lena M, et al. Adjuvant vinorelbine plus cisplatin versus observation in patients with completely resected stage IB-IIIA non-small-cell lung cancer (Adjuvant Navelbine International Trialist Association [ANITA]): a randomised controlled trial. *Lancet Oncol.* 2006;7:719–727.
17. Butts CA, Ding K, Seymour L, et al. Randomized phase III trial of vinorelbine plus cisplatin compared with observation in completely resected stage IB and II non-small-cell lung cancer: updated survival analysis of JBR-10. *J Clin Oncol.* 2009;28:29–34.
18. Strauss GM, Herndon JE 2nd, Maddaus MA, et al. Adjuvant paclitaxel plus carboplatin compared with observation in stage IB non-small-cell lung cancer: CALGB 9633 with the Cancer and Leukemia Group B, Radiation Therapy Oncology Group, and North Central Cancer Treatment Group Study Groups. *J Clin Oncol.* 2008;26:5043–5051.
19. Arriagada R, Bergman B, Dunant A, et al. Cisplatin-based adjuvant chemotherapy in patients with completely resected non-small-cell lung cancer. *N Engl J Med.* 2004;350:351–360.
20. Hanna N, Neubauer M, Yiannoutsos C, et al. Phase III study of cisplatin, etoposide, and concurrent chest radiation with or without consolidation docetaxel in patients with inoperable stage III non-small-cell lung cancer: the Hoosier Oncology Group and U.S. Oncology. *J Clin Oncol.* 2008;26:5755–5760.
21. Albain KS, Swann RS, Rusch VW, et al. Radiotherapy plus chemotherapy with or without surgical resection for stage III non-small-cell lung cancer: a phase III randomised controlled trial. *Lancet.* 2009;374:379–386.
22. Schiller JH, Harrington D, Belani CP, et al. Comparison of four chemotherapy regimens for advanced non-small-cell lung cancer. *N Engl J Med.* 2002;346:92–98.
23. Scagliotti GV, Parikh P, von Pawel J, et al. Phase III study comparing cisplatin plus gemcitabine with cisplatin plus pemetrexed in chemotherapy-naive patients with advanced-stage non-small-cell lung cancer. *J Clin Oncol.* 2008;26:3543–3551.
24. Reck M, von Pawel J, Zatloukal P, et al. Phase III trial of cisplatin plus gemcitabine with either placebo or bevacizumab as first-line therapy for nonsquamous non-small-cell lung cancer: AVAil. *J Clin Oncol.* 2009;27:1227–1234.
25. Mok TS, Wu YL, Thongprasert S, et al. Gefitinib or carboplatin-paclitaxel in pulmonary adenocarcinoma. *N Engl J Med.* 2009;361:947–957.
26. Giaccone G, Herbst RS, Manegold C, et al. Gefitinib in combination with gemcitabine and cisplatin in advanced non-small-cell lung cancer: a phase III trial—INTACT 1. *J Clin Oncol.* 2004;22:777–784.
27. Herbst RS, Giaccone G, Schiller JH, et al. Gefitinib in combination with paclitaxel and carboplatin in advanced non-small-cell lung cancer: a phase III trial—INTACT 2. *J Clin Oncol.* 2004;22:785–794.
28. Ciuleanu T, Brodowicz T, Zielinski C, et al. Maintenance pemetrexed plus best supportive care versus placebo plus best supportive care for non-small-cell lung cancer: a randomised, double-blind, phase 3 study. *Lancet.* 2009;374:1432–1440.
29. Cappuzzo F, Ciuleanu T, Stelmakh L, et al. Erlotinib as maintenance treatment in advanced non-small-cell lung cancer: a multicentre, randomised, placebo-controlled phase 3 study. *Lancet Oncol.* 2010;11:521–529.
30. Shepherd FA, Rodrigues Pereira J, Ciuleanu T, et al. Erlotinib in previously treated non-small-cell lung cancer. *N Engl J Med.* 2005;353:123–132.
31. Hanna N, Shepherd FA, Fossella FV, et al. Randomized phase III trial of pemetrexed versus docetaxel in patients with non-small-cell lung cancer previously treated with chemotherapy. *J Clin Oncol.* 2004;22:1589–1597.
32. Temel JS, Greer JA, Muzikansky A, et al. Early palliative care for patients with metastatic non-small-cell lung cancer. *N Engl J Med.* 2010;363:733–742.
33. Kwak EL, Bang YJ, Camidge DR, et al. Anaplastic lymphoma kinase inhibition in non-small-cell lung cancer. *N Engl J Med.* 2010;363:1693–1703.
34. Govindan R, Bogart J, Vokes EE. Locally advanced non-small cell lung cancer: the past, present, and future. *J Thorac Oncol.* 2008;3:917–928.
35. Govindan R, Page N, Morgensztern D, et al. Changing epidemiology of small-cell lung cancer in the United States over the last 30 years: analysis of the surveillance, epidemiologic, and end results database. *J Clin Oncol.* 2006;24:4539–4544.

36. Vallieres E, Shepherd FA, Crowley J, et al. The IASLC Lung Cancer Staging Project: proposals regarding the relevance of TNM in the pathologic staging of small cell lung cancer in the forthcoming (seventh) edition of the TNM classification for lung cancer. *J Thorac Oncol.* 2009;4:1049–1059.
37. Turrisi AT, Kim K, Blum R, et al. Twice-daily compared with once-daily thoracic radiotherapy in limited small-cell lung cancer treated concurrently with cisplatin and etoposide. *N Engl J Med.* 1999;340:265–271.
38. Arriagada R, Le Chevalier T, Borie F, et al. Prophylactic cranial irradiation for patients with small-cell lung cancer in complete remission. *J Natl Cancer Inst.* 1995;87:183–190.
39. Slotman B, Faivre-Finn C, Kramer G, et al. Prophylactic cranial irradiation in extensive small-cell lung cancer. *N Engl J Med.* 2007;357:664–672.
40. http://www.nccn.org/professionals/physician_gls/PDF/sclc.pdf. Accessed on 12/01/10.

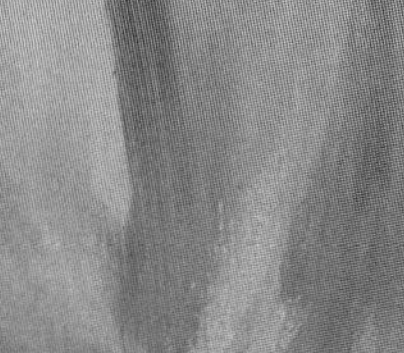

Colorectal Cancer

20

Aruna Rokkam

GENERAL PRINCIPLES

Lower gastrointestinal tract tumors are the third most commonly diagnosed cancers in the United States, and second leading cause of cancer death. Surgery cures a high percentage of these cases (50% of all diagnosed cases). This chapter gives an overview of colorectal and anal cancer presentation, pathophysiology, staging, and general principles of treatment.

Epidemiology

Colorectal cancer (CRC) is the fourth most frequently diagnosed cancer and the second leading cause of cancer death in the United States. It accounts for 9% of all cancers deaths. In the United States, the estimated number of new cases and deaths from colorectal cancer in 2010 are 142,570 and 51,370, respectively. The overall incidence of CRC in the United States has been declining for unclear reasons. The current incidence of CRC is ~60.4 per 100,000 population. Incidence increases with age, with ~90% of cases diagnosed in those >50 years old. Peak incidence occurs in the eighth decade of life. The lifetime risk for CRC is 6% in average-risk persons living in the United States.[1]

Pathophysiology

Most CRCs are thought to develop from adenomatous polyps that arise from the colonic mucosa. Studies have shown that adenomatous polyps can become malignant over a period of 5 to 20 years. The common histologies of a polyp are tubular, tubulovillous, and villous. Villous adenomas are most likely to become malignant. Other characteristic polyps to develop into malignancies are a size >1 cm in diameter and a high grade of dysplasia. Adenomatous polyps are found in ~35% of persons in autopsy studies. Up to 5% of polyps are believed to become malignant over time. More than 95% of CRCs are adenocarcinomas. Of these, >80% are moderately differentiated. Other histologic types seen are undifferentiated, squamous, carcinoid, leiomyosarcomas, and lymphoid neoplasias. *Poor prognosis* is associated with colloid and signet ring subtypes of adenocarcinoma, which together represent ~20% of tumors.

Risk Factors

Risk factors for CRC are listed below.

- First-degree relative with CRC
- Personal history of CRC
- History of other malignancies
- History of radiation therapy to the abdomen or pelvis
- Increasing age

- Ureterosigmoidostomies
- Inflammatory bowel disease, especially ulcerative colitis but also Crohn disease
- Family history of a CRC syndrome
- **Familial adenomatous polyposis** (FAP) is an autosomal dominant disease caused by a defect in the APC gene that leads to colon cancer in 100% of patients by the age of 40 years if they are left untreated. Affected persons will have up to thousands of adenomatous polyps with malignant potential in their bowel. Persons with FAP should have a prophylactic subtotal colectomy by age 30 years. Aggressive precolectomy screening for the development of cancer is also indicated. Other cancers such as medulloblastoma, papillary thyroid carcinoma, hepatoblastoma, pancreatic cancer, and gastric cancer are also associated with this syndrome.
- **Hereditary nonpolyposis colorectal cancer** (HNPCC) is inherited in an autosomal dominant manner and often leads to malignancies with mucinous histology in the right side of the colon. Often these tumors may arise without going through a polyp phase and, therefore, are seen as flat adenomas. HNPCC is also associated with cancers of the endometrium, ovary, stomach, and hepatobiliary system. Prophylactic subtotal colectomy is also recommended for persons with HNPCC.
- Other inherited syndromes associated with an increased risk of CRC include MYH-associated polyposis, Gardner's syndrome, Turcot's syndrome, Muir–Torre syndrome, and Peutz–Jeghers syndrome.

Prevention/Screening

Screening methods used to detect CRC include fecal occult blood testing (FOBT), endoscopy, and barium enema. Early detection improves survival through detection of more curable lesions, and CRC incidence is high enough that screening can be cost-effective with an acceptable positive predictive value. Patients with warning signs of CRC require more aggressive investigations, typically colonoscopy.

For the *asymptomatic* patient:

- **FOBT** is the least expensive and most widely used screening test for the detection of CRC. There are problems with its sensitivity, which has been reported to be from 25% to 80% with a specificity of >90%. Sensitivity will be affected by polyp size and frequency of bleeding. Specificity is affected by NSAID use, other sources of gastrointestinal bleeding, consumption of red meat, and consumption of certain vegetables in the diet. Hydration of samples before testing them is not recommended, as this worsens the specificity of the test.
- **Flexible sigmoidoscopy** examines up to 60 cm of the rectum and distal colon and can detect ~50% of CRC cases. Its advantages are that it can be performed in the primary care physician's office and that it has a specificity of nearly 100%. However, it has the disadvantage of not assessing the entire colon, and biopsies cannot be obtained during the procedure. Abnormalities necessitate a follow-up colonoscopy for biopsy.
- **Double-contrast barium enema** is a radiologic method for detection of CRC and is the safest of the visualization methods. It also requires a bowel preparation and, like FOBT, has the disadvantage of requiring subsequent endoscopy for biopsy of identified lesions.
- **Colonoscopy** is considered the **gold standard for detection of CRC** but is associated with a higher complication rate and a higher cost than the other

methods. It also involves more extensive preparation before the procedure and sedation during it. For the general population after age 50 years, National Comprehensive Cancer Network (NCCN) guidelines recommend colonoscopy every 10 years or annual FOBT combined with flexible sigmoidoscopy every 5 years. If risk factors such as a history of inflammatory bowel disease, family members with CRC, or a known defect such as HNPCC or FAP are present, then more frequent and earlier testing is recommended. For patients with a familial history of colorectal cancer, screening begins 10 years before the age of cancer diagnosis of the affected family member.

DIAGNOSIS

Colonoscopy with biopsy is the diagnostic procedure of choice and is potentially curative for benign polyps and carcinoma in situ. Diagnosis depends on tissue pathology consistent with invasive colon cancer.

Clinical Presentation

History

- CRC may present with symptoms such as fatigue, anorexia, failure to thrive, lower gastrointestinal bleeding, and right upper quadrant pain associated with liver metastasis, although it is often asymptomatic until the tumor is large in size. Patients may also present due to a positive screen test.
- Symptoms associated with CRC are often related to the location of the tumor within the bowel. Therefore, ***right-sided lesions*** often present with symptoms of anemia and, occasionally, of melena. ***Left-sided lesions*** commonly cause obstruction, tenesmus, constipation, bright-red blood per rectum, and other changes in bowel habits. Patients often have an iron-deficiency anemia and may have symptoms of pica.
- Because CRC is a cause of anemia, it is important to evaluate any person who presents with unexplained anemia for CRC, especially men and postmenopausal women.
- CRC most often metastasizes to the liver, lung, adrenals, ovaries, and bone, so symptoms of organ compromise such as abdominal discomfort, shortness of breath, and bone pain may be present in metastatic disease.

Physical Exam

Signs of CRC on physical exam include gross blood or melanotic stool in the rectal vault, pallor in the conjunctivae and the nail beds, or a palpable mass in the abdomen or the rectum. If liver metastases are present, patients may have hepatomegaly and be tender to palpation in the right upper quadrant. On barium enema, an **apple core** lesion may be seen, which suggests colon cancer. Bacteremia or endocarditis with *Streptococcus bovis* is also a sign of CRC, and these findings should trigger an evaluation for colon cancer.

Diagnostic Testing

Laboratories

- CBC to evaluate for associated iron-deficiency anemia
- Chemistry and liver function tests to evaluate for liver involvement

- Carcinoembryonic antigen (CEA): if initially elevated, then a rise in CEA after treatment may indicate a recurrence

Imaging Studies

- Chest/abdomen/pelvis CT scan to rule out metastasis

Diagnostic Procedures

- All patients should have the entire colon evaluated by **colonoscopy** or barium enema to rule out synchronous lesions. Up to 5% of patients have another focus of CRC in their bowels. Patients should have a tissue biopsy before therapy to confirm the diagnosis.

Staging

- Surgery is important for accurate staging of CRC. The preferred staging system for CRC is the American Joint Committee on Cancer (AJCC) TNM (tumor, node, metastases) system (Table 20-1). TNM uses the degree of tumor invasion, the presence of positive lymph nodes, and the presence of distant metastasis to

TABLE 20-1 AMERICAN JOINT COMMITTEE ON CANCER TNM SYSTEM FOR COLORECTAL CANCER STAGING

Tumor	
Tis:	Carcinoma in situ: intraepithelial or invasion of the lamina propria
T1:	Invasion of the submucosa
T2:	Invasion into the muscularis propria
T3:	Invasion through the muscularis propria into the perocolorectal tissues
T4a:	Invasion through visceral peritoneum
T4b:	Invasion or adherence to other organs or structures.
Node	
N0:	No lymph node metastases
N1:	Metastasis in one to three lymph nodes
N1a:	Metastasis in one regional lymph node
N1b:	Metastasis in two to three regional lymph nodes
N1c:	Tumor deposit (s) in the subserosa, mesentery, or nonperitonealized pericolic or perirectal tissues without regional nodal metastasis.
N2:	Metastases in four or more lymph nodes
N2a:	Metastasis in four to six regional lymph nodes
N2b:	Metastasis in seven or more regional lymph nodes.
Metastases	
M0:	No distant metastases
M1:	Distant metastases present
M1a:	Metastasis confined to one organ or site (e.g.: liver, ovary lung, nonregional node)
M1b:	Metastasis in more than one organ/site or the peritoneum.

TNM, tumor, node, metastases.

Adapted from American Joint Committee on Cancer. *AJCC Cancer Staging Manual.* 7th ed. New York: Springer; 2010.

TABLE 20-2 STAGING OF COLORECTAL CANCER BY AMERICAN JOINT COMMITTEE ON CANCER TNM SYSTEM (AND DUKE STAGE EQUIVALENTS)

Stage	Tumor	Node	Metastases	Duke stage/MAC
0	Tis	N0	M0	—
I	T1	N0	M0	A
	T2	N0	M0	B1
IIA	T3	N0	M0	B2
IIB	T4a	N0	M0	B2
IIC	T4b	N0	M0	B3
IIIA	T1–T2	N1/N1c	M0	C1
IIIB	T1	N2a	M0	C1
IIIC	T3–T4a	N1/N1c	M0	C2
IVA	T2–T3	N2a	M0	C1/C2
IVB	T1–T2	N2b	M0	C1
	T4a	N2a	M0	C2
	T3–T4a	N2b	M0	C2
	T4b	N1–N2	Mo	C3
	Any T	Any N	M1a	—
	Any T	Any N	M1b	—

TNM, tumor, node, metastases; MAC, modified Astler–Coller classification.

classify the disease in one of four stages. Although the AJCC TNM staging system is the preferred staging system today, the Duke staging system with the Astler–Coller modification is often referred to in older literature (Table 20-2).

TREATMENT

The goals of therapy need to be clearly delineated from the beginning and reevaluated throughout the patient's course. Colon cancer that has not metastasized is a curable disease with surgery. Chemotherapy can be added to improve cure rates for stage II or III tumors or as palliation for incurable tumors (Table 20-3).

- **Surgery** is undertaken with intent to cure in 75% of those with colon cancer. Many of the remainder will require surgery to prevent obstruction, perforation,

TABLE 20-3 TREATMENT FOR VARIOUS STAGES OF COLON CANCER

Stage	Treatment
0	Polypectomy/surgical resection
I	Surgery alone
II	Surgery ± chemotherapy
III	Surgery + chemotherapy
IV	Palliative chemotherapy, metastasis resection (limited cases)

or bleeding. Wide excision of the tumor with a distal margin of ~5 cm is recommended for curative surgery. The length of colon and mesentery resected is determined by vascular anatomy. If the tumor is adherent to or invades another organ, an en bloc excision must be done to prevent seeding to allow for the possibility of cure. If the surgical intent is palliation instead of cure, a simple resection or diversion is used to lessen morbidity from the procedure. In stage IV cancer, some patients may benefit from resection of metastases. Five-year survival rates of up to 40% have been obtained with resection of limited liver metastases.[3]

- **Adjuvant chemotherapy** is administered to patients who have undergone potentially curative resection of colon cancer. The goal of adjuvant therapy is to eradicate micrometastases, thereby reducing the likelihood of disease recurrence. 5-Fluorouracil (5-FU), leucovorin, and oxaliplatin (FOLFOX) is preferred but may consider 5-FU with leucovorin or capecitabine for patients who cannot tolerate oxaliplatin after resection of stage III colon cancer. Capecitabine is an oral prodrug that is converted to 5-FU in tumor tissues. Adjuvant chemotherapy has demonstrated approximately a 30% reduction in the risk of disease recurrence and 10% reduction in mortality. However, controversy remains over adjuvant chemotherapy for stage II disease. Because there seems to be only a small benefit from treating stage II colon cancer, chemotherapy should be considered for high-risk disease, including those patients who present with a total obstruction, T4 tumors (stage IIB), perforation, poor histological grade, lymphovascular invasion, or positive surgical margins and inadequately sampled nodes (<12 lymph nodes).[4–9] In patients with stage II disease, a deficiency in MMR (mismatch repair) protein expression or high levels of microsatellite instability protein (MSI-H) are markers of a more favorable outcome with decreased benefit (possibly detrimental impact) from adjuvant therapy with 5-FU alone.[10]
- Palliative treatment for metastatic disease depends on the functional status of the patient. It typically involves 5-FU with leucovorin, capecitabine alone, or 5-FU and leucovorin in combination with either the topoisomerase I inhibitor irinotecan (the FOLFIRI regimen) or oxaliplatin (the FOLFOX regimen).[11–16] Both of the combination regimens have improved efficacy by the addition of the vascular endothelial growth factor antibody, bevacizumab (Avastin)[17,18] or endothelial growth factor receptor inhibitory antibodies, cetuximab (Erbitux), or panitumumab (Vectibix) in patients with K-Ras wild-type gene. After disease progression, patients are usually switched to another one of the primary regimens and may also receive either of the endothelial growth factor receptor inhibitory antibodies, cetuximab (Erbitux), or panitumumab (Vectibix)[19–21] if the tumors are K-Ras wild type. Patients with stage IV disease should be referred for clinical trials when possible.

Treatment of Rectal Cancer

- **Surgery** is used in rectal cancer to cure the disease, and it also plays a role in palliative therapy. The most important feature of the rectum is the lack of a serosa for these tumors. Because of this anatomy, local recurrence for rectal cancer is high, and neoadjuvant therapy may be needed to make a tumor resectable. Accordingly, surgery is used in conjunction with radiation or chemoradiation,[22–24] and this multimodality approach has been associated with decreased recurrence. Approaches aimed at sphincter preservation, obviating the need for colostomy, can often be performed if a 2-cm margin can be obtained.

- Compared to colon cancer, rectal cancer is much more likely to recur locally than distally. Adjuvant chemoradiation is therefore tailored to prevent local recurrence in stage II and III cancers.[22,23] Currently, **stage II** rectal cancer is treated with surgery along with FOLFOX, 5-FU, or capecitabine and radiation, leading to significant improvements in overall survival compared to treatment with surgery alone.[25,26] For **stage III** tumors, part of the systemic chemotherapy and radiation therapy may be given before surgery to increase resectability.[24–26]

COMPLICATIONS

Tumor Related

Complications that can result from CRC include bowel obstruction, anemia, and abdominal pain. More serious complications can include peritonitis after perforation, fistula formation, and malnutrition. Complications can also result from sites of metastatic disease. Liver metastases can lead to hyperbilirubinemia and coagulopathies. Pulmonary metastases, when advanced, may result in cough or shortness of breath. Patients may also develop pain at sites of metastases.

Treatment Related

Complications of treatment are commonly related to surgery and chemotherapy but can also occur with radiation therapy. Postoperative mortality rates are 1% to 5%. Major morbidity includes bowel and bladder dysfunction, sexual dysfunction, anastomotic leaks, and bowel obstruction. The need for a permanent colostomy can be psychologically upsetting. Chemotherapy complications may include neuropathy (possibly long term), nausea, diarrhea, and hand-foot syndrome. Radiation may cause local radiation dermatitis with pain, desquamation, and color changes.

MONITORING/FOLLOW-UP

Current recommendations are for a history, physical, and CEA every 3 months for 2 years, and then every 6 months for another 3 years. At 1 year, a colonoscopy should be performed to look for local recurrence and synchronous disease. If the colonoscopy is negative, then it should be repeated in 3 years and then every 5 years. If the patient had a high-grade tumor or lymphovascular invasion, then a CT of the chest, abdomen, and pelvis should be repeated annually for the first 3 years to monitor for metastatic spread.

OUTCOMES/PROGNOSIS

Stage has great significance in the prognosis and treatment of the disease. In the United States between 1996 and 2002, the overall 5-year survival rate for patients with CRC was 65.1%. The 5-year survival for stages I/II, III, and IV was 90.4%, 68.1%, and 9.8%, respectively. Other prognostic factors include the number of positive lymph nodes and if the tumor invasion was through the bowel wall into adjacent organs or into veins.

ANAL CANCER

GENERAL PRINCIPLES

Epidemiology

Anal cancer accounts for ~1.6% of all alimentary malignancies in the United States. Its incidence generally increases with age, with the peak incidence in the sixth and seventh decades of life. The incidence is increasing in men <40 years old due to increased risk in the HIV+ population. Histologically, 63% of anal cancers are squamous cell carcinomas. Basaloid transitional cell carcinomas (cloacogenic) make up 23% of cases. More rare types of anal cancers are adenocarcinoma, basal cell carcinoma, and melanoma.

Risk Factors

- The risk factor most commonly associated with anal cancer is **human papilloma virus** (HPV) infection particularly with serotypes 16 and 18. In women, increased anal cancers are seen with HPV-associated cervical cancer. In men, anal cancer is more frequently associated with receptive anal intercourse and HPV. As many as 70% of anal cancers are positive for HPV.
- Other risk factors include immunosuppression, such as that seen after renal transplant or HIV infection. Current cigarette smoking is also a risk factor for anal cancer, with a relative risk of seven- to ninefold for smokers.

DIAGNOSIS

Clinical Presentation

History

Anal cancers present with bleeding 50% of the time. Other symptoms include pain, mass, constipation, diarrhea, and pruritus. Often the symptoms are ascribed to hemorrhoids, which may delay diagnosis. Approximately 25% of people are asymptomatic when the cancer is discovered.

Physical Exam

Physical exam findings include an anal mass and lymphadenopathy. On palpation, an anal mass will often be firm and indurated. Anoscopy, proctoscopy, and transrectal ultrasonography are used to visualize the mass. Diagnosis is made by incisional biopsy of the mass and any suspicious inguinal lymphadenopathy.

Diagnostic Testing

Procedures

Digital rectal exam and **inguinal lymph node exam** should be accompanied by **anoscopy.** Notes should be made of the location of the mass, including its position relative to the dentate line. Anal cancers are divided into those of the anal margin and those of the anal canal. The line of demarcation is a zone approximately halfway between the dentate line and the anal verge. Women should have a pelvic exam for **cervical cancer screening** due to the association with HPV. Men and women should be tested for **HIV,** especially if any risk factors are present.

TABLE 20-4 STAGING OF ANAL CANCER

Tumor	
Tis:	Carcinoma in situ
T1:	Tumor ≤2 cm in diameter
T2:	Tumor between 2 and 5 cm in diameter
T3:	Tumor ≥5 cm in diameter
T4:	Tumor of any size that invades adjacent organs such as the vagina, urethra, or bladder
Node	
N0:	No regional lymph nodes involved
N1:	Metastases in perirectal lymph nodes
N2:	Metastases in unilateral internal iliac or inguinal lymph node
N3:	Metastases in perirectal and inguinal lymph node(s) and/or bilateral internal iliac and/or inguinal lymph nodes
Metastases	
M0:	No distant metastases present
M1:	Distant metastases present
Stage	
I:	T1, N0, M0
II:	T2 or T3, N0, M0
IIIA:	T1–T3, N1, M0 or T4, N0, M0
IIIB:	T4, N1, M0 or any T, N2–N3, M0
IV:	Any T, any N, M1

Imaging

Imaging may include chest x-ray or chest CT, abdominal/pelvic CT or MRI, and possible PET scan to rule out metastatic disease.

Staging

Staging is based on the TNM system (Table 20-4).

TREATMENT

Very small tumors at the anal margin may be treated with wide local excision. Larger (T2-T4) and node positive cancers should be treated similar to anal canal carcinomas with concurrent chemoradiation (5-FU and Mitomycin).[27,28] In several trials, 5-year survival varied between 64% and 83% with combined-modality therapy. After treatment, close medical follow-up is needed to screen for recurrence. Recurrences may be treated surgically if resectable, or if unresectable consider cisplatin-based chemotherapy or clinical trial.

OUTCOME/PROGNOSIS

Prognosis is related to the size of the primary tumor and the presence of lymph node metastases.

The 5-year survival rate for patients with tumors that are treated with chemoradiation and that are ≤2 cm is 80%, whereas if they are ≥5 cm it is less than 50%.[29,30] Tumors in the anal margin have a more favorable prognosis than those in the canal.

REFERENCES

1. Jemal A, Siegal R, Xu J, et al. Cancer statistics 2010. *CA Cancer J Clin.* 2010;60:277–300.
2. Edge SB, Byrd DR, Compton CC, et al. AJCC (*American Joint Committee on Cancer*) *Cancer Staging Manual.* 7th ed. New York: Springer; 2010.
3. Choti MA, Sitzmann JV, Tiburi MF, et al. Trends in long term survival following liver resection for hepatic colorectal metastases. *Ann Surg.* 2002;235(6):759–766.
4. Benson AB, Schrag D, Somerfield MR, et al. American society of clinical oncology recommendations on adjuvant chemotherapy for stage II colon cancer. *J Clin Oncol.* 2004;22: 3408–3419.
5. Andre T, Boni C, Navarro M, et al. Improved survival with oxaliplatin, fluorouracil, and leucovorin as adjuvant treatment in stage II or III colon cancer in the mosaic trial. *J Clin Oncol.* 2009;27:3109–3116.
6. National Comprehensive Cancer Network (NCCN) guidelines. www.nccn.org (accessed on 12/02/10)
7. O'Connell MJ, Mailliard JA, Kahn MJ, et al. Controlled trial of fluorouracil and low dose leucovorin given for 6 months as postoperative adjuvant therapy for colon cancer. *J Clin Oncol.* 1997;15:246–250.
8. Gill S, Loprinzi CL, Sargent DJ, et al. Pooled analysis of flurouracil-based adjuvant therapy for Stage II and Stage III colon cancer: who benefit and by how much? *J Clin Oncol.* 2004; 22:1797–1806.
9. Quasar Collaborative group, Gray R, Barnwell J, et al. Adjuvant chemotherapy versus observation in patients with colorectal cancer: a randomised study. *Lancet.* 2007;370:2020–2029.
10. Sargent DJ, Marsoni S, Monges G, et al. Defective mismatch repair as a predictive marker for lack of efficacy of fluorouracil-based adjuvant therapy in colon cancer. *J Clin Oncol.* 2010;28:3219–3223.
11. Van Custem E, Twelves C, Cassidy J, et al. Oral capecitabine compared with intravenous flurouracil plus leucovorin in patients with metastatic colorectal cancer: results of a large phase III study. *J Clin Oncol.* 2001;19:4097–4106.
12. Saltz LB, Cox JV, Blanke C, et al. Irinotecan plus fluorouracil and leucovorin for metastatic colorectal cancer. *N Engl J Med.* 2000;343:905–914.
13. De Gramont A, Figer A, Seymour M, et al. Leucovorin and flurouracil with or without oxaliplatin as first-line treatment in advanced colorectal cancer. *J Clin Oncol.* 2000;18:2938–2947.
14. Goldberg RM, Sargent DJ, Morton RF, et al. A randomized controlled trial of fluorouracil plus leucovorin, irinotecan and oxaliplatin combinations in patients with previously untreated metastatic colorectal cancer. *J Clin Oncol.* 2004;22:23–30.
15. Tournigand C, Andre T, Achille E, et al. FOLFIRI followed by FOLFOX6 or the reverse sequence in advanced colorectal cancer: a randomized GERCOR study. *J Clin Oncol.* 2004; 22:229–237.
16. Cassidy J, Clarke S, Diaz–Rubio E, et al. Randomized phase III study of capecitabine plus oxaliplatin compared with fluorouracil/folinic acid plus oxaliplatin as first line therapy for metastatic colorectal cancer. *J Clin Oncol.* 2008;26:2006–2012.
17. Hurwitz H, Fehrenbacher L, Novotny W, et al. Bevacizumab plus irinotecan, fluorouracil and leucovorin for metastatic colorectal cancer. *N Engl J Med.* 2004;350:2335–2342.
18. Saltz LB, Clarke S, Diaz–Rubio E, et al. Bevacizumab in combination with oxaliplatin based chemotherapy as first line therapy in metastatic colorectal cancer: a randomized phase III study. *J Clin Oncol.* 2008;26:2013–2019.
19. Van Custem E, Kohne CH, Hitre E, et al. Cetuximab and chemotherapy as initial treatment for metastatic colorectal cancer. *N Engl J Med.* 2009;360:1408–1417.
20. Bokemeyer C, Bondarenko I, Makhson A, et al. Fluorouracil, leucovorin and oxaliplatin with and without cetuximab in the first-line treatment of metastatic colorectal cancer. *J Clin Oncol.* 2009;27:663–671.
21. Cunningham D, Humblet Y, Siena S, et al. Cetuximab monotherapy and cetuximab plus irinotecan in irinotecan-refractory metastatic colorectal cancer. *N Engl J Med.* 2004;351: 337–345.

22. Roh MS, Colangelo LH, O'Connell MJ, et al. Preoperative multimodality therapy improves disease-free survival in patients with carcinoma of the rectum: NSABP R-03. *J Clin Oncol.* 2009;27(31):5124–5130.
23. Bosset JF, Collette L, Calais G, et al. Chemotherapy with preoperative radiotherapy in rectal cancer. *N Engl J Med.* 2006;355(11):1114–1123.
24. Sauer R, Becker H, Hohenberger W, et al. Preoperative versus postoperative chemoradiotherapy for rectal cancer. *N Engl J Med.* 2004;351(17):1731–1740.
25. Krook JE, Moertel CG, Gunderson LL, et al. Effective surgical adjuvant therapy for high-risk rectal carcinoma. *N Engl J Med.* 1991;324(11): 709–715.
26. Douglass HO, Moertel CG, Mayer RJ, et al. Survival after postoperative combination treatment of rectal cancer. *N Engl J Med.* 1986;315:1294–1295.
27. Ajani JA, Winter KA, Gunderson LL, et al. Fluorouracil, mitomycin, and radiotherapy vs fluorouracil, cisplatin, and radiotherapy for carcinoma of the anal canal: a randomized controlled trial. *JAMA.* 2008;299:1914–1921.
28. Faivre C, Rougier P, Ducreux M, et al. 5-Fluorouracil and cisplatin combination chemotherapy for metastatic squamous–cell anal cancer. *Bull Cancer.* 1999;86:861–865.
29. Cummings BJ, Ajani JA, Swallow CJ. Cancer of the anal region. In: DeVita VT, Lawrence TS, Rosenberg SA, eds. *Cancer: Principles and Practice of Oncology.* 8th ed. Philadelphia, PA: Lippincott, Williams & Wilkins; 2008:1301–1313.
30. Bilimoria KY, Bentrem DJ, Rock CE, et al. Outcomes and prognostic factors for squamous-cell carcinoma of the anal cancer: analysis of patients from the national cancer data base. *Dis Colon Rectum.* 2009;52:624–631.

Other Gastrointestinal Malignancies

21

Kian-Huat Lim

ESOPHAGEAL CANCER

GENERAL PRINCIPLES

Definition

- Primary carcinoma that arises from the cricopharyngeal sphincter to the gastroesophageal junction

Classification

- Site: divided into upper, middle, and lower third.
- Histology: most commonly adenocarcinoma (occurs predominantly at lower third of esophagus) and squamous cell carcinoma (occurs predominantly at middle and upper third); other less common types include mucoepidermoid carcinoma, small-cell carcinoma, sarcoma, leiomyosarcoma, and primary lymphoma.

Epidemiology

- The incidence in the United States is ~5 per 100,000, although in African American men it may be as high as 18 per 100,000. China and Iran have an incidence of 20 per 100,000.
- In the United States, 16,640 new cases and 14,500 deaths from this cancer were estimated in 2010. It is the seventh leading cause of cancer death in men.
- Age: 6th to 7th decades.
- Sex: M:F, 3 to 4:1.
- Race: in the United States, esophageal adenocarcinomas are more common in white males, whereas squamous cell carcinomas are more common in African Americans.
- Socioeconomic status: Lower socioeconomic status as defined by income, occupation, and education are associated with higher risk for squamous cell carcinoma.
- Histology: in the United States, squamous cell carcinoma used to be the more prominent type until the early 1990s when it was surpassed by adenocarcinoma. Such shift is believed to be due to increased incidence of GERD, Barrett's esophagus, and obesity.

Etiology and Pathophysiology

- The exact etiology of esophageal carcinoma remains unclear but likely is an evolution of oncogenic changes within the esophageal epithelium following chronic exposure to known carcinogens or chronic irritation by gastric acid in patients with GERD. Conversely, patients with chronic atrophic gastritis caused by cagA-positive *Helicobacter pylori* are associated with decreased risk of esophageal adenocarcinoma.

Risk Factors

- Alcohol, tobacco, nitrosamines, GERD, Barrett's esophagus, obesity, Plummer–Vinson syndrome, history of head and neck cancer
- High-fat, low-calorie, and low-protein diet

Prevention

- Cessation from smoking and alcohol consumption
- Raw fruits and vegetables, fibers, selenium, as well as vitamins A, C, and E

Associated Conditions

- Barrett's esophagus (30- to 125-fold increased risk of developing adenocarcinoma), Howel–Evans syndrome

DIAGNOSIS

Clinical Presentation

History

- Due to the lack of initial symptoms, most cases are diagnosed at advanced stage. Typical presenting symptoms are dysphagia (95%), which typically progressed from solid to liquid, body weight loss (50%), odynophagia (20%), and gastric reflux (40%). Extraesophageal spread can cause pain, cough (20%), hoarseness (secondary to recurrent laryngeal nerve involvement), aspiration, tracheal narrowing, or tracheoesophageal fistula.

Physical Examination

- Most patients lack obvious physical findings, but cervical or supraclavicular adenopathy may be appreciated in patients with nodal metastasis.

Diagnostic Criteria

- Histopathologic diagnosis from endoscopic biopsy and/or transcutaneous lymph node biopsy (if applicable) is required.

Differential Diagnosis

- Barrett's esophagus, esophageal stricture, achalasia, gastric cancer

Diagnostic Testing

Laboratories

- Complete blood count (CBC), comprehensive metabolic panel (CMP), prothrombin time (PT), partial thromboplastin time (PTT), and iron studies

Initial Diagnostic Test

- **Upper endoscopy with directed biopsy** is the current gold standard.
- Barium studies may show strictures or intraluminal lesions, but they are less sensitive and do not allow for biopsy.

Imaging Studies

- Once the diagnosis is established, an initial **CT scan of chest, abdomen with IV and oral contrast** should be obtained to assess extent of primary disease, nodal and distant organ metastasis.
- Bone scan is indicated in patients with bone pain or elevated alkaline phosphatase.

- If no distant metastasis is seen from the initial CT scan, more sensitive diagnostic tests should be performed to provide more accurate staging. A positron emission tomography (PET) or PET-CT scan (preferred by the NCCN guideline) should be obtained. They have a higher sensitivity and specificity than conventional CT scan in detecting nodal and distant metastasis. In many medical centers, this PET scan has become part of the standard preoperative workup. If indicated, FDG-avid lymph nodes should be biopsied to confirm metastasis.

Diagnostic Procedures

- Once distant metastasis is excluded by PET scan, an **endoscopic ultrasonography** (EUS) should be performed. This procedure allows the most precise assessment of tumor depth, length of esophagus affected, and magnitude of lymph node metastases, particularly paraesophageal and celiac nodes. A fine-needle aspiration of suspicious lymph nodes can be done during the study.
- Patients presenting with cough, symptoms or radiographic evidence of aspiration pneumonia, tumor abutting/invading the trachea at or above carina should receive bronchoscopy to assess tracheal invasion or tracheoesophageal fistula.

TREATMENT

Treatment is based on TNM stage (Table 21-1):

- **Stage 0.** Endoscopic mucosal resection followed by periodic surveillance
- **Stage I.**
  - Esophagectomy if patients are medically fit, with esophageal carcinoma at mid or lower third esophagus, or if they have adenocarcinoma.
  - Concurrent chemoradiation is preferred for cancer in the upper third esophagus and is an alternative for patients who are not surgical candidates.
- **Stage II, III, or Iva.**
  - Esophagectomy with regional lymphadenectomy is the main treatment, but is inadequate.
  - Neoadjuvant therapies with chemotherapy, radiation, or in combination have been studied, and conflicting results have been obtained.[1] Current NCCN guidelines support the use of neoadjuvant chemoradiation in medically fit patients. Patients with adenocarcinoma of distal esophagus or gastroesophageal junction should receive neoadjuvant chemotherapy (epirubicin, cisplatin, and 5-FU) before esophagectomy.
  - Adjuvant chemoradiotherapy clearly has a role in the treatment of esophageal cancer. The most common regimen is cisplatin plus 5-FU with daily irradiation.
    - Patients with gross (R2 resection) or microscopic (R1 resection) residual disease following surgery should receive combined chemoradiation.
  - Adjuvant chemoradiotherapy in patients without residual disease (R0 resection) is less defined. In the current NCCN guidelines, observation is recommended for those with squamous cell carcinoma. Patients with adenocarcinoma, lymph node–positive disease, or large tumors (≥T3) should receive chemoradiotherapy.
  - Patients with localized unresectable disease or who are medically unfit for surgery should be considered for definitive chemoradiation consisting of cisplatin, 5-FU, plus daily irradiation.[2]

TABLE 21-1 STAGING CLASSIFICATION OF ESOPHAGEAL CANCER (AJCC TNM 2002)

Primary Tumor (T)	Regional Lymph Nodes (N)	Distant Metastasis (M)	Stage
TX: primary tumor cannot be assessed	NX: regional lymph node involvement cannot be assessed	MX: presence of metastasis cannot be assessed	Stage 0: Tis N0 M0
T0: no evidence of primary tumor	N0: no regional lymph node metastasis	M0: no distant metastasis	Stage 1: T1a/b N0 M0
Tis: carcinoma in situ	N1: regional lymph node metastasis	M1: distant metastasis	Stage IIA: T2 N0 M0, T3 N0 M0
T1: tumor invades lamina propria or submucosa	N1a: 1–3 nodes involved	Tumors of the lower thoracic esophagus: M1a, metastasis to celiac lymph nodes; M1b, other distant metastasis	Stage IIB: T1a/b N1 M0, T2 N1 M0
T1a: tumor invades mucosa or lamina propria	N1b: 4–7 nodes involved	Tumors of the midthoracic esophagus: M1a, n/a; M1b, nonregional lymph nodes and/or other distant metastasis	Stage III: T3 N1 M0, T4 any N M0
T1b: tumor invades submucosa	N1c: >7 nodes involved	Tumors of the upper thoracic esophagus: M1a, metastasis to cervical lymph nodes; M1b, other distant metastasis	Stage IVA: any T any N M1a
T2: tumor invades muscularis propria			Stage IVB: any T any N M1b
T3: tumor invades adventitia			
T4: tumor invades adjacent structures			

- **Stage IVb.** Metastatic esophageal cancer is incurable with a median survival of 9 months. Several chemotherapeutic agents including cisplatin, carboplatin, 5-FU, paclitaxel, docetaxel, vinorelbine, oxaliplatin, and irinotecan are commonly used.
  - In general, platinum-based doublets have the highest response rate and are typically used as first-line therapy.
  - Addition of cetuximab to platinum-based doublets can be considered in patients with epidermal growth factor receptor (EGFR)-overexpressing tumor.
  - Targeted therapies such as erlotinib and gefitinib as second-line monotherapy have been shown to offer some benefit to a small number of patients and can be considered for patients who cannot tolerate cytotoxic chemotherapy.

Other Non-Pharmacologic Therapies

- **Palliative care in swallowing and nutritional support** is especially important. This includes esophageal dilation, stent placement, brachytherapy, external-beam radiation, and laser therapy. Patients with metastatic esophageal cancer frequently require a gastrostomy tube.

Lifestyle/Risk Modification

- All patients should be encouraged to **cease smoking and consuming alcohol.** Patients with gastroesophageal reflux should be managed by dietary modification, exercise, and, if necessary, treated medically with H2-blockers or proton pump inhibitors.

Diet

- Increase consumption of fresh fruits and vegetables and dietary fibers, and abstain from alcohol and high-fat diet.

Activity

- Overweight or obese patients should be encouraged to exercise and lose weight.

COMPLICATIONS

- Hemorrhage, obstruction, tracheoesophageal fistula, aspiration pneumonia, and mediastinitis.

REFERRAL

- Nutritional consult should be obtained for all patients undergoing treatment of esophageal cancer.

MONITORING/FOLLOW-UP

- Patients with Barrett's metaplasia should receive surveillance endoscopy at least every 12 months with biopsy taken.
- After definitive treatment, asymptomatic patients should typically be evaluated by history and physical examination every 3 months for 2 years, and then every 6 months for 3 additional years. CBC and CMP should be obtained during each routine follow-up, and imaging studies such as CT scan should be

obtained at least every 6 months in the first 1 to 3 years or when clinically indicated.

OUTCOME/PROGNOSIS

- The most important prognostic factor is initial staging; others include age, performance status, and weight loss (>10%). Neither histology nor grade has been shown to affect prognosis. Molecular profiling of tumor cells is an area of active investigation.
- Five-year survival rates are >90% (stage 0), 70% to 80% (stage I), 10% to 30% (stage II), 5% to 10% (stage III), and rare in stage IV disease.

GASTRIC CANCER

GENERAL PRINCIPLES

Definition

- Cancer that arises between the gastroesophageal junction and pylorus

Classification

- Histology:
  - Adenocarcinoma (95%), primary lymphoma such as non-Hodgkin's lymphoma, MALToma, GI stromal tumor (GIST), leiomyosarcoma, squamous cell carcinoma, small cell carcinoma, and carcinoid
- Lauren classification of gastric adenocarcinoma:
  - Intestinal type: more common in Japan, associated with diet and possibly *H. pylori* infection
  - Diffuse type: more common in the United States, not associated with diet, associated with poorer outcome
  - Mixed type
- Borrmann classification of gastric adenocarcinoma:
  - Type 1 (polypoid), II (ulcerated), III (ulcerated infiltrating), IV (diffusely infiltrating or *linitis plastica*)

Epidemiology

- Gastric cancer is a relatively less common cancer in the United States but much more common in eastern Asia, especially Japan. It is the second most common cause of cancer deaths in the world.
- In the United States, 21,000 new cases and 10,570 deaths from this cancer were estimated in 2010. Incidence and mortality of gastric cancer have been declining in the United States.
- Age: 7th decade.
- Sex: M:F, 2 to 3:1.
- Race: slightly more frequent in African American than Caucasian.

Etiology and Pathophysiology

- Oncogenic mutation of *K-Ras* and *H-Ras,* overexpression of *Her2/neu* and *c-met,* and loss of *p53* are among the common genetic changes found in gastric adenocarcinoma.

- *C-kit* (90% to 95%) or *PDGFR* (5%) mutations are found in most GISTs. MALT lymphomas are frequently associated with *H. pylori* infection and can be cured with antibiotics alone.

Risk Factors

- History of atrophic gastritis or pernicious anemia, cigarette smoking, alcohol, *H. pylori* infection, chronic gastric ulcer, Barrett's esophagitis, high salt, nitrate intake, smoked or pickled food, family history of gastric cancer.
- Patients with germline E-cadherin (*CDH1* gene) mutation are at extremely high risk of developing gastric cancer at young age.

Prevention

- Because ***H. pylori* infection** is associated with 40% to 50% of gastric adenocarcinomas, it **should be actively eradicated when diagnosed.** Patients diagnosed with gastric ulcer should undergo repeat endoscopic surveillance in 3 to 6 months.

DIAGNOSIS

Clinical Presentation

History

- Most gastric carcinomas are diagnosed at an advanced stage due to the lack of early warning symptoms. Most patients present with nonspecific constitutional symptoms such as weight loss (~80%), anorexia, fatigue, vague stomach pain, hematemesis (~15%), dysphagia (from gastroesophageal junction tumors), and vomiting (from gastric outlet obstruction).
- Patients with GIST typically present with bleeding such as hematemesis, tarry stools or melena, epigastric pain, and nausea.

Physical Examination

- The physical findings in gastric carcinoma are typically manifestations of metastatic disease. **Virchow node** describes metastasis to the left supraclavicular node. **Sister Mary Joseph node** is a periumbilical lymph node metastasis. A **Krukenberg tumor** is a gastric cancer metastatic to the ovaries. **Blumer shelf** describes a "drop metastasis" into the perirectal pouch. Other common physical findings in patients with metastatic gastric cancer include cachexia, palpable abdominal masses, and malignant ascites.

Diagnostic Criteria

- Histopathologic diagnosis from endoscopic biopsy and/or transcutaneous lymph node biopsy (if applicable) is required.
- In the case of GIST, tumor size and mitotic index are important factors in risk stratification.

Differential Diagnosis

- Gastric ulcer, gastritis, non-Hodgkin's lymphoma, GIST, esophageal cancer

Diagnostic Testing

Laboratories

- CBC, CMP, PT, PTT, CEA, and iron studies

Initial Diagnostic Test

- **Upper endoscopy with directed biopsy** is the current gold standard.
- Barium studies with double contrast provide information on size of ulcerated lesion and gastric motility but are less sensitive and do not allow for biopsy.

Imaging

- CT scans or PET/CT is frequently used to evaluate for extent of disease.

Diagnostic Procedures

- In the absence of metastasis by CT, endoscopic ultrasound can be used to gauge tumor depth and involvement of local lymph nodes.
- Metastatic peritoneal deposits may not be seen on routine imaging, and a diagnostic laparoscopy is necessary to rule this out before definitive resection.

TREATMENT

For gastric adenocarcinoma, treatment is based on TNM stage (Table 21-2):

- **Stage 0 and Ia.** Endoscopic mucosal resection
- **Stage Ib.** Subtotal gastrectomy if at distal stomach, otherwise total gastrectomy with at least D1 resection
- **Stage II to IV,** but without distant metastasis.
    - For potentially resectable disease, either perioperative chemotherapy (such as ECF) for three cycles before and after total gastrectomy or adjuvant 5-FU-based chemoradiation can be considered.[3,4]
    - For medically unfit or unresectable localized gastric adenocarcinoma, 5-FU-based chemoradiation (45 to 50 cGy) is the standard of care. Only a very small percentage of patients can be cured with chemoradiation alone.
- **Metastatic disease.** Incurable with median survival of 9 months. Chemotherapy offers improved life quality and survival. No clear standard of care first-line regimen exists, but commonly used regimens are ECF, DCF, EOX, EOF, ECF, FOLFIRI, and CF. Addition of trastuzumab to chemotherapy improves median survival in patients with Her2-positive gastric cancer.[5]

For GIST

- Surgical resection is the treatment of choice. Adjuvant imatinib for 1 year is recommended by the NCCN for patients with intermediate or high risk (based on tumor size and mitotic index).
- For advanced or metastatic GIST, imatinib should be used until disease progression.[6] Upon progression, increased imatinib dosage or switching to sunitinib can be considered.

SPECIAL CONSIDERATIONS

- Given the rarity of gastric cancer in the United States, there is no justification for routine screening for esophageal or stomach cancer at this time. However, in countries of high incidence (e.g., Japan), screening for stomach cancer via

TABLE 21-2 STAGING CLASSIFICATION OF GASTRIC CANCER

Primary Tumor (T)	Regional Lymph nodes (N)	Distant Metastasis (M)	Stage
TX: primary tumor cannot be assessed	NX: regional lymph node involvement cannot be assessed	MX: presence of metastasis cannot be assessed	Stage 0: Tis N0 M0
T0: no evidence of primary tumor	N0: no regional lymph node metastasis	M0: no distant metastasis	Stage IA: T1 N0 M0
Tis: intraepithelial tumors without invasion of lamina propria	N1: regional lymph node metastasis in 1–6 nodes	M1: distant metastasis	Stage IB: T1 N1 M0, T2a/b N0 M0
T1: tumor invades lamina propria or submucosa	N2: regional lymph node metastasis in 7–15 nodes		Stage II: T1 N2 M0, T2a/b N1 M0, N3 N0 M0
T2: tumor invades lamina propria/ submucosa	N3: regional lymph node metastasis in >15 nodes		Stage IIIA: T2a/b N2 M0, T3 N1 M0, T4 N0 M0
T2a: tumor invades muscularis propria			Stage IIIB: T3 N2 M0
T2b: tumor invades submucosa			Stage IV: T4 any N M0, any T N3 M0, any T any N M1
T3: tumor penetrates serosa (visceral peritoneum)			
T4: tumor invades adjacent structures			

endoscopy or upper gastrointestinal imaging is standard for those >50 years old.

COMPLICATIONS

- Include hemorrhage, gastric obstruction, and malignant ascites.
- Disseminated intravascular coagulation (DIC) is a rare complication that may occur in patients with advanced gastric carcinoma and bone marrow metastasis.

Mortality is high at 1 to 4 weeks of onset and requires aggressive supportive management and, if possible, chemotherapy.
- Patients who underwent total gastrectomy often develop dumping syndrome, vitamin B_{12} deficiency, and reflux esophagitis.

MONITORING/FOLLOW-UP

- After definitive treatment, asymptomatic patients should typically be evaluated by history and physical examination every 3 months for 2 years, and then every 6 months for 3 additional years. CBC, CMP, and, if applicable, CEA should be obtained during each routine follow-up, and imaging studies such as CT scan should be obtained at least every 6 months in the first 1 to 3 years or when clinically indicated.

OUTCOME/PROGNOSIS

- Five-year survival rates are stage I 60% to 80%, stage II 20% to 40%, and stage III 10% to 20%.

PANCREATIC CANCER

GENERAL PRINCIPLES

Definition

- Cancer that arises from either the exocrine or the endocrine tissue of the pancreas

Classification

- Site: Two-thirds of the cases originate from pancreatic head.
- Histology: 95% of pancreatic cancers are exocrine ductal carcinoma, with the rest being acinar carcinoma or neuroendocrine tumors.

Epidemiology

- Pancreatic cancer is the fourth leading cause of cancer death in the United States, with an annual incidence of ~12.3/100,000.
- Up to 43,140 new cases and 36,800 deaths were anticipated in 2010.
- Age: 6th to 7th decades.
- Sex: slightly higher in males.
- Race: higher in African Americans.

Etiology and Pathophysiology

- Activation mutation of *K-Ras* and loss of tumor suppressor *INK4a* are found in >90% of pancreatic cancer. Recently, activation of Sonic hedgehog signaling pathway has been shown to be important in oncogenesis of pancreatic cancer.
- Chronic inflammation is believed to accelerate mutagenesis and cancer formation.

Risk Factors

- Cigarette smoking, positive family history, chronic pancreatitis, obesity, diabetes mellitus

Associated Conditions

- Lynch syndrome, ataxia-telangiectasia, *BRCA2* mutation, familial atypical mole melanoma syndrome, Peutz–Jeghers syndrome, HNPCC.

DIAGNOSIS

Clinical Presentation

History

- Most patients are asymptomatic until advanced stage. Presenting symptoms may include abdominal or back pain, weight loss, nausea, vomiting, painless jaundice, fatigue, and depression.

Physical Examination

- Palpable abdominal mass, jaundice, ascites, Courvoisier sign (painless palpable gallbladder), Virchow node, and Sister Mary Joseph node may occasionally be found.
- Paraneoplastic syndromes, such as Trousseau syndrome (migratory superficial phlebitis), idiopathic deep venous thrombosis, myositis syndromes, and Cushing syndrome, are rarely seen.

Diagnostic Testing

Laboratories

- CBC, CMP, PT, and PTT
- CEA, CA19–9 levels should be obtained as a baseline and followed for response/recurrence.

Imaging

- Initial imaging studies are usually **abdominal CT scan** or **ultrasonography**.
- **Dynamic-phase spiral CT of the abdomen** ("pancreatic protocol") is the current most accurate imaging modality in assessing pancreatic tumor. It allows detailed evaluation of the pancreas, extent of local invasion, and common sites of metastasis such as peripancreatic lymph nodes and the liver.
- Patients with confirmed pancreatic cancer should complete staging workup with chest and pelvic CT scan.

Diagnostic Procedures

- Further tumor staging with an endoscopic ultrasound or endoscopic retrograde cholangiopancreatography (ERCP) may be necessary.
- **Tissue diagnosis** can be obtained by percutaneous ultrasound or CT-guided-needle biopsy, laparoscopy, ERCP, or ascitic fluid cytology.
- Staging can be done by TNM system (Table 21-3), or more commonly by resectability (localized/resectable, borderline resectable, locally advanced/unresectable and metastatic stages).

TABLE 21-3 STAGING CLASSIFICATION OF PANCREATIC CANCER

Primary Tumor (T)	Regional Lymph Nodes (N)	Distant Metastasis (M)	Stage
TX: primary tumor cannot be assessed	NX: regional lymph node involvement cannot be assessed	MX: presence of metastasis cannot be assessed	Stage 0: Tis N0 M0
T0: no evidence of primary tumor	N0: no regional lymph node	M0: no distant metastasis	Stage IA: T1 N0 M0
Tis: Carcinoma in situ	N1: regional lymph node metastasis	M1: distant metastasis	Stage IB: T2 N0 M0
T1: tumor limited to the pancreas, ≤2 cm in greatest dimension			Stage IIA: T3 N0 M0
T2: tumor limited to the pancreas, >2 cm in greatest dimension			Stage IIB: T1 N1 M0, T2 N1 M0, T3 N1 M0
T3: tumor extends beyond the pancreas but without involvement of the celiac axis or the superior mesenteric artery			Stage III: T4 any N M0
T4: tumor involves the celiac axis or the superior mesenteric artery			Stage IV: any T any N M1

TREATMENT

- In the absence of metastatic disease, surgical consult should always be obtained to assess resectability, which is the basis for subsequent management.
- **Localized, resectable disease**
  - The standard procedure is a pancreaticoduodenectomy with choledochojejunostomy, cholecystectomy, and gastrojejunostomy (**Whipple procedure**). Surgical mortality is 1% to 4% even at high volume centers.
  - Adjuvant therapy is necessary after resection of the primary, since close to 80% of these patients later develop locoregional recurrence or distant metastases. Patients should be enrolled in clinical trials if available. Commonly used regimens include concurrent chemoradiation with 5-FU or gemcitabine, or gemcitabine followed by 5-FU-based chemoradiation.

- **Borderline resectable disease**
  - This new category was introduced in 2009 and is defined by certain radiographic features in which upfront surgery is likely to result in positive surgical margin.
  - Neoadjuvant chemotherapy (5-FU or gemcitabine) with or without radiation have been proposed with hopes to downstage the tumor and improve the likelihood of complete resection, to exclude patients with rapidly progressive disease who may not benefit from surgery, and to avoid delay in chemoradiation due to prolonged postoperative recovery. While this approach is gaining popularity, its benefit has not been convincingly shown by large randomized-control studies.
- **Locally advanced disease**
  - 5-FU or gemcitabine-based concurrent chemoradiation is the standard therapy and yields comparable results. A minority of patients can become resectable using this approach.
- **Metastatic pancreatic cancer.**
  - Metastatic pancreatic cancer is incurable. Chemotherapy has a low objective response rate (6% to 12%) but has been shown to improve quality of life and overall survival.
  - Clinical trials should be recommended if available.
  - Current recommended first-line chemotherapy is gemcitabine-based regimens. Gemcitabine plus erlotinib showed a marginal survival benefit over gemcitabine alone, but at the expense of more toxicity.[7] Combinations with other agents such as capecitabine, pemetrexed, irinotecan, cisplatin, cetuximab, or bevacizumab did not show additional benefit than gemcitabine alone. The combination of drugs in the **FOLFIRINOX** regiment does increase survival over gemcitabine alone.
  - Second-line chemotherapies include capecitabine and 5-FU/oxaliplatin.

Lifestyle/Risk Modification

- All patients should be encouraged to cease smoking and consuming alcohol.

Diet

- Most patients undergoing treatment suffer from pancreatic insufficiency and, therefore, should be prescribed pancreatic enzymes and told to avoid high-fat diet.

SPECIAL CONSIDERATIONS

- Routine **preoperative biliary stenting for obstructive jaundice** secondary to localized pancreatic head cancer was recently shown to be associated with higher postoperative complications compared to patients who received early surgery. Therefore, discussion should be made between hepatobiliary surgeon and gastroenterologist before stenting.

COMPLICATIONS

- **Pain management** is paramount in pancreatic cancer patients. In addition to standard analgesics, celiac plexus block may be an option in selected patients.
- **Biliary obstruction and subsequent cholangitis** should be relieved by stenting or draining procedures.
- Patients who undergo Whipple procedure will develop **diabetes.**

MONITORING/FOLLOW-UP

- After definitive treatment, asymptomatic patients should typically be evaluated by history and physical examination every 3 months for 2 years, and then every 6 months for 3 additional years. CBC, CMP, and, if applicable, CA19–9 or CEA and CT scan of chest/abdomen/pelvis should be obtained during each routine follow-up.

OUTCOME/PROGNOSIS

- Overall 5-year survival is 5%. Upon diagnosis, >50% of cases were metastatic, 25% locally advanced, and <20% were potentially resectable.
- Most important prognostic factors include surgical margin, lymph node status, and tumor size. However, even patients who underwent curative resection have a 15% to 20% 5-year survival rate.
- Median survival for unresectable disease has been as short as 6 months, but many trials are now reporting median survivals of treated patients closer to 12 months.

HEPATOCELLULAR CARCINOMA

GENERAL PRINCIPLES

Definition

- Primary cancer that arises from hepatocytes

Epidemiology

- Hepatocellular carcinoma (HCC) is the fifth most common cancer worldwide, but it is rare in the United States. The incidence in the United States is around 5 per 100,000, but this has been rising over the last few decades due to the increase in hepatitis B and C infections.
- Age: 7th decade.
- Sex: M:F, 3:1.
- Race: higher incidence in African Americans and Asians.

Etiology and Pathophysiology

- Chronic inflammation, necrosis, and liver regeneration likely predispose hepatocytes to acquire mutations.
- Integration of HBV DNA into hepatocyte genome can contribute to cancer formation.

Risk Factors

- Hepatitis B, hepatitis C, and cirrhosis from any cause such as alcohol and nonalcoholic steatohepatitis, alpha1-antitypsin deficiency, hemochromatosis

Prevention

- Vaccination against hepatitis B.
- Treatment of chronic hepatitis B with lamivudine has been shown to decrease the risk of developing hepatocellular carcinoma (HCC).

- Treatment of hepatitis C with interferon may decrease the subsequent risk of hepatocellular carcinoma. Patients with hepatitis C should be screened with annual alpha-fetoprotein levels and liver ultrasound.
- Retinoids may have a role in secondary prevention of HCC.

Associated Conditions

- Twenty percent to 30% of patients with chronic hepatitis C eventually develop cirrhosis. Cirrhotic patients have 2% to 6% per year risk of developing hepatocellular carcinoma.

DIAGNOSIS

Clinical Presentation

History

- Patients may have nonspecific complaints of abdominal pain, malaise, weight loss, or fever. Most patients have history of liver cirrhosis.

Physical Examination

- Patients may occasionally have a palpable liver mass. Most patients have physical **findings of cirrhosis,** such as ascites, splenomegaly, spider angiomata, and collateral circulation muscle wasting.

Diagnostic Criteria

- **Alpha-fetoprotein (AFP) level** of >200 ng/mL (in absence of chronic hepatitis B) or >400 ng/mL (in chronic hepatitis B), and presence of hepatic mass >2 cm with classic arterial enhancement by CT scan or MRA, is adequate for diagnosis.
- **Percutaneous needle biopsy** (FNA or core biopsy) should be performed in uncertain cases (low AFP, small liver lesion or without vascular enhancement).

Differential Diagnosis

- Adenoma, hemangioma, metastatic cancer

Diagnostic Testing

Laboratories

- CBC, CMP, PT, PTT, and AFP (elevated in 85% cases)

Imaging studies

- **Abdominal ultrasound** or **CT scan with contrast** is usually done initially.
- If primary hepatocellular cancer is strongly suspected, more detailed imaging studies including **triple-phase contrast enhanced CT scan or MRI** are used to define anatomic relationships and vascular anatomy. Conventional angiography, CT or MR-angiography is usually needed to completely reveal the anatomy and characteristics of the tumor vasculature.

TREATMENT

- Many staging systems have been proposed, which include the Okuda, CLIP, BCLC, and TNM staging.

- The Barcelona Clinic Liver Cancer (BCLC) staging system integrates Okuda staging and Child–Pugh score and treatment recommendations, and is currently endorsed by the American Association for Study of Liver Disease.[8]
  - **Stage 0.** Solitary lesion <2 cm with preserved liver function. Surgical resection is the primary treatment. Unfortunately, <5% of patients are resectable because of advanced disease or cirrhosis at presentation. Recurrent local disease may also be treated surgically, with potential for cure.
  - **Stage A.** Patients who are not eligible for resection (primarily due to insufficient liver reserve) or who meet the Milan criteria (one tumor ≤5 cm or up to three tumors ≤3 cm, no extrahepatic manifestations, or vascular invasion). Liver transplantation is the treatment of choice with 5-year survival up to 75%. Patients who are not transplant candidates should be referred for percutaneous ethanol injection or radiofrequency ablation.
  - **Stage B.** Patients typically have multinodular disease. Transarterial chemoembolization (TACE) is the treatment of choice. This therapy involves catheter-guided embolization of tumor-feeding hepatic artery using materials such as Lipiodol or Gelfoam with or without chemotherapeutic agents such as cisplatin or doxorubicin. It may provide a survival benefit. Due to risk of liver failure, TACE is contraindicated in patients with portal vein thrombosis and most patients with Child C liver disease.
  - **Stage C.** Sorafenib was found to provide a survival benefit versus supportive care for unresectable hepatocellular carcinoma with Child A disease.[9] The median overall survival improved from 7.9 to 10.7 months. Clinical trials should be recommended if available. Chemotherapeutic agents such as doxorubicin and capecitabine have a 10% response rate. Response rate is slightly higher (18% to 20%) with combinations such as cisplatin/capecitabine and oxaliplatin/gemcitabine.
  - **Stage D.** Best supportive care.

COMPLICATIONS

- Liver decompensation is of major concern after surgical resection or TACE.
- Complications of liver cirrhosis such as ascites, jaundice, bleeding diathesis, and variceal bleed are commonly seen.

MONITORING/FOLLOW-UP

- Patients with chronic HCV or liver cirrhosis should be screened with AFP and liver ultrasonography every 6 to 12 months.
- Due to high risk of recurrence, patients should be followed closely. A repeat CT scan should be obtained 1 month after surgical resection or local therapy. CBC, CMP, PT, serum AFP and abdominal CT/ultrasonography should be obtained every 3 months afterward.
- Patients who underwent liver transplantation should be followed by a liver transplant team regularly.

OUTCOME/PROGNOSIS

- Overall 5-year survival for stage 0 and A is 50% to 70%, 3-year survival of stage B/C is 20% to 40%, and 1-year survival for stage D disease is <10%, with median survival of 6 months.

GALLBLADDER CANCER

GENERAL PRINCIPLES

Classification

- Histology: 85% adenocarcinoma, the rest being squamous cell carcinoma or mixed type

Epidemiology

- Gallbladder cancer is a rare cancer of the biliary system, with ~5000 cases diagnosed per year in North America.
- Age: 7th decade.
- Sex: M:F, 1:1.7.

Risk Factors

- Chronic cholecystitis, cholelithiasis, typhoid carriers. Seventy-five percent to 98% of patients with gallbladder cancer will have gall stones. Incidence of gallbladder cancer in patients with "Porcelain gallbladder" is up to 25%.

Prevention

- Due to high risk of developing cancer, patients with porcelain gallbladder or gallbladder polyp >1 cm should be referred for surgery.

Associated Conditions

- Gall stones, chronic cholecystitis, gallbladder polyp, typhoid carrier, inflammatory bowel disease

DIAGNOSIS

Clinical Presentation

History

- These tumors may present with symptoms of acute or chronic cholecystitis, although jaundice and weight loss are more common.

Physical Examination

- Scratch marks for pruritus, jaundice, hepatomegaly, right upper quadrant tenderness, or symptoms/signs of acute cholecystitis

Diagnostic Criteria

- Histopathology diagnosis, usually after cholecystectomy, is required.

Differential Diagnosis

- Cholecystitis, cholangitis, cholangiocarcinoma, biliary colic, choledocholithiasis, gallbladder polyp, primary HCC, metastatic cancer, primary sclerosing cholangitis

Diagnostic Testing

Laboratories

- CBC, LFT, GGT, BMP, PT, PTT, AFP, and CEA

Imaging

- **Right upper quadrant ultrasonography** is usually the first imaging modality to be ordered.
- When gallbladder tumor is suspected, further imaging modalities such as **liver MRI** or **abdominal CT** should be obtained. **MRCP** is recommended to delineate tumor extent and nodal status in more details.

Diagnostic Procedures

- Tissue diagnosis can be made by ERCP if the tumor is distal. However, diagnosis is often made at the time of surgery.

TREATMENT

- The only curative treatment for gallbladder cancer is **surgical resection,** but <30% of patients have resectable disease at the time of presentation. Surgery typically involves cholecystectomy, en bloc hepatic resection, lymphadenectomy, and possible bile duct resection. Adjuvant therapy with 5-FU-based concurrent chemoradiation is recommended for most patients with resected gallbladder cancer, except for those with very small tumors (T1 N0).
- For patients with **unresectable but nonmetastatic gallbladder cancer,** therapy with **5-FU-based concurrent chemoradiation** is recommended, provided that the patient has an adequate performance status and is not jaundiced (total bilirubin ≤3 mg/dL is commonly used). Jaundiced patient should receive biliary decompression before chemotherapy.
- For patients with **metastatic disease,** choices of chemotherapy include **cisplatin plus gemcitabine,**[10] **5-FU, or capecitabine.** Cisplatin can be omitted in patients with poorer performance status.

COMPLICATIONS

- Obstructive jaundice, cholecystitis, and cholangitis are commonly seen.

MONITORING/FOLLOW-UP

- After definitive treatment, asymptomatic patients should typically be evaluated by history and physical examination every 3 months for 2 years, and then every 6 months for 3 additional years. CBC, CMP, and, if applicable, CA19–9 or CEA and CT scan of chest/abdomen/pelvis should be obtained during each routine follow-up.

OUTCOME/PROGNOSIS

- Five-year survival rates for localized, regional, and distant disease are 40%, 15%, and <10%, respectively. The median survival for advanced disease is 2 to 4 months.

CHOLANGIOCARCINOMA

GENERAL PRINCIPLES

Definition

- Cancers that arise from the biliary duct and before the ampulla of Vater

Classification

- Site: intrahepatic (<10%) and extrahepatic origin (>90%). Intrahepatic cholangiocarcinomas arise in the small intrahepatic ductules or the large intrahepatic ducts proximal to the bifurcation of the right and left hepatic ducts. Extrahepatic cholangiocarcinomas originate in any of the major hepatic or biliary ducts. **Klatskin's tumor** refers to extrahepatic cholangiocarcinoma that arises in the hilum of left and right hepatic duct.
- Histology: >95% adenocarcinoma, further subtyped into sclerosing, nodular, and papillary variants; <5% squamous cell carcinoma.

Epidemiology

- Cholangiocarcinoma is a rare cancer of the biliary tree, accounting for ~2500 new cases each year in the United States.
- Age: 6th decade.
- Sex: M:F, ~1:1.

Etiology and Pathophysiology

- Largely unknown but chronic inflammation may result in accelerated mutagenesis and dysplastic change.

Risk Factors

- Primary sclerosing cholangitis, hepatolithiasis, choledochal cysts, ulcerative colitis, and liver fluke infection

DIAGNOSIS

Clinical Presentation

History

- Up to 98% of patients with cholangiocarcinomas present with jaundice, and quite frequently right upper quadrant pain, fever, pruritus, and body weight loss.

Physical Examination

- Jaundice, hepatomegaly, or right upper quadrant mass.

Diagnostic Criteria

- Histopathology diagnosis is required.

Differential Diagnosis

- Cholecystitis, cholangitis, gallbladder cancer, primary HCC, pancreatic cancer, cancer of ampulla of Vater, metastatic cancer, primary sclerosing cholangitis

Diagnostic Testing

Laboratories

- CBC, BMP, LFT, PT, PTT, CA19–9, and CEA

Imaging

- **Abdominal CT** or **ultrasonography** is usually the first imaging studies performed.
- When cholangiocarcinoma is suspected, further imaging modalities such as liver MRI should be obtained. MRCP is recommended to delineate tumor extent and nodal status in more details.

Diagnostic Procedures

- Tissue diagnosis can be made by ERCP if the tumor is distal or by CT-guided biopsy if proximal or intrahepatic. Occasionally, diagnosis is often made at the time of surgery.

TREATMENT

- Complete surgical resection offers the only chance of cure. Overall management depends on location and stage of the disease.
- **Proximal third including intrahepatic cholangiocarcinoma:** hilar resection, lymphadenectomy, and possibly en bloc hepatic resection. If surgical margin is positive, adjuvant 5-FU- or gemcitabine-based chemoradiation, radiofrequency ablation, or repeat surgery should be recommended.
- **Mid-ductal lesion:** bile duct resection and portal lymphadenectomy followed by adjuvant 5-FU- or gemcitabine-based chemoradiation. Further chemotherapy with gemcitabine or 5-FU can be considered.
- **Distal ductal lesion:** Pancreaticoduodenectomy plus lymphadenectomy followed by adjuvant 5-FU- or gemcitabine-based chemoradiation. Further chemotherapy with gemcitabine or 5-FU can be considered.
- Due to lack of standard adjuvant therapy, **participation in clinical trials** should be recommended.
- **Unresectable cholangiocarcinomas** or **medically unfit patients** can be treated with 5-FU- or gemcitabine-based chemoradiation, or chemotherapy with 5-FU or gemcitabine alone. The prognosis is poor, with a median survival of 7 to 12 months.
- **Metastatic disease** is typically treated with chemotherapy such as cisplatin plus gemcitabine.[10] In these patients, priority should be palliation of obstructive jaundice and pain.

COMPLICATIONS

- Obstructive jaundice, cholecystitis, and cholangitis are commonly seen.

MONITORING/FOLLOW-UP

- After definitive treatment, asymptomatic patients should typically be evaluated by history and physical examination every 3 months for 2 years, and then every 6 months for 3 additional years. CBC, CMP, and, if applicable, CA19–9 or CEA and CT scan of chest/abdomen/pelvis should be obtained during each routine follow-up.

OUTCOME/PROGNOSIS

- Prognosis depends on stage and performance status. However, >70% of patients presented with advanced stage and <10% patients are surgical candidate.
- Patients with distal extrahepatic tumors that are completely resected have a 5-year survival rate of up to 40%. Overall median survival duration in patients with localized disease who undergo resection and adjuvant chemoradiation is 17 to 27.5 months.
- Patients who are not surgical candidates and received chemoradiation alone have a median survival 7 to 17 months.
- Patients who can tolerate biliary stenting alone have median survival of a few months.

REFERENCES

1. Bosset JF, Gignoux M, Triboulet JP, et al. Chemoradiotherapy followed by surgery compared with surgery alone in squamous-cell cancer of the esophagus. *N Engl J Med.* 1997;337:161–167.
2. Herskovic A, Martz K, al-Sarraf M, et al. Combined chemotherapy and radiotherapy compared with radiotherapy alone in patients with cancer of the esophagus. *N Engl J Med.* 1992;326:1593–1598.
3. Cunningham D, Allum WH, Stenning SP, et al. Perioperative chemotherapy versus surgery alone for resectable gastroesophageal cancer. *N Engl J Med.* 2006;355:11–20.
4. Macdonald JS, Smalley SR, Benedetti J, et al. Chemoradiotherapy after surgery compared with surgery alone for adenocarcinoma of the stomach or gastroesophageal junction. *N Engl J Med.* 2001;345:725–730.
5. Bang YJ, Van Cutsem E, Feyereislova A, et al. Trastuzumab in combination with chemotherapy versus chemotherapy alone for treatment of HER2-positive advanced gastric or gastro-oesophageal junction cancer (ToGA): a phase 3, open-label, randomised controlled trial. *Lancet.* 2010;376:687–697.
6. Demetri GD, von Mehren M, Blanke CD, et al. Efficacy and safety of imatinib mesylate in advanced gastrointestinal stromal tumors. *N Engl J Med.* 2002;347:472–480.
7. Moore MJ, Goldstein D, Hamm J, et al. Erlotinib plus gemcitabine compared with gemcitabine alone in patients with advanced pancreatic cancer: a phase III trial of the National Cancer Institute of Canada Clinical Trials Group. *J Clin Oncol.* 2007;25:1960–1966.
8. Llovet JM, Bru C, Bruix J. Prognosis of hepatocellular carcinoma: the BCLC staging classification. *Semin Liver Dis.* 1999;19:329–338.
9. Llovet JM, Ricci S, Mazzaferro V, et al. Sorafenib in advanced hepatocellular carcinoma. *N Engl J Med.* 2008;359:378–390.
10. Valle J, Wasan H, Palmer DH, et al. Cisplatin plus gemcitabine versus gemcitabine for biliary tract cancer. *N Engl J Med.* 2010;362:1273–1281.

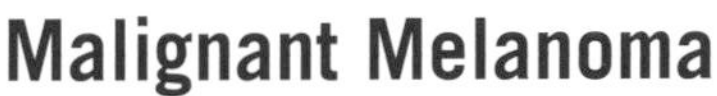

22 Malignant Melanoma

Gregory H. Miday and Yee Hong Chia

GENERAL PRINCIPLES

Definition

Malignant melanoma is an aggressive neoplasm that arises from melanocytes, which are long-lived pigment–producing cells.[1] Melanocytes are located in the basal layer of the epidermis, hair bulb, eyes, ears, and meninges. Melanoma most commonly arises in the skin; however, melanoma can also arise in non-cutaneous sites as well. Intraocular melanoma of the choroid and ciliary body is the most common ocular malignant tumor in adults, and the most common non-cutaneous melanoma.[2]

Classification

Malignant melanoma is traditionally classified into superficial spreading melanoma (estimated 50% to 75% of melanomas), nodular melanoma (15% to 35%), lentigo maligna melanoma (5% to 15%), acral lentiginous melanoma (5% to 10%), desmoplastic melanoma (uncommon) and a miscellaneous group (rare).[1] ***Superficial spreading melanoma*** (SSM) is the most common form of melanoma. In SSM, the melanoma cells demonstrate pagetoid spread in the epidermis, and the lesions classically show variation in pigmentation. ***Nodular melanoma*** (NM) can appear nodular, polypoid, or pedunculated. ***Lentigo maligna melanoma*** (LMM) is a variant of melanoma that affects the sun-exposed skin, face, and upper extremities of elderly patients. Lentigo maligna (LM) is a subtype of melanoma in situ and should be distinguished from LMM. LM typically presents on sun-exposed areas of middle-aged and elderly individuals, and appears as centrifugally expanding large patch with variable shades ranging from tan to black.[3] The lifetime risk of progression to LMM is approximately 5%. ***Acral lentiginous melanoma*** (ALM) arises in the palmar, plantar, or ungual skin. Most mucosal melanomas, including those affecting the oral cavity, vulva, vagina, and cervix, share histological features of ALM.

Epidemiolgy

In the United States, an estimated 68,130 new cases of melanoma will be diagnosed in 2010, and an estimated 8700 deaths will result from the disease.[4] Overall, the incidence of melanoma increased 3.1% annually over the last two decades.[5] The incidence of melanoma rises with increasing age, and is significantly lower in non-Caucasian populations. About 10% of malignant melanomas present in familial clusters.

Etiology

- The transformation of benign melanocytes to melanoma results from a collection of genetic changes. Hereditary melanoma typically demonstrates an autosomal-dominant pattern within multiplex families [reviewed in[6]]. Germline mutations in the cyclin-dependent kinase inhibitor 2A (*CDKN2A*) gene located on chromosome 9p21 conferred susceptibility to melanoma with high penetrance. Subsequently, a second high penetrance gene, the cyclin-dependent kinase 4 (*CDK4*) gene located on chromosome 12q14, was identified in certain kindreds that lacked hereditable *CDKN2A* mutations. Together, these foci account for about 20% to 57% of disease susceptibility. Two proteins, p14Arf and p16Ink4a, are encoded by splice variants of the *CDKN2A* locus. The p14Arf protein regulates the p53 tumor suppressor network, and loss of p14Arf results in the indirect loss of p53 function, thereby leading to dysregulation of cell cycling and DNA damage response. The p16Ink4a mutant proteins are unable to inhibit Cdk4 and Cdk6, thereby leading to the inability to suppress phosphorylation of the retinoblastoma (Rb) protein. Hyperphosphorylation of Rb allows the cell to transition from G1 to S-phase of the cell cycle, and to proliferate. A key pigmentation gene, the melanocortin-1-receptor (MC1R), has also been implicated as a low to moderate penetrance melanoma susceptibility gene.

- Activating mutations in the *BRAF* gene have been found in 60% to 80% of melanoma cases.[7] The *BRAF* gene encodes a serine/threonine protein kinase that plays an important role in regulating signaling pathways, such as the mitogen activated protein kinase (MAPK) pathway. Dysregulated BRAF signaling is thought to promote dysregulated cell division and differentiation. Curtin et al. postulated that the clinical heterogeneity seen in melanoma could be explained by genetically distinct types of melanoma, and used array-based comparative genomic hybridization to interrogate four groups of melanomas, namely, melanoma on skin without chronic sun-induced damage, melanoma on skin with chronic sun-induced damage, mucosal melanoma and acral melanoma.[8] Acral or mucosal melanoma had significantly higher degree of chromosomal aberrations. While amplifications were found in the majority of acral and mucosal melanomas, they involved different genomic regions. On the other hand, amplifications were infrequent in the other two groups. Melanomas on mucosal membranes, acral skin, and skin with chronic sun-induced damage were found to have infrequent mutations in *BRAF* and *NRAS,* two genes involved with the MAPK pathway, in contrast to melanomas on skin without chronic sun-induced damage. On the other hand, somatic activation of KIT was found in a fraction of melanomas on mucosal membranes (39%), acral skin (36%), and skin with chronic sun-induced damage (28%), but not in melanomas on skin without chronic sun-induced damage.[9] These findings have implications for the development of targeted therapies.

Risk Factors

Risk factors for melanoma include environmental factors such as **sun exposure** and **exposure to artificial ultraviolet (UV) rays** via indoor tanning [reviewed in[5] and[10]]. Persons with fair skin, freckles, and inability to tan are more likely to develop melanoma. Family history of malignant melanoma in a first or second-degree relative confers increased risk. Persons with large numbers of nevi (>100) or atypical nevi of any number have a higher risk of developing melanoma. Large congenital nevi pose a risk of melanoma of approximately 5% to 10%. Organ-transplant patients on chronic immunosuppression have a higher risk of developing skin cancers, including melanoma.

Prevention

Given the association between UV radiation and the development of melanoma, the use of **sunscreen** and **avoidance of UV rays** have been advocated as means of reducing the risk of developing melanoma. For secondary prevention, patients at risk for developing melanoma might benefit from education on self skin examinations. Patients should be encouraged to report any unusual or changing nevus.

DIAGNOSIS

Clinical Presentation

- The "ABCDE" **mnemonic** in melanoma diagnosis refers to **asymmetry, border irregularity, color variations, dimension, and evolution.** The clinical history should include queries about risk factors for melanoma (as outlined earlier in this chapter) and changing nevi[10]. Changes in the color or an increase in size in a new mole are usually the early signs noted by patients. Later changes include bleeding, itching and tenderness. A global evaluation of the skin is necessary to assess the degree of sun damage, number of nevi, distribution of nevi, and the presence of atypical or dysplastic nevi.
- When a lesion suspicious for melanoma is identified, the next key step is an appropriate biopsy. If melanoma is suspected, a **complete excisional removal** into adipose tissue, with a 2-mm margin of adjacent normal-appearing skin, is preferred. **Shave biopsies should be avoided** as they may not provide an accurate Breslow depth, which is an important part of melanoma staging. For large lesions that are not easily amenable to complete excision, an incisional full-thickness biopsy or multiple representative punch biopsies might be acceptable.
- Once a diagnosis of melanoma is made, a thorough history and physical examination will help guide further testing. Lymph nodes should be carefully examined, and patients with clinically palpable suspicious lymph nodes should be referred for a lymph node aspirate or open biopsy. Patients with symptoms suspicious for metastatic disease should be worked up as appropriate. In patients with distant metastases, a serum lactate dehydrogenase (LDH) is of prognostic value.

Staging

- Staging of melanoma is based on the thickness of the tumor and the presence of nodal or distant metastases. The absolute depth of invasion (millimeters) is referred to as the Breslow thickness. The Clark level refers to the depth of invasion into the layers of the skin. Tables 22-1 and 22-2 summarize the 2009 American Joint Committee on Cancer (AJCC) melanoma staging and classification.[11] The AJCC Melanoma Staging Committee recommends that a sentinel lymph node (SLN) biopsy be discussed with otherwise healthy patients who have T2, T3, and T4 melanomas and clinically uninvolved lymph nodes. Select patients with T1b melanomas (mitotic rate $\geq 1/mm^2$ and a thickness of ≥ 0.76 mm) may also benefit from a SLN biopsy as such melanomas are associated with an approximately 10% risk of occult metastases in their sentinel lymph nodes.[11]

TABLE 22-1 TNM STAGING CATEGORIES FOR CUTANEOUS MELANOMA

Classification	Thickness (mm)	Ulceration Status/ Mitoses
T (primary tumor)		
Tis	NA	NA
T1	≤1.00	a: Without ulceration and mitosis <1/mm^2 b: With ulceration or mitoses ≥1/mm^2
T2	1.01–2.00	a: Without ulceration b: With ulceration
T3	2.01–4.00	a: Without ulceration b: With ulceration
T4	>4.00	a: Without ulceration b: With ulceration
N	**(No. of Metastatic Nodes)**	**Nodal Metastatic Burden**
N0	0	Not applicable
N1	1	a: Micrometastasis[a] b: Macrometastasis[b]
N2	2–3	a: Micrometastasis[a] b: Macrometastasis[b] c: In transit metastases/ satellites without metastatic nodes
N3	4+ metastatic nodes, or matted nodes, or in transit metastases/ satellites with metastatic nodes	
M	**Site**	**Serum LDH**
M0	No distant metastases	NA
M1a	Distant skin, subcutaneous, or nodal metastases	Normal
M1b	Lung metastases	Normal
M1c	All other visceral metastases	Normal
	Any distant metastasis	Elevated

[a]Micrometastases are diagnosed after sentinel lymph node biopsy.

[b]Macrometastases are defined as clinically detectable nodal metastases confirmed pathologically.

- In the Multicenter Selective Lymphadenectomy Trial (MSLT), patients with intermediate thickness melanomas (1.2 to 3.5 mm in thickness) were randomized to SLN biopsy or observation.[12] All patients underwent wide excision of the primary melanoma. For those randomized to the biopsy group, an immediate complete lymphadenectomy was performed only on those with a positive

TABLE 22-2 ANATOMIC STAGE GROUPINGS FOR CUTANEOUS MELANOMA

Clinical Staging				Pathologic Staging			
	T	N	M		T	N	M
0	Tis	N0	M0	0	Tis	N0	M0
IA	T1a	N0	M0	IA	T1a	N0	M0
IB	T1b	N0	M0	IB	T1b	N0	M0
	T2a	N0	M0		T2a	N0	M0
IIA	T2b	N0	M0	IIA	T2b	N0	M0
	T3a	N0	M0		T3a	N0	M0
IIB	T3b	N0	M0	IIB	T3b	N0	M0
	T4a	N0	M0		T4a	N0	M0
IIC	T4b	N0	M0	IIC	T4b	N0	M0
III	Any T	N > N0	M0	IIIA	T1-4a	N1a	M0
					T1-4a	N2a	M0
				IIIB	T1-4b	N1a	M0
					T1-4b	N2a	M0
					T1-4a	N1b	M0
					T1-4a	N2b	M0
					T1-4a	N2c	M0
				IIIC	T1-4b	N1b	M0
					T1-4b	N2b	M0
					T1-4b	N2c	M0
					Any T	N3	M0
IV	Any T	Any N	M1	IV	Any T	Any N	M1

Adapted from Balch CM, Gershenwald JE, Soong SJ, et al. Fain version of 2009 AJCC melanoma staging and classification. *J Clin Oncol.* 2009;27:6199–6206.

SLN biopsy. In the observation group, a delayed complete lymphadenectomy was performed when nodal recurrence was observed. Among patients with nodal metastases, the 5-year survival rate was higher among those who underwent immediate lymphadenectomy compared to those in whom lymphadenectomy was delayed, with a hazard ratio (HR) of death of 0.51 (95% confidence interval (CI) of 0.32 to 0.18, $p = 0.004$), supporting the use of SLN biopsy as a tool for identifying patients with nodal metastases in whom early intervention may be beneficial.[12]

TREATMENT

Local and Locoregional Disease (Stage I to III)

- **Surgical excision,** when feasible, is the primary treatment for cutaneous melanoma[10]. Recommended excision margins depend on the Breslow depth. For melanoma in situ (excluding LM), the recommended margin is 0.5 to 1.0 cm. For stage Ia (<1 mm) melanomas, a margin of 1 cm is considered adequate.

For melanomas that are 1 to 2 mm deep, the recommended margin is at least 1 cm, but up to 2 cm is recommended if feasible. For melanomas >2 mm deep, the recommended margin is 2 cm.[10] Dissection should be sufficiently deep, typically to the level of the deep subcutaneous tissue at the level of the fascia. As discussed above, SLN biopsy, followed by an immediate lymphadenectomy if positive, may be appropriate in select patients. For patients with in-transit melanoma, local excision of isolated metastases is sometimes feasible. For in-transit melanoma patients with more widespread cutaneous disease not amenable to resection, nonsurgical modalities including localized immune therapy, heated limb perfusion, and external beam radiation may offer reasonable control.[13]

- **Adjuvant systemic therapy with interferon alpha-2b** (IFN α2b) has been extensively evaluated in high-risk stage II and stage III melanoma after definitive surgical resection. The Eastern Cooperative Group (ECOG) E1684 trial randomized patients to either high-dose interferon (20 MIU/m^2/d intravenously for 1 month then 10 MIU/m^2 3 times per week subcutaneously for 48 weeks) or observation. All patients in this trial underwent a complete regional lymphadenectomy. Earlier reports of this trial indicated a significant prolongation of relapse free survival (RFS) and overall survival (OS) in favor of adjuvant high-dose interferon.[14] However, with longer term follow-up, whilst the benefit in RFS is maintained, the improvement in OS reported earlier was diminished.[15] A pooled analysis of ECOG and Intergroup trials of high-dose interferon (HDI) in melanoma (which included E1684) failed to demonstrate an OS survival benefit in the pooled population. Different dosing[16,17] and duration of interferon treatment[18] have been evaluated, with largely similar results. Toxicities of HDI include constitutional symptoms, neurologic toxicities, myelosuppression, and hepatotoxicity. The nontrivial toxicities of HDI and the absence of unequivocal benefit led to controversy regarding its appropriateness in this setting. Other investigations into systemic adjuvant therapies were reviewed by Algazi et al.[13]

Distant Metastatic Disease (Stage IV)

- Survival in patients with distant metastases is poor. Resection of solitary skin, lung, or brain metastases can be considered. As treatment options for metastatic melanoma are limited, **enrollment in a clinical trial,** whenever feasible, is recommended for patients with stage IV disease. **Dacarbazine,** an alkylating agent, is the only chemotherapy approved by the Federal Food and Drug Administration (FDA) for treatment of metastatic melanoma. **Temozolomide,** a close analog of dacarbazine, is more commonly used because it can be administered orally. In a randomized Phase III trial comparing temozolomide to dacarbazine, the response rates were similar at 13.1% and 12.1%, respectively.[19] The median OS was similar in both arms, although temozolomide has a marginally longer median progression free survival of 1.9 months versus 1.5 months. High dose interleukin-2 (IL-2) is also FDA-approved for treatment of metastatic melanoma. Atkins et al. reported on 270 assessable patients with metastatic melanoma who were entered onto eight clinical trials involving IL-2 conducted between 1985 and 1993.[20] The overall objective response rate was 16% (95% CI of 12% to 21%), with 17 complete responses (CRs) (6%) and 26 partial responses (PRs) (10%). In this series, high dose IL-2 appeared to produce durable CRs or PRs in a small subset of patients. Unfortunately, high dose IL-2 is a highly toxic regimen that is challenging to administer. Some patients receiving high dose IL-2 will even require vasopressor support in an intensive care unit.

- Two recently published trials provided encouraging results for systemic treatment of metastatic melanoma. Hodi et al.[21] reported on a Phase III trial evaluating ipilimumab, an antibody that blocks cytotoxic T-lymphocyte-associated antigen 4 (CTLA-4), and the gp100 vaccine, a synthetic peptide cancer vaccine consisting of amino acid residues 209 through 217 of the glycoprotein 100 (gp100) melanoma antigen. In this study, 676 patients with unresectable stage III or IV malignant melanoma were randomly assigned, in a 3:1:1 ratio, to receive ipilimumab plus gp100 ($n = 403$ patients), ipilimumab alone ($n = 137$), or gp100 alone ($n = 136$).[16] The median OS was 10.0 months among patients receiving ipilimumab plus gp100, compared to 6.4 months among patients receiving gp100 alone (HR for death, 0.68; $P < 0.001$). Median OS with ipilimumab alone was 10.1 months (HR for death in the comparison with gp100 alone, 0.66; $P = 0.003$). These data demonstrated the efficacy of ipilimumab in metastatic melanoma. In another study, Flaherty et al.[22] reported on a phase I dose-escalation trial of PLX4032, an oral inhibitor of mutated BRAF. In the dose-escalation cohort, of the 16 patients with melanoma whose tumors carried the V600E BRAF mutation, there were 10 PRs and 1 CR. Among the 32 patients in the extension cohort of melanoma patients whose tumors carried the V600E BRAF mutation, 24 had a PR and 2 had a CR. The estimated median progression-free survival among all patients was more than 7 months, suggesting that BRAF inhibition may be a viable therapeutic strategy in BRAF mutated melanoma. Another potential therapeutic target is c-kit. Hodi et al. reported a major response to imatinib mesylate, an oral tyrosine kinase inhibitor which inhibits c-kit, in a patient with a c-kit-mutated melanoma, suggesting that targeting of this pathway may also represent a therapeutic avenue worth evaluating in select patients.[23]

PROGNOSIS

Prognosis is dependent on stage of disease.[11] In patients with localized melanomas (stage I and II), 10-year survival ranges from 93% for stage IA to 39% for stage IIC. In these patients, increasing tumor thickness and mitotic rate are associated with declining survival rates. Patients with ulcerated melanomas have proportionately lower survival rates than those with equivalent T staged non-ulcerated tumors. In patients with regional metastatic melanoma (stage III), the 5-year survival rates were 78%, 59%, and 40% for patients with stage IIIA, IIIB, and IIIC melanoma, respectively. In patients with distant metastatic melanoma (stage IV), the site(s) of metastases and serum LDH levels delineate the M1 stage into M1a, M1b, and M1c (as shown in Table 22-1). The 1-year survival rates were 62%, 53%, and 33% for M1a, M1b, and M1c melanomas, respectively.

REFERENCES

1. Bandarchi B, Ma L, Navab R, et al. From melanocyte to metastatic malignant melanoma. *Dermatol Res Pract.* Epub Aug 11, 2010;2010:1–8.

2. Laver NV, McLaughlin ME, Duker JS. Ocular melanoma. *Arch Pathol Lab Med.* 2010; 134:1778–1784.
3. McKenna JK, Florell SR, Goldman GD, et al. Lentigo maligna/lentigo maligna melanoma: current state of diagnosis and treatment. *Dermatol Surg.* 2006;32:493–504.
4. Jemal A, Siegel R, Xu J, et al. Cancer statistics, 2010. *Ca Cancer J Clin.* 2010;60:277–300.
5. Rigel DS. Epidemiology of melanoma. *Semin Cutan Med Surg.* 2010;29:204–209.
6. Udayakumar D, Mahato B, Gabree M, et al. Genetic determinants of cutaneous melanoma predisposition. *Semin Cutan Med Surg.* 2010;29:190–195.
7. Davies H, Bignell GR, Cox C, et al. Mutations of the BRAF gene in human cancer. *Nature.* 2002;417:949–954.
8. Curtin JA, Fridlyand J, Kageshita T, et al. Distinct sets of genetic alterations in melanoma. *N Engl J Med.* 2005;353:2135–2147.
9. Curtin JA, Busam K, Pinkel D, et al. Somatic activation of KIT in distinct subtypes of melanoma. *J Clin Oncol.* 2006;24:4340–4346.
10. Brown MD. Office management of melanoma patients. *Semin Cutan Med Surg.* 2010; 29:232–237.
11. Balch CM, Gershenwald JE, Soong SJ, et al. Final version of 2009 AJCC melanoma staging and classification. *J Clin Oncol.* 2009;27:6199–6206.
12. Morton DL, Thompson JF, Cochran AJ, et al. Sentinel-node biopsy or nodal observation in melanoma. *N Engl J Med.* 2006;355:1307–1317.
13. Algazi AP, Soon CW, Daud AI. Treatment of cutaneous melanoma: current approaches and future prospects. *Cancer Manag Res.* 2010;2:197–211.
14. Kirkwood JM, Strawderman MH, Ernstoff MS, et al. Interferon alfa-2b adjuvant therapy of high-risk resected cutaneous melanoma: the Eastern Cooperative Oncology Group Trial EST 1684. *J Clin Oncol.* 1996;14:7–17.
15. Kirkwood JM, Manola J, Ibrahim J, et al. A pooled analysis of eastern cooperative oncology group and intergroup trials of adjuvant high-dose interferon for melanoma. *Clin Cancer Res.* 2004;10:1670–1677.
16. Eggermont AM, Suciu S, MacKie R, et al. Post-surgery adjuvant therapy with intermediate doses of interferon alfa 2b versus observation in patients with stage IIb/III melanoma (EORTC 18952): randomised controlled trial. *Lancet.* 2005;366:1189–1196.
17. Kirkwood JM, Ibrahim JG, Sondak VK, et al. High- and low-dose interferon alfa-2b in high-risk melanoma: first analysis of intergroup trial E1690/S9111/C9190. *J Clin Oncol.* 2000;18:2444–2458.
18. Pectasides D, Dafni U, Bafaloukos D, et al. Randomized phase III study of 1 month versus 1 year of adjuvant high-dose interferon alfa-2b in patients with resected high-risk melanoma. *J Clin Oncol.* 2009;27:939–944.
19. Middleton MR, Grob JJ, Aaronson N, et al. Randomized phase III study of temozolomide versus dacarbazine in the treatment of patients with advanced metastatic malignant melanoma. *J Clin Oncol.* 2000;18:158–166.
20. Atkins MB, Lotze MT, Dutcher JP, et al. High-dose recombinant interleukin 2 therapy for patients with metastatic melanoma: analysis of 270 patients treated between 1985 and 1993. *J Clin Oncol.* 1999;17:2105–2116.
21. Hodi FS, O'Day SJ, McDermott DF, et al. Improved survival with ipilimumab in patients with metastatic melanoma. *N Engl J Med.* 2010;363:711–723.
22. Flaherty KT, Puzanov I, Kim KB, et al. Inhibition of mutated, activated BRAF in metastatic melanoma. *N Engl J Med.* 2010;363:809–819.
23. Hodi FS, Friedlander P, Corless CL, et al. Major response to imatinib mesylate in KIT-mutated melanoma. *J Clin Oncol.* 2008;26:2046–2051.

Head and Neck Cancer

23

George Ansstas

GENERAL PRINCIPLES

Squamous cell carcinoma of the head and neck (SCCHN) represents 5% of newly diagnosed cancers in adult patients in the United States. There are more than 500,000 new cases that are diagnosed annually worldwide.[1] While there are many similarities between head and neck cancers arising from different sites, there are particular differences in anatomy, natural history, and functional consequence that present unique treatment challenges for each site.

Classification

Malignancies of the head and neck are classified by their anatomic location, which is divided into (a) lip and oral cavity, (b) oropharynx, (c) larynx and hypopharynx, (d) nasopharynx, (e) nasal cavity and sinuses, and (f) salivary glands. With the exception of salivary gland tumors, squamous cell carcinoma accounts for >90% of head and neck tumors. As nasopharyngeal cancer and neck masses with unknown primary have different epidemiology and/or management, they are discussed separately.

SQUAMOUS CELL CARCINOMA OF THE HEAD AND NECK

GENERAL PRINCIPLES

Epidemiology

Head and neck cancers have a significant male predominance, with a male-to-female ratio of 3:1. These tumors are estimated to account for ~45,000 new cases per year, with an estimated 11,000 deaths per year. Incidence and mortality are higher in African-Americans.

Pathophysiology

SCCHN is an example of the multistep process of carcinogenesis with accumulated genetic mutations that result in changes ranging from hyperplasia to dysplasia to carcinoma in situ to invasive cancer. Statistical analysis based on the age-specific incidence of head and neck cancer suggests that HNSCC tumors arise after the accumulation of 6 to 10 independent genetic events. These studies demonstrated consistent chromosomal abnormalities and the presence of important alterations. Loss of chromosomes 3p, 5q, 8p, 9p, 18q, and 21q were commonly identified, and data also suggest that loss of 18q may indicate the presence of a tumor with a poor prognosis.[2] Moderate increases in epidermal growth factor receptor (EGFR) copy number are observed in SCCHN, and EGFR signaling is a key pathway in HNSCC tumorigenesis.[3] In some tumors, an alternately translated EGFR variant (EGFRvIII) contributes to head and neck growth and resistance to EGFR targeting.

Risk Factors

- The main risk factors for development of these malignancies are **tobacco in any form** and **alcohol use**. Tobacco and alcohol are sources of carcinogens that increase the risk of cancer in a dose-dependent fashion and are synergistic in their effects. Field cancerization is a key concept in the natural history of head and neck cancer. Exposure of the mucosa to carcinogens in tobacco is diffuse across the aerodigestive tract. Consequently, tumors may be surrounded by areas of dysplasia or carcinoma in situ. Patients diagnosed with a head and neck cancer are at an increased risk of developing new primary tumors in the head and neck, lung, and esophagus. The risk is estimated to be 3% to 4% per year. Sun exposure has been associated with an increased risk of carcinoma of the lip.
- Approximately 20% of head and neck cancers, however, occur in people without these established risk factors. A subset of these cancers includes **human papilloma virus** (HPV)-associated tumors of the oropharynx.[4] Risk factors for HPV-associated tumors of the oropharynx include an increasing number of sexual partners, the practice of oral sex, a history of genital warts, and a younger age at first sexual intercourse. As in cervical cancer, HPV-16 and HPV-18 are thought to play an important role. These HPV-positive oropharyngeal cancers were less likely to occur among heavy smokers and drinkers, less likely to harbor a p53 mutation, and had an improved disease-specific survival. Another group suggested that HPV-positive tumors may also inactivate Rb and harbor a better prognosis.

DIAGNOSIS

Clinical Presentation

- The clinical presentation of these malignancies varies depending on the anatomic location of the tumor. **Cancers of the lip and oral cavity** often present with nonhealing lesions in the mouth, pain in the mouth or ear, trismus, weight loss, and "hot potato speech." Leukoplakia and erythroplakia are premalignant lesions of the mucosa and are frequently seen in conjunction with dysplastic changes or invasive carcinoma.
- **Cancers of the nasal cavity** can present with epistaxis, nonhealing ulcers, or obstruction.
- **Cancers of the oropharynx** present with many of the features associated with cancers of the lip and oral cavity. Bleeding from the mouth, alterations in speech, dysphagia, odynophagia, otalgia, and weight loss can be symptoms of oropharyngeal cancers.
- **Cancers of the larynx and hypopharynx** can present challenges in management, as these anatomic structures are intricately associated with the key functions of speech and swallowing. Symptoms include dysphagia, odynophagia, weight loss, dyspnea (including dyspnea with speech), and hoarseness. Symptoms of aspiration should also be elucidated in the history. However, the time of presentation of these cancers varies greatly with their primary site. Supraglottic tumors or tumors in the pyriform sinus may be diagnosed only after cervical metastases occur because symptoms of dysphagia may not become

significant until the tumors are quite advanced. On the other hand, glottic carcinomas are associated with symptoms of hoarseness even when they are small, which may lead to earlier detection.

Diagnostic Testing

- The initial workup of suspected head and neck cancers includes a detailed history and physical examination. Assessment should include a cranial nerve exam, assessment of status of dentition, and examination of tongue movement and atrophy. Lymph nodes in the neck should be palpated, and measurements taken of palpable nodes. Suspicious lesions should be biopsied for histologic confirmation and grading.
- **Imaging studies** should include a chest radiograph, Panorex x-ray for mandibular bony involvement for cancers that abut the mandible, and computed tomography (CT) or magnetic resonance imaging (MRI) of the head and neck to help further delineate disease extent at presentation. **Panendoscopy**, including esophagoscopy with direct laryngoscopy, helps characterize the primary lesion and evaluates for possible second tumors, as there is a 10% to 15% incidence of synchronous primary tumors. A CT scan of the chest should also be performed to rule out pulmonary metastases. Positron emission tomography (PET) or CT may also be helpful in the staging of head and neck cancers and are used at some centers. The staging for head and neck cancer is according to the American Joint Committee on Cancer TNM system, with different staging for SCCHN (Tables 23-1 through 23-6).

TABLE 23-1 AJCC STAGING OF LIP AND ORAL CAVITY CANCER: PRIMARY TUMOR (T)

TX	Primary tumor cannot be assessed.
T0	No evidence of primary tumor
Tis	Carcinoma in situ
T1	Tumor ≤2 cm in greatest dimension
T2	Tumor >2 cm but ≤4 cm in greatest dimension
T3	Tumor >4 cm in greatest dimension
T4 (lip)	Tumor invades adjacent structures (e.g., through cortical bone, inferior alveolar nerve, floor of mouth, skin of face).
T4a (oral cavity)	Tumor invades adjacent structures (e.g., through cortical bone, into deep [extrinsic] muscle of tongue, maxillary sinus, skin). (Superficial erosion of bone/tooth socket by gingival primary alone is not sufficient to classify as T4.)
T4b (oral cavity)	Tumor invades masticator space, pterygoid plates, or skull base and/or encases internal carotid artery.

From American Joint Committee on Cancer. *AJCC Cancer Staging Manual.* 7th ed. New York: Springer-Verlag; 2002, with permission.

TABLE 23-2 AJCC STAGING OF LIP AND ORAL CAVITY CANCER, OROPHARYNX, HYPOPHARYNX, AND LARYNX: REGIONAL LYMPH NODES (N), DISTANT METASTASIS (M)

NX	Regional lymph nodes cannot be assessed.
N0	No regional lymph node metastasis
N1	Metastasis in a single ipsilateral lymph node, ≤3 cm in greatest dimension
N2	Metastasis in a single ipsilateral lymph node, >3 cm but not ≤6 cm in greatest dimension; or in multiple ipsilateral lymph nodes, none >6 cm in greatest dimension; or in bilateral or contralateral lymph nodes, none >6 cm in greatest dimension
N2a	Metastasis in a single ipsilateral lymph node >3 cm but not ≤6 cm in greatest dimension
N2b	Metastasis in multiple ipsilateral lymph nodes, none >6 cm in greatest dimension
N2c	Metastasis in bilateral or contralateral lymph nodes, none >6 cm in greatest dimension
N3	Metastasis in a lymph node >6 cm in greatest dimension
MX	Distant metastasis cannot be assessed.
M0	No distant metastasis
M1	Distant metastasis

From American Joint Committee on Cancer. *AJCC Cancer Staging Manual.* 7th ed. New York: Springer-Verlag; 2002, with permission.

TABLE 23-3 AJCC STAGE GROUPING: ORAL CAVITY AND LIP, OROPHARYNX, LARYNX, AND HYPOPHARYNX

Stage 0	Tis	N0	M0
Stage I	T1	N0	M0
Stage II	T2	N0	M0
Stage III	T3	N0	M0
	T1–T3	N1	M0
Stage IVA	T4a	N0–N1	M0
	Any T	N2	M0
Stage IVB	Any T	N3	M0
	T4b	Any N	M0
Stage IVC	Any T	Any N	M1

From American Joint Committee on Cancer. *AJCC Cancer Staging Manual.* 7th ed. New York: Springer-Verlag; 2002, with permission.

TABLE 23-4 AJCC STAGING OF OROPHARYNX CANCER: PRIMARY TUMOR (T)

TX	Primary tumor cannot be assessed.
T0	No evidence of primary tumor
Tis	Carcinoma in situ
T1	Tumor ≤2 cm in greatest dimension
T2	Tumor >2 cm but ≤4 cm in greatest dimension
T3	Tumor >4 cm in greatest dimension
T4a	Tumor invades the larynx, deep/extrinsic muscle of tongue, medial pterygoid, hard palate, or mandible.
T4b	Tumor invades lateral pterygoid muscle, pterygoid plates, lateral nasopharynx, or skull base or encases carotid artery.

—
From American Joint Committee on Cancer. *AJCC Cancer Staging Manual.* 7th ed. New York: Springer-Verlag; 2002, with permission.

TREATMENT

- Management of patients requires a multidisciplinary approach, including head and neck surgeons and radiation and medical oncologists, along with allied health professionals including speech language pathologists and nutritionists. Radiation and surgery are the mainstays of treatment with head and neck cancers. Chemotherapy is reserved for patients with regionally advanced disease or metastatic disease.

TABLE 23-5 AJCC STAGING HYPOPHARYNX CANCER: PRIMARY TUMOR (T)

TX	Primary tumor cannot be assessed.
T0	No evidence of primary tumor
Tis	Carcinoma in situ
T1	Tumor limited to one subsite of hypopharynx and ≤2 cm in greatest dimension
T2	Tumor involves more than one subsite of hypopharynx or an adjacent site, or measures >2 cm but ≤4 cm in greatest dimension without fixation of hemilarynx.
T3	Tumor measures >4 cm in greatest dimension or with fixation of hemilarynx.
T4a	Tumor invades thyroid/cricoid cartilage, hyoid bone, thyroid gland, esophagus, prelaryngeal strap muscles, or subcutaneous fat.
T4b	Tumor invades prevertebral fascia, encases carotid artery, or involves mediastinal structures.

—
From American Joint Committee on Cancer. *AJCC Cancer Staging Manual.* 7th ed. New York: Springer-Verlag; 2002, with permission.

TABLE 23-6 AJCC STAGING LARYNX CANCER: PRIMARY TUMOR (T)

TX	Primary tumor cannot be assessed.
T0	No evidence of primary tumor
Tis	Carcinoma in situ
T1 supraglottis	Tumor limited to one subsite of supraglottis with normal vocal cord mobility
T1 glottis	Tumor limited to vocal cord(s) (may involve anterior or posterior commissure) with normal mobility
T1a	Tumor limited to one vocal cord
T1b	Tumor involves both vocal cords.
T1 subglottis	Tumor limited to the subglottis
T2 supraglottis	Tumor invades mucosa of more than one adjacent subsite of supraglottis or glottis or region outside the supraglottis (e.g., mucosa of base of tongue, vallecula, medial wall of pyriform sinus) without fixation of the larynx.
T2 glottis	Tumor extends to supraglottis and/or subglottis, and/or with impaired vocal cord mobility.
T2 subglottis	Tumor extends to vocal cord(s), with normal or impaired mobility.
T3 supraglottis	Tumor limited to larynx with vocal cord fixation and/or invades either of the following: postcricoid area, pre-epiglottic tissues.
T3 glottis	Tumor limited to the larynx with vocal cord fixation
T3 Subglottis	Tumor limited to the larynx with vocal cord fixation
T4a supraglottis	Tumor invades through the thyroid cartilage and/or extends into soft tissues of the neck, thyroid, and/or esophagus.
T4a glottis	Tumor invades through the thyroid cartilage and/or to other tissues beyond the larynx (e.g., trachea, soft tissues of neck, including thyroid, pharynx).
T4a subglottis	Tumor invades through cricoid or thyroid cartilage, and/or extends to other tissues beyond the larynx (e.g., trachea, soft tissues of neck, including thyroid, esophagus).
T4b supraglottis	Tumor invades prevertebral space, encases carotid artery, or invades mediastinal structures.
T4b glottis	Tumor invades prevertebral space, encases carotid artery, or invades mediastinal structures.
T4b subglottis	Tumor invades prevertebral space, encases carotid artery, or invades mediastinal structures.

From American Joint Committee on Cancer. *AJCC Cancer Staging Manual.* 7th ed. New York: Springer-Verlag; 2002, with permission.

- Patients with **stage I and stage II SCCHN** as a group have survival rate of 70% to 80% with standard therapy, which includes either surgery or radiotherapy alone. Surgery is generally the preferred approach in operable patients, because it is typically associated with less morbidity than RT. Definitive RT is reserved for patients who cannot tolerate surgery or for whom surgical resection would result in particularly significant functional loss. Chemotherapy is unproven as first-line curative treatment for early SCCHN and should not be used outside the setting of a clinical trial. Although outcomes with primary surgery and definitive RT are comparable, neither surgery nor RT has been compared in a randomized trial. Thus, outcomes are based upon retrospective reviews or uncontrolled case series.
- Unfortunately, patients often present with **advanced locoregional disease** and carry poor prognosis with survival rate of 50% to 60% at 2 years with standard therapy.[5] Failure to control the tumor occurs via two biologically distinct pathways: local recurrence and/or metastatic spread. This makes the treatment of locoregionally advanced SCCHN complex as it continues to evolve. Patients with tumors amenable to surgical resection undergo surgery followed by adjuvant therapy with postoperative radiation or concurrent chemoradiation. For patients with locally advanced, unresectable disease, the standard of care is definitive concurrent chemoradiation for patients who can tolerate such therapy because an 8% survival advantage for concurrent chemoradiation compared to radiation alone, particularly with the use of platinum chemotherapy, was shown by meta-analyses of more than 10,000 patients from 63 randomized trials. Usually this entails the use of cisplatin, 100 mg/m^2, on days 1, 22, and 43 of a 7-week course of 70 Gy of radiation. More recently, an epidermal growth factor receptor (EGFR) inhibitor, cetuximab (Erbitux), has demonstrated benefits when used concurrently with radiation. In patients who do not achieve a complete tumor response after definitive chemoradiation, surgical resection of residual tumor may improve survival.
- In patients with **distant metastases,** several standard chemotherapeutic agents have significant activity against SCCHN and can provide palliation of symptoms. These include cisplatin, carboplatin, 5-fluorouracil (5-FU), paclitaxel, docetaxel, pemetrexed, methotrexate, ifosfamide, and gemcitabine. The most commonly used first-line therapy is a platinum compound combined with a second agent, usually a taxane or 5-FU. First-line therapy typically has a tumor response rate of ~20% to 30%. Targeted therapy also has a significant role in the management of SCCHN. Cetuximab has recently been found to extend survival in recurrent and/or metastatic SCCHN when added to chemotherapy. Cetuximab is also a reasonable option for platinum-resistant disease.

COMPLICATIONS

- A multidisciplinary approach is essential to minimize the complications of the malignancy and treatment. **Complications of disease** include weight loss, aspiration, and airway compromise. Nutritional support in the form of oral supplements or enteral feedings may be needed when caloric intake is inadequate. Tracheostomy may be needed in cases of airway compromise. Head and neck tumors may also invade into key structures, such as the carotid artery, leading to major bleeding, which may be a terminal event. Invasion into neural structures may lead to neuropathic pain syndromes. Amitriptyline or gabapentin may be helpful in such cases. The limitation to swallowing imposed by some head and neck cancers can make pain management difficult. In such cases, transdermal fentanyl patches or methadone elixir can be used in conjunction with concentrated opiate elixirs (breakthrough) for pain relief.

- **Complications of treatment** include complications of surgery, acute radiation toxicity, late radiation effects, and complications of chemotherapy. **Acute radiation toxicity** may include severe mucositis, with resulting pain and difficulties with swallowing. Concurrent chemoradiation increases the risk of severe mucositis beyond radiation alone. Oral candidiasis complicating mucositis may be treated with topical or systemic antifungal agents. Many patients find a cocktail of equal volume of diphenhydramine suspension, nystatin, viscous lidocaine, and aluminum hydroxide/magnesium hydroxide ("magic mouthwash") as a topical oral swish-and-swallow solution to be helpful. Opiates can also help in pain management, especially in severe cases. Skin toxicity should be treated with emollients. **Late radiation effects** include xerostomia, dental caries, osteoradionecrosis, and fibrosis of neck tissues resulting in trismus, lymphedema, and loss of range of motion. Xerostomia can be treated with cholinergic stimulants such as pilocarpine to improve salivary flow. Other measures, including topical lubricants, lozenges, coating agents, and artificial saliva, may provide some transient relief. The risk of dental caries should be minimized with good dental care. Osteoradionecrosis may be treated conservatively with antibiotics, hyperbaric oxygen therapy, or surgical debridement. Exercises may help in prevention of trismus associated with radiation therapy. With neck irradiation, hypothyroidism may occur, which can be treated with thyroid replacement therapy.
- The **complications of chemotherapy** are dependent on the agents used. Platinum compounds, a mainstay of chemotherapy in head and neck cancer, are known to cause significant nausea, nephrotoxicity, ototoxicity, myelosuppression, and peripheral neuropathy. 5-FU, another commonly used agent, is associated with mucositis and myelosuppression. Cetuximab, a newer agent, is associated with rash, diarrhea, hypomagnesemia, paronychial inflammation, and hypersensitivity infusion reactions.

MONITORING/FOLLOW-UP

Patients should have close follow-up for evaluation of local recurrence and distant metastases, as well as physical therapy and speech pathology follow-up if needed. In addition, patients should be advised on tobacco and alcohol cessation.

PROGNOSIS

Patients with recurrent or metastatic squamous cell carcinomas of the head and neck have a median survival of 6 to 9 months, and a 1-year survival rate of 20% to 40% when treated with chemotherapy alone.[6] Common sites of distant metastases include the bone, lung, and liver.

NASOPHARYNGEAL CARCINOMA

GENERAL PRINCIPLES

Epidemiology

Nasopharyngeal carcinoma has a different epidemiology and a separate set of risk factors from the other head and neck cancers. Although rare in the United States, it is endemic in the Far and Middle East and in Africa, especially in Southern China and Southeast Asia. It accounts for 18% of newly diagnosed malignancies in Southeast China.

Risk Factors

In Southeast Asia, nasopharyngeal cancer is associated with **Epstein–Barr virus infection** in genetically predisposed individuals. Other risk factors have been implicated, including diet (consumption of salted fish and low intake of fresh fruits and vegetables) and smoking.

DIAGNOSIS

Clinical Presentation

Nasopharyngeal cancer can present with a painless neck mass, but other symptoms include nasal obstruction, epistaxis, dysphagia, odynophagia, and Eustachian tube obstruction with otitis media. Tumors may extend through the foramen ovale to access the middle cranial fossa and the cavernous sinus to involve the oculomotor, trochlear, trigeminal, and abducens nerves leading to cranial neuropathy. In advanced cases, the optic nerve and orbital invasion can occur. Headaches, weight loss, trismus, and referred pain to the ear and neck can also be symptoms. Physical examination should include a thorough examination of the nares and oral cavity and the cranial nerves. Proptosis suggests orbital invasion by the tumor.

Diagnostic Testing

Workup of patients with nasopharyngeal cancer should include a thorough physical evaluation and diagnostic imaging with **CT** or **MRI** from the skull down to the clavicles. **Endoscopy** should also be performed. A **chest x-ray** or CT scan should be done to assess for pulmonary metastases. The staging for nasopharynx is according to the American Joint Committee on Cancer TNM system (Tables 23-7 and 23-8).

TREATMENT

Nasopharyngeal carcinoma is very sensitive to **chemoradiation. Early-stage disease (stages I and II)** is typically treated with radiation therapy alone. For local recurrences, surgical resection or repeat irradiation are options for treatment. For **advanced disease (stages III and IV),** concurrent chemoradiation followed by adjuvant cisplatin and 5-FU has demonstrated benefit in terms of overall survival, progression-free survival, and control of local disease and distant metastases.[7] **Metastatic disease** is managed with chemotherapeutic agents such as cisplatin, carboplatin, and 5-FU.

TABLE 23-7 STAGING OF NASOPHARYNX CANCER

Primary tumor (T)	
TX	Primary tumor cannot be assessed.
T0	No evidence of primary tumor
Tis	Carcinoma in situ
T1	Tumor confined to the nasopharynx
T2	Tumor extends to soft tissues of oropharynx and/or nasal fossa.
T2a	Without parapharyngeal extension
T2b	With parapharyngeal extension
T3	Tumor invades bony structures and/or paranasal sinuses.
T4	Tumor with intracranial extension and/or involvement of cranial nerves, infratemporal fossa, hypopharynx, or orbit
Regional lymph nodes (N)	
NX	Regional lymph nodes cannot be assessed.
N0	No regional lymph node metastasis
N1	Unilateral metastasis in lymph node(s), ≤6 cm in greatest dimension, above the supraclavicular fossa
N2	Bilateral metastasis in lymph node(s), ≤6 cm in greatest dimension, above the supraclavicular fossa
N3	Metastasis in a lymph node(s)
N3a	>6 cm in dimension
N3b	Extension to the supraclavicular fossa
Distant metastasis (M)	
MX	Distant metastasis cannot be assessed.
M0	No distant metastasis
M1	Distant metastasis

—
From American Joint Committee on Cancer. *AJCC Cancer Staging Manual.* 7th ed. New York: Springer-Verlag; 2002, with permission.

SALIVARY GLAND TUMORS

GENERAL PRINCIPLES

Salivary gland tumors may arise either in the major glands, namely, the parotid, submandibular, and sublingual glands, or in the minor glands located in the oral mucosa, palate, uvula, floor of the mouth, posterior tongue, retromolar area and peritonsillar area, pharynx, larynx, and paranasal sinuses. Salivary gland tumors account for ~5% of all head and neck cancers and are varied in their histologic patterns as low- or high-grade malignancies. Approximately 80% arise from the parotid gland, but of those, 80% are benign. In contrast, 95% to 100% of tumors arising from the sublingual gland are malignant.

TABLE 23-8 AJCC STAGE GROUPING: NASOPHARYNX

Stage 0	Tis	N0	M0
Stage I	T1	N0	M0
Stage IIA	T2a	N0	M0
Stage IIB	T1	N1	M0
	T2	N1	M0
	T2a	N1	M0
	T2b	N0	M0
	T2b	N1	M0
Stage III	T1	N2	M0
	T2a	N2	M0
	T2b	N2	M0
	T3	N0	M0
	T3	N1	M0
	T3	N2	M0
Stage IVA	T4	N0	M0
	T4	N1	M0
	T4	N2	M0
Stage IVB	Any T	N3	M0
Stage IVC	Any T	Any N	M1

From American Joint Committee on Cancer. *AJCC Cancer Staging Manual*. 7th ed. New York: Springer-Verlag; 2002, with permission.

TREATMENT

Treatment usually involves **surgical resection** of the gland. Prognosis is more favorable for low-grade tumors and those located in major glands, especially in the parotid. For aggressive or bulky tumors, resection is often combined with postoperative radiation.

NECK MASS WITH AN UNKNOWN PRIMARY

DIAGNOSIS

Differential Diagnosis

The differential diagnosis for a malignant neck mass includes squamous cell carcinoma, adenocarcinoma, lymphoma, thyroid neoplasms, and melanoma.

Diagnostic Testing

As cancers that originate elsewhere in the body can also present with a neck mass, a thorough history and physical should be performed, along with evaluation for potential primary sites. A **fine-needle biopsy for cytology** may be pursued as the initial step for evaluation of a neck mass without a clear primary. Open biopsy may be helpful if the suspicion for lymphoma is high. If the cytology shows squamous cell carcinoma, then endoscopy with blind biopsy of potential sites in the nasopharynx, tonsils, base of tongue, and pyriform sinus should be performed.

TREATMENT

If no primary site is found and the tumor is amenable to resection, surgical resection may be the primary therapy. If the surgical pathology shows extracapsular extension or involvement of multiple nodes, postoperative radiation may be given. If the tumor is not amenable to surgical resection, radiation therapy is the primary treatment modality.

REFERENCES

1. Haddad RI, Shin DM. Recent advances in head and neck cancer. *N Engl J Med.* 2008; 359:1143–1154.
2. Van Dyke DL, Worsham MJ, Benninger MS, et al. Recurrent cytogenetic abnormalities in squamous cell carcinomas of the head and neck region. *Genes Chromosomes Cancer.* 1994;9(3):192–206.
3. Chung CH, Ely K, McGavran L, et al. Increased epidermal growth factor receptor gene copy number is associated with poor prognosis in head and neck squamous cell carcinomas. *Clin Oncol.* 2006;24(25):4170–4176.
4. D'Souza G, Kreimer AR, Viscidi R, et al. Case-control study of human papillomavirus and oropharyngeal cancer. *N Engl J Med.* 2007;356:1944–1956.
5. Forastiere AA, Goepfert H, Maor M, et al. Concurrent chemotherapy and radiotherapy for organ preservation in advanced laryngeal cancer. *N Engl J Med.* 2003;349:2091–2098.
6. Colevas AD. Chemotherapy options for patients with metastatic or recurrent squamous cell carcinoma of the head and neck. *J Clin Oncol.* 2006;24:2644–2652.
7. Al-Sarraf M, LeBlanc M, Shanker Giri PG, et al. Chemoradiotherapy versus radiotherapy in patients with advanced nasopharyngeal cancer: phase III randomized intergroup study 0099. *J Clin Oncol.* 1998;16:1310–1317.

Sarcoma

24

Brian A. Van Tine

GENERAL PRINCIPLES

Sarcomas (from the Greek *sarx* for flesh) are a rare group of malignancies of the connective tissue. They represent over 100 different histologies of tumors derived from the mesenchymal or ectodermal germ layers. The presenting signs and symptoms depend on the anatomic site of origin and can vary markedly. In general, sarcomas can be divided into two large groups: soft tissue tumors and bone tumors.

Epidemiology

Sarcomas are rare tumors, comprising 1% of adult malignancies and 7% of pediatric malignancies. Sarcomas occur with equal frequency in both genders.[1] In the United States in 2010, the estimated incidence of soft tissue sarcomas (STSs) and bone sarcomas is 13,170 cases per year, with 5380 deaths expected.[1] Compared to other rare tumors, sarcomas carry a high mortality rate.

Risk Factors

Most cases of sarcoma are sporadic; however, a number of etiologic factors have been identified, as detailed below.

- **Radiation**
  Sarcomas have been found to originate in or near tissues that have received prior external-beam radiation therapy and tend to develop at least 2 years after radiation therapy, but can develop decades after radiation.[2–4] The majority of these lesions are high grade, and they are typically osteosarcomas, malignant fibrous histiocytomas, and angiosarcomas. The relative risk of radiation-induced sarcoma is 0.6 for patients that receive 10 Gy of radiation and 38.3 for patients that receive 60 Gy.[5]
- **Chemical exposure**
  Thorotrast, an IV contrast dye, has been found to cause hepatic angiosarcomas.[6] Other agents such as vinyl chloride,[7] arsenic,[8] and dioxin in chemical workers and farmers but not in Vietnam Veterans (i.e., dioxin is in Agent Orange) has also been linked to sarcomas.[9] Alkylating chemotherapy, particularly when used to treat childhood malignancies, has also been associated with the development of sarcomas in adulthood.[5]
- **Genetic conditions**
  Patients with neurofibromatosis type I have a 10% risk of developing a malignant peripheral nerve sheath tumor.[10] Sarcomas also occur in patients with Li-Fraumeni syndrome.[11] Familial retinoblastoma is linked to the development of osteosarcoma[5] and Werner syndrome is a risk factor for multiple types of sarcomas.[12]

- **Other risks associated with sarcomas**
  Lymphangiosarcomas have been known to develop in a lymphedematous arm after mastectomy (Stewart-Treves syndrome).[13] Kaposi sarcoma is associated with co-infection with the human immunodeficiency virus and the human herpes virus 8.[14] Paget disease of bone is a risk factor for the development of osteosarcoma or fibrosarcoma.[15]

SPECIAL CONSIDERATIONS

The treatment of sarcoma is complex because sarcoma is an ever growing group of many very rare diseases that are historically treated as large group in clinical trials. As many of specific subtypes are driven by known translocations, the treatment and understanding of each individual subtype is rapidly evolving.[16–18] Translocation-based treatment of sarcoma is the reason patients with **sarcomas should be treated by physicians that specifically sub-specialize in the treatment of sarcoma.**

SOFT TISSUE SARCOMAS

DIAGNOSIS

Clinical Presentation

Soft tissue sarcomas represent greater than 75% of all sarcomas diagnosed each year.[1] Patients typically present with an asymptomatic mass. Pain may be present if there is entrapment of neurovascular structures or involvement of bone. Sarcomas may grow quite large before they become obvious on physical exam.[19]

- **Extremity sarcomas**
  Approximately half of all soft tissue sarcomas arise in the extremities. The majority are first seen as a painless soft tissue mass.
- **Retroperitoneal sarcomas**
  Most patients have an abdominal mass and approximately half have abdominal pain that is vague and nonspecific. Weight loss is seen less frequently, with early satiety, nausea, and emesis occurring in <40% of patients. Neurologic symptoms, particularly paresthesia, occur in up to 30% of patients.[20,21]

Physical Examination

Physical examination of a patient presenting with a soft tissue mass should include an assessment of the size of the mass and its mobility with respect to the underlying tissue. If a mass is >5 cm and deep, it should be presumed to be sarcoma until proven otherwise. High-grade sarcomas may have significant necrosis and can be confused with a hematoma or abscess. A site-specific neurovascular examination should also be performed.

Differential Diagnosis

The differential diagnosis includes benign soft tissue tumors as well as carcinoma, lymphoma, and melanoma. The most common benign tumors include lipoma, desmoid tumor, neurofibroma, hemangioma, and schwannoma.

Diagnostic Testing

Imaging

Patients with masses suspicious for sarcoma should undergo **radiologic evaluation and biopsy.** The studies needed for adequate staging vary depending on the site of disease. Sarcoma of the head and neck or extremities should be evaluated with **plain films** and **MRI.** Plain films may reveal soft tissue mineralization (which is typical for synovial sarcoma) or may reveal skeletal reaction to the tumor. MRI is valuable for assessing fat and distinguishing it from surrounding tissues. This may assist in the diagnosis of the lesion and allows for planning of the biopsy and subsequent surgery. For retroperitoneal and abdominal sarcomas, CT is the imaging modality of choice, as this provides the best anatomic definition of the tumor.

In addition to evaluating the primary lesion with imaging, **distant metastatic disease** may also be assessed. STS spreads *hematogenously,* and the **lung** is the **most common site** of metastasis. Chest x-ray may be sufficient for small, low-grade lesions, but in patients with high-grade tumors or tumors larger than 5 cm, a staging CT of the chest should be performed.

Diagnostic Procedures

- An accurate biopsy diagnosis is essential for STS. Any lesion >5 cm or any rapidly growing lesion should be biopsied. The placement of the biopsy tract is also critical, as it can be seeded with tumor and must be excised at the time of resection. Generally, the preferred technique is open incisional biopsy performed by a surgeon with experience in resection of STS. Hemostasis is also very important, as a hematoma may require enlarging radiation fields or may interfere with resection planning.
- **Histologic evaluation** should be performed at an experienced center, as **grade is critically important to determining prognosis.** STSs are named for their tissue of origin based on light microscopy examination, and there are many possible histological types (Table 24-1). Tumors are also carefully evaluated for grade, which takes into account cellularity, mitotic activity, nuclear atypia, and necrosis. In general, the *grade, size,* and *depth* are more important factors than the histologic type. Immunohistochemistry and FISH studies are used to subclassify STS. The three most common types of STS are malignant fibrous histiocytoma, liposarcoma, and leiomyosarcoma.

TABLE 24-1 GUIDELINES TO THE HISTOLOGIC GRADING OF SARCOMAS

Low-Grade Sarcomas	High-Grade Sarcomas
Good differentiation	Poor differentiation
Hypocellularity	Hypercellularity
Increased stroma	Minimal stroma
Hypovascularity	Hypervascularity
Minimal necrosis	Much necrosis
<5 mitoses per high-power field	>5 mitoses per high-power field

Adapted from Hajdu SI, Shiu MH, Brennan MF. The role of the pathologist in the management of soft tissue sarcomas. *World J Surg.* 1988;12:326–331, with permission.

TREATMENT

Early-Stage Disease (Stages I to III)

- **Extremity soft tissue sarcomas**
  - **Surgery.** Surgery is the mainstay of therapy for early-stage STSs of the extremities. Sarcomas grow along planes and grossly appear to be well encapsulated. However, they usually extend into the pseudocapsule (an area around the tumor that is composed of tumor fimbriae and normal tissue), and "shelling-out" of lesions is associated with high local recurrence rates, 37% to 63%. In the past, radical excision and amputation were utilized to avoid this problem. Over the past 20 years, there has been a gradual shift in the surgical management of extremity soft tissue sarcomas away from radical ablative surgery toward limb-sparing surgery. Amputation is only required in ~5% of patients today.
  - **Radiation therapy.** Wide local excision alone is all that is necessary for small (T1), low-grade, STSs of the extremities, with a local recurrence rate of <10%. **Adjuvant radiation therapy,** however, is required in a number of situations: (a) virtually all high-grade extremity sarcomas, (b) lesions larger than 5 cm (T2), and (c) positive or equivocal surgical margins in patients for whom re-excision is impractical. When adjuvant radiation is planned, metal clips should be placed at margins of resection to facilitate radiation field planning. **Neoadjuvant radiation** may be needed prior to definitive resection. This is most commonly performed for tumors that are borderline resectable or for tumors located adjacent to the joint capsule. A phase III National Cancer Institute of Canada trial comparing adjuvant (postoperative) and neoadjuvant (preoperative) radiation demonstrated similar local control rates, metastatic outcome, and overall survival rates between the two arms. However, patients receiving preoperative radiation had a significantly higher incidence of wound complications (35% vs. 17%).[22]
    - **Radiation as definitive therapy** alone in the treatment of unresectable or medically inoperable soft tissue sarcoma patients yields a 5-year survival rate of 25% to 40% and a local control rate of 30%. Radiation doses should be at least 65 Gy, if feasible, given the site of the lesion.
    - **Brachytherapy** also has been used in treatment for sarcomas. Iridium-192 is the most commonly used agent. It has similar local control rates to adjuvant external beam radiation and has the advantage of a decrease in the patient's entire treatment from 10 to 12 weeks to 10 to 12 days. In addition, smaller volumes of tissues are irradiated, which may be useful if important structures, such as joints, are nearby.
  - **Adjuvant chemotherapy.** The benefit of adjuvant chemotherapy for extremity STSs is controversial. The only exception to this is rhabdomyosarcomas, in which adjuvant chemotherapy is accepted as standard of care.
    - A formal meta-analysis of individual data from 1568 patients who participated in 13 trials was performed by the Sarcoma Meta-Analysis Collaboration. The analysis demonstrated a significant reduction in the risk of local or distant recurrence in patients who received adjuvant chemotherapy. There also was a decrease in the risk of distant relapse (metastasis) by 30% in treated patients. Overall survival, however, did not meet criteria for statistical significance between the control group

and adjuvant chemotherapy arm, with a hazard ratio of 0.89.[23] Most of the randomized trials examined in this meta-analysis were limited by patient numbers, inclusion of all subtypes of STS and of low-grade tumors, heterogeneous patient and disease characteristics, and varied chemotherapy regimens.

- Certain subgroups of patients, such as those with high-grade lesions, may benefit from adjuvant chemotherapy, but further studies are needed.

- **Retroperitoneal sarcomas**
  - **Surgery.** As with other soft tissue sarcomas, surgery is the primary treatment of retroperitoneal sarcomas. Tumors that are <5 cm and that not located close to adjacent viscera or critical neurovascular structures are considered resectable. If a tumor is thought to be a sarcoma and is resectable, a preoperative biopsy is not necessary. One should consider a preoperative CT-guided core biopsy if an incomplete resection is a reasonable possibility to allow neoadjuvant therapy.
    - Unfortunately, only 50% of patients with early-stage retroperitoneal sarcomas are able to undergo complete surgical resection. Of the tumors removed, approximately half will develop a local recurrence. Adjuvant therapy, therefore, plays an important role in the management of retroperitoneal sarcomas.
  - **Radiation therapy. Adjuvant radiation** therapy is most frequently recommended for patients with high-grade tumors or positive margins. The radiation is typically started 3 to 8 weeks following surgery to allow wound healing. Two-year local control rates of 70% have been reported with the addition of postoperative radiation therapy. **Neoadjuvant radiation therapy** can be given to patients with marginally resectable tumors and to those in whom one would expect postoperative radiotherapy to be required. It has a number of advantages over postoperative radiotherapy including smaller radiation portals and reduction of the extent of the surgical procedure.
  - **Management of unresectable, locally advanced retroperitoneal sarcomas.** Unresectable retroperitoneal sarcomas can be managed in a number of ways. Radiation therapy can be given for palliation and with the hope that the tumor could be made resectable. Palliative surgery to reduce local symptoms can be performed. Chemotherapy can also be administered (see management of metastatic patients for specific regimens).

Stage IV Metastatic Soft Tissue Sarcomas

Metastatic STSs can be divided into limited metastasis and extensive metastasis. **Limited metastatic disease** is defined as resectable metastasis involving one organ system. The prognosis of these two subsets of patients is very different. **It is possible to cure limited metastatic disease,** whereas patients with extensive metastatic disease can only be palliated.

- **Management of limited metastatic disease.** For patients with a limited number of pulmonary metastases, metastasectomy has been performed with some improvement in survival compared with no surgery. In patients with visceral sarcomas and limited liver metastasis, it is sometimes possible to perform a metastasectomy by surgery, chemoembolization, or radiofrequency ablation.

- **Management of extensive metastatic disease.** The goal of therapy for patients with metastatic sarcoma is palliation and prolongation of survival. Cure is no longer a viable goal. Systemic chemotherapy is the primary modality of treatment. Radiation and surgery may be used with a goal of palliation.

  Numerous chemotherapy agents have been used as single agents or in combination for the treatment of soft tissue sarcomas. These include epirubicin, doxorubicin, ifosfamide, cyclophosphamide, dacarbazine, gemcitabine, and taxanes amongst others.

PROGNOSIS

- The most important prognostic factors for STS are **size, grade, depth,** and **relationship to fascial planes.** The American Joint Committee on Cancer (AJCC) staging system for STSs incorporates histologic grade (G), size of the primary (T), nodal involvement (N), and distant metastasis (M) (Table 24-2).[24]
- Grade of the tumor is the predominant feature predicting early metastatic recurrence and death. Beyond 2 years of follow-up, the size of the lesion becomes as important as the histologic grade.
- Nomograms exist for the relapse-free survival prediction by histology.

BONE SARCOMAS

GENERAL PRINCIPLES

Bone sarcoma may arise from any tissue within the bones. The most common bone sarcomas are osteosarcoma, chondrosarcoma, and Ewing sarcoma.

Classification

- **Osteosarcoma**

  Osteosarcoma is the most common primary bone tumor, accounting for 40% to 50% of bone sarcomas.[25] It usually presents with pain and swelling. Approximately 60% occur in adolescents and children. Ten percent may occur in the third decade. There is a second peak in the fifth and sixth decades, which is frequently due to radiation-associated osteosarcomas or transformation of existing lesions. They are spindle cell neoplasms that produce bone and are more common in long bones. Most osteosarcomas occur in the metaphyseal region, near the growth plate, of skeletally immature long bones. The distal femur, proximal tibia, and proximal humerus are common sites. The majority is classified as "classic," and this type is more common at between 10 and 20 years of age. Most of these lesions are high grade and highly vascular.
- **Chondrosarcoma**

  Chondrosarcoma is the second most frequent malignant primary bone tumor, representing approximately 20% of bone sarcomas. They generally occur between the fourth and the sixth decades. They tend to develop in flat bones, including the shoulder and pelvic girdles. They may arise de novo or from pre-existing lesions. They are indolent and are generally low grade. Chondrosarcoma may arise peripherally or centrally. Imaging studies may be bland, particularly in central lesions, which may make it difficult to distinguish between benign

TABLE 24-2 AJCC STAGING SYSTEM FOR SOFT TISSUE SARCOMA

Primary Tumor (T)	Regional Lymph Nodes (N)	Distant Metastasis (M)	Grade (G)	Stage
TX: primary tumor cannot be assessed	NX: regional lymph node involvement cannot be assessed		GX: grade cannot be assessed G1: low, well differentiated	Stage IA: T1a,b N0 M0 G1, GX T2a,b N0 M0, G1, GX Stage IB: T2a, bN0 M0 G1, GX T2a,b N0 M0, G1, GX
T0: no evidence of primary tumor	N0: no regional lymph node metastasis	M0: no distant metastasis	G2: intermediate, moderately well differentiated	Stage IIA: T1a,b N0 M0, G2–3; T2a N0 M0, G2–3
T1: tumor is <5 cm in greatest dimension T1a: tumor is located above and without invasion of the superficial fascia T1b: tumor is located below and/or with invasion of the superficial fascia T2: tumor is >5 cm in greatest dimension T2a: tumor is located above and without invasion of the superficial fascia T2b: tumor is located below and/or with invasion of the superficial fascia	N1: regional lymph node metastasis	M1: distant metastasis	G3: high; poorly differentiated	Stage III: T2a, T2b N0 M0, G3 Any T, N1, Mo, Any G Stage IV: any T, any N M1, any G

From American Joint Committee on Cancer. *AJCC Cancer Staging Manual.* 7th ed. New York: Springer-Verlag, 2010, with permission.

and malignant lesions. New pain, increasing size, and signs of inflammation point toward malignant lesions. In general, these malignancies are resistant to chemotherapy and radiation.

- **Ewing sarcoma**
  Ewing sarcoma accounts for 10% to 15% of bone sarcomas, and incidence peaks in the second decade. It is the second most common malignant tumor of the bone in childhood and adolescence. It tends to occur in the diaphysis of long bones. The femoral diaphysis is the most common location. These are highly aggressive tumors and are best considered a systemic disease. A characteristic chromosomal translocation, *t*(11:22), is associated with this sarcoma and with peripheral primitive neuroectodermal tumor (PNET). Ewing sarcoma is one of the small, round, blue cell tumors.

DIAGNOSIS

An accurate tissue biopsy is needed for diagnosis. Imaging studies may be suggestive of tumor type; however, it can be difficult to distinguish benign and malignant bone tumors. Biopsy specimens are used to determine the histologic type of tumor as well as the grade. As with STSs, **open incisional biopsy is preferred for bone sarcomas.** The biopsy should be performed by a surgeon experienced in sarcoma so that it does not compromise the definitive surgical procedure.

Clinical Presentation

History

Localized pain and swelling are the hallmark clinical features of bone sarcomas. The pain is initially insidious but can become unremitting. Occasionally, a pathologic fracture will bring the patient to medical attention. If the tumor arises in the lower extremities, the patient may have a limp. Constitutional symptoms are rare but can be observed in patients with Ewing sarcoma or patients with metastatic disease. A pertinent history should note how long a lesion has been present and any change in it. Rapid growth or change in a lesion favors a malignant etiology.

Physical Exam

Physical exam may reveal a palpable mass. A joint effusion may be observed, and range of motion of the joint may be limited, with stiffness or pain. Neurovascular and lymph node examinations are usually normal.

Diagnostic Testing

Imaging

- Patients who are suspected to have bone sarcoma should undergo imaging studies, including plain films, MRI, and biopsy.
- **Plain films** may demonstrate characteristic lesions for bone sarcoma. Osteosarcoma is associated with destructive lesions showing a moth-eaten appearance. In addition, a spiculated periosteal reaction and cuff of periosteal new bone may be seen. Plain films in chondrosarcoma show lesions with a lobulated appearance with punctate or annular calcification of cartilage. Ewing sarcoma is associated with an "onion peel" periosteal reaction and soft tissue mass. Metastatic disease may be associated with either osteolytic or osteoblastic lesions, depending on the type of primary malignancy.

- **MRI** is the imaging modality of choice to evaluate the relationship of the tumor to surrounding structures and determine resectability. CT scan of the primary site may be considered in place of MRI to demonstrate cortical destruction more accurately and for evaluation of pelvic tumors. CT scan of the chest is used to evaluate for pulmonary metastases. **Bone scan** helps to evaluate for the local extent of the tumor as well as to evaluate for other lesions.

Diagnostic Procedures

- Tissue biopsy, preferably open incisional biopsy, is essential for diagnosis.
- Bone sarcomas are staged using the American Joint Committee on Cancer staging system based on grade, tumor size, and metastatic disease as reported in Table 24-3. Adverse prognostic indicators include elevated lactate dehydrogenase (LDH), elevated alkaline phosphatase, and an axial primary. Patients with Ewing sarcoma should have bilateral bone marrow biopsies as part of staging.

TREATMENT

The treatment of bone sarcoma is dependent on histologic subtype.

- **General principles of local therapy**
  - **Surgical excision is the mainstay of treatment for patients with low-grade bone sarcomas. For high-grade tumors, multimodality therapy is indicated.** As an example, for high-grade osteosarcomas, preoperative multiagent chemotherapy is followed by surgical removal of the tumor and then further adjuvant chemotherapy. **Physical therapy** and **prosthetics** are of great importance in these patients because of the highly invasive nature of the treatment.
  - The Musculoskeletal Tumor Society and the National Comprehensive Cancer Network (NCCN) recognize wide excision, either by amputation or by a limb-salvage procedure, as the recommended surgical approach for all high-grade bone sarcomas. This type of resection is predicated on complete tumor removal, effective skeletal reconstruction, and adequate soft tissue coverage.
- **Osteosarcoma therapy.** The 5-year survival for osteosarcoma with surgery alone is <20%. This occurs because microscopic metastatic dissemination is likely to be present in 80% of patients at the time of diagnosis. The addition of adjuvant chemotherapy has improved survival for high-grade osteosarcoma, permitting long-term survival as high as 80% is selected patients.
  - **Neoadjuvant and adjuvant chemotherapy.** Neoadjuvant chemotherapy began as a strategy to permit limb-sparing surgery, allows time for creation of custom-made prosthetics. Since its acceptance, other advantages have been recognized with this approach. It permits earlier treatment of occult micrometastatic disease, preventing emergence of resistant clones and potentially allows for the debulking of the primary to improve chances for limb-sparing surgery.
    - Chemotherapeutic agents active in osteosarcomas include doxorubicin, cisplatin, ifosfamide, and high-dose methotrexate with leucovorin rescue. These agents are typically used in combination to improve response, although the optimal combination and duration of therapy remain controversial.
    - Histologic response to preoperative therapy is recognized as a significant prognostic factor. Various systems have been developed for grading histologic

TABLE 24-3 AJCC STAGING SYSTEM FOR BONE SARCOMA

Primary Tumor (T)	Regional Lymph Nodes (N)	Distant Metastasis (M)	Grade (G)	Stage
TX: primary tumor cannot be assessed	NX: regional lymph node involvement cannot be assessed		GX: grade cannot be assessed G1: low, well differentiated	Stage IA: T1 N0 M0, G1; G2 low grade, GX
T0: no evidence of primary tumor	N0: no regional lymph node metastasis	M0: no distant metastasis	G2: low, moderately differentiated	Stage IB: T2 N0 M0, G1; G2 low grade, GX T3 N0 M0, G1; G2 low grade, GX
T1: tumor ≤8 cm in greatest dimension	N1: regional lymph node metastasis	M1: distant metastasis	G3: high; poorly differentiated	Stage IIA: T1 N0 M0, G3; G4
T2: tumor is >8 cm in greatest dimension		M1a: lung metastasis	G4: undifferentiated (Ewing sarcoma)	Stage IIB: T2 N0 M0, G3; G4
T3: discontinuous tumors in the primary bone site		M2b: other sites of metastasis		Stage III: T3 N0 M0, any G Stage IVA: any T N0 M1a, any G Stage IVB: any T N1, any M, any G Any T, any N M1b, any G

From American Joint Committee on Cancer. *AJCC Cancer Staging Manual*. 7th ed. New York: Springer-Verlag, 2010, with permission.

response to chemotherapy, but >90% necrosis of tumor cells is associated with the best prognosis. If the tumor has been resected to negative margins and had a good histologic response to chemotherapy, the patient continues on chemotherapy for an additional 2 to 12 cycles. If the tumor was fully resected but has <90% necrosis, salvage chemotherapy with agents not used in induction is attempted, but the effect of this change in chemotherapy on outcomes is unclear. If the tumor margins are positive, additional local surgery should be attempted.

- **Radiation therapy.** Radiation is not routinely used in the therapy of osteosarcoma, but it may prove helpful in patients who refuse definitive resection or in palliation of patients with metastatic disease.
- **Management of metastatic disease.** Approximately 10% to 20% of patients with osteosarcoma have evidence of metastatic disease at presentation. Some of these patients may be candidates for the surgical resection of pulmonary metastases. For patients with more extensive metastatic disease, chemotherapy is used to provide control of disease and palliation of symptoms.

- **Ewing sarcoma**

Therapy for Ewing sarcoma and the related primitive peripheral neuroectodermal tumors uses a combined-modality approach.[26]

- **Treatment of the primary tumor.** The optimal treatment for local tumor control is not well defined. Historically, radiation therapy has been the mainstay of local therapy, but there has been a recent trend toward surgery. No prospective randomized trials have been performed to compare the two modalities, but retrospective data suggest improvements in local control and survival when surgery is done with a complete resection of the tumor. Patients with unresectable disease or positive margins require radiation therapy to improve local control.
- **Chemotherapy.** Before the availability of effective chemotherapeutic agents, <10% of patients with Ewing sarcoma survived beyond 5 years, despite the fact that only 15% to 35% of patients with Ewing sarcoma/primitive peripheral neuroectodermal tumors had evidence of metastatic disease at presentation. This suggests that many patients with Ewing sarcoma have occult microscopic dissemination of the disease at the time of diagnosis. The current standard regimen is to use vincristine, actinomycin D, and cyclophosphamide (VAC) alternating with ifosfamide and etoposide (IE).
- **Recurrent metastatic Ewing sarcoma.** In this setting, cure is not a realistic goal. Palliation and prolongation of survival are more realistic expectations. Fortunately, aggressive combination chemotherapy (VAC or IE) and radiation therapy can still lead to prolonged progression-free survival.

REFERENCES

1. Jemal A, Siegel R, Xu J, et al. Cancer Statistics, 2010. *CA Cancer J Clin.* 2010;60:277–300.
2. Brady MS, Gaynor JJ, Brennan MF. Radiation-associated sarcoma of bone and soft tissue. *Arch Surg.* 1992;127:1379–1385.
3. Robinson E, Neugut AI, Wylie P. Clinical aspects of postirradiation sarcomas. *J Natl Cancer Inst.* 1988;80:233–240.
4. Pitcher ME, Davidson TI, Fisher C, et al. Post irradiation sarcoma of soft tissue and bone. *Eur J Surg Oncol.* 1994;20:53–56.

5. Tucker MA, D'Angio GJ, Boice JD Jr, et al. Bone sarcomas linked to radiotherapy and chemotherapy in children. *N Engl J Med.* 1987;317:588–593.
6. Da Horta JS, Da Motta LC, Abbatt JD, et al. Malignancy and other late effects following administration of thorotrast. *Lancet.* 1965;1:201–205.
7. Creech JL Jr, Johnson MN. Angiosarcoma of liver in the manufacture of polyvinyl chloride. *J Occup Med.* 1974;16:150–151.
8. Falk H, Caldwell GG, Ishak KG, et al. Arsenic-related hepatic angiosarcoma. *Am J Ind Med.* 1981;2:43–50.
9. Steenland K, Bertazzi P, Baccarelli A, et al. Dioxin revisited: developments since the 1997 IARC classification of dioxin as a human carcinogen. *Environ Health Perspect.* 2004;112: 1265–1268.
10. Sorensen SA, Mulvihill JJ, Nielsen A. Long-term follow-up of von Recklinghausen neurofibromatosis. Survival and malignant neoplasms. *N Engl J Med.* 1986;314:1010–1015.
11. Schneider K, Garber J. Li-Fraumeni syndrome. *Gene Reviews Online Journal.* 2010. Last accessed 3/27/2011 <http://www.ncbi.nlm.nih.gov/books/NBK1311/>.
12. Yu CE, Oshima J, Fu YH, et al. Positional cloning of the Werner's syndrome gene. *Science.* 1996;272:258–262.
13. Chung KC, Kim HJE, Jeffers LLC. Lymphangiosarcoma (Stewart-Treves syndrome) in postmastectomy patients. *J Hand Surg Am.* 2000;25:1163–1168.
14. Mesri EA, Cesarman E, Boshoff C. Kaposi's sarcoma and its associated herpesvirus. *Nat Rev Cancer.* 2010;10:707–719.
15. Mankin HJ, Hornicek FJ. Paget's sarcoma: a historical and outcome review. *Clin Orthop Relat Res.* 2005;438:97–102.
16. Osuna D, de Alava E. Molecular pathology of sarcomas. *Rev Recent Clin Trials.* 2009;4:12–26.
17. Jain S, Xu R, Prieto VG, et al. Molecular classification of soft tissue sarcomas and its clinical applications. *Int J Clin Exp Pathol.* 2010;3:416–428.
18. Ordonez JL, Osuna D, Garcia-Dominguez DJ, et al. The clinical relevance of molecular genetics in soft tissue sarcomas. *Adv Anat Pathol.* 2010;17:162–181.
19. Luis AM, Aguilar DP, Martin JA. Multidisciplinary management of soft tissue sarcomas. *Clin Transl Oncol.* 2010;12:543–553.
20. Jaques DP, Coit DG, Hajdu SI, et al. Management of primary and recurrent soft-tissue sarcoma of the retroperitoneum. *Ann Surg.* 1990;212:51–59.
21. Alvarenga JC, Ball AB, Fisher C, et al. Limitations of surgery in the treatment of retroperitoneal sarcoma. *Br J Surg.* 1991;78:912–916.
22. O'Sullivan B, Davis AM, Turcotte R, et al. Preoperative versus postoperative radiotherapy in soft-tissue sarcoma of the limbs: a randomised trial. *Lancet.* 2002;359:2235–2241.
23. Sarcoma Meta-analysis Collaboration. Adjuvant chemotherapy for localised resectable soft-tissue sarcoma of adults: meta-analysis of individual data. Sarcoma meta-analysis collaboration. *Lancet.* 1997;350:1647–1654.
24. Edge S, Byrd D, Compton C, et al. *AJCC (American Joint Committee on Cancer) Cancer Staging Manual.* New York: Springer; 2010:291.
25. Maki RG. Pediatric sarcomas occurring in adults. *J Surg Oncol.* 2008;97:360–368.
26. Schiffman JD, Wright J. Ewing's sarcoma and second malignancies. *Sarcoma.* 2011:736841. Epub 2010 Oct 13.

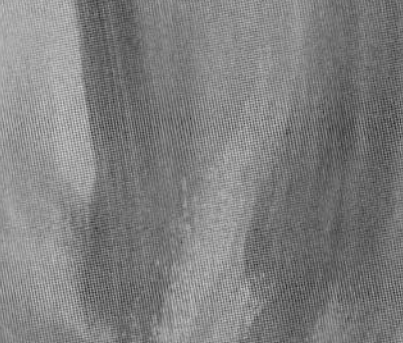

Endocrine Malignancies 25

Parvin F. Peddi

GENERAL PRINCIPLES

In 1954, a family was described with hyperparathyroidism and tumors of the pituitary and pancreatic islet cells. Now known as multiple endocrine neoplasia type I (MEN I), it is one of the most well-known hereditary endocrine neoplastic syndromes. Since then, our knowledge about the genetics and pathology of endocrine tumors has grown tremendously and has led to various new diagnostic and therapeutic measures. Endocrine neoplasms are a heterogenous group of tumors. This chapter will cover the most common types, including pituitary, thyroid, parathyroid, adrenal cortex, gastroenteropancreatic neuroendocrine, and pheochromocytoma, as well as the MEN syndromes.

THYROID CARCINOMA

GENERAL PRINCIPLES

Multiple histologic subtypes of thyroid cancer exist (Table 25-1), and together they account for >90% of all endocrine malignancies. The normal thyroid is composed of two main cell types. One is the follicular cell type that concentrates iodine and produces thyroid hormone. The other cell type is the parafollicular cell that produces calcitonin. Follicular cells give rise to well-differentiated cancers (papillary, follicular, and Hürthle) and anaplastic tumors. Parafollicular cells give rise to medullary thyroid carcinoma (MTC).

Epidemiology

According to American Cancer Society, 44,670 patients were diagnosed with thyroid cancer in 2010 and 1,690 died from it. Thyroid cancer is nearly twice as common in women as in men.

Risk Factors

Previous radiation exposure is the main risk factor with an average lag time of 25 years to cancer presentation. Other risk factors include female sex and family history. MTCs are different in that radiation exposure is not a risk factor and can occur sporadically (two-thirds) or in individuals who have either MEN II syndrome or familial MTC (one-third).

DIAGNOSIS

Clinical Presentation

Initial presentation is typically a solitary thyroid nodule. The majority of thyroid nodules are benign, and the history and physical exam assist in directing further

TABLE 25-1 THYROID CANCER HISTOLOGIC SUBTYPES AND KEY FEATURES

Histologic Subtype	% of Thyroid Cancers	Characteristics
Well-differentiated		Younger patients, relatively benign, indolent course. Metastases occur late and to bone, lungs, cervical lymph nodes, and skin. Surgery and radioactive iodine are treatments of choice.
Papillary	80	Psammoma bodies present on histology in 50%.
Follicular	12–20	Hürthle cell variety (3%) is more aggressive form.
Anaplastic (spindle cell)	2	Older patients, aggressive tumors with local invasion common and always considered stage IV. Metastases to lung common and advanced diseases are uniformly fatal. External-beam radiation is marginally effective.
Medullary thyroid carcinoma	5–9	Neoplasia of the parafollicular/C cells. Sporadic and inherited forms exist. Secrete calcitonin and occasionally ACTH. May cause diarrhea in advanced disease. Metastases to inferior surface of liver capsule typical. Treatment is surgical.

investigation. The probability of malignancy is higher if the nodule is found in men, individuals younger than 15 or older than 60 years, those with a positive family history, those with other diseases associated with MEN II (hyperparathyroidism, pheochromocytoma, or mucosal neuromas), and those with previous radiation exposure. A solitary, firm, immobile nodule or a rapid change in size is also of greater concern, as are symptoms of hoarseness, dyspnea, dysphagia, or new Horner syndrome. Symptoms of diarrhea and flushing are occasionally seen in advanced MTC due to hormone secretion.

Physical Examination

Exam should evaluate nodule size, firmness, mobility, and local lymphadenopathy. Nodules <1 cm in a patient without other risk factors may be followed with a repeat exam in 6 to 12 months. However, nodules >1 cm or a nodule of any size in a patient with one of the previously listed risk factors warrants further evaluation.

Diagnostic Testing

- **Ultrasound of the thyroid** is recommended; central hypervascularity, irregular borders, and/or microcalcifications suggest malignancy. Fine-needle aspiration

(FNA) is combined with ultrasound as the initial approach to establish diagnosis. If malignancy cannot be excluded by FNA, a lobectomy is usually performed to obtain adequate tissue for determining the correct diagnosis.

- Radioactive isotope scans and serologic testing with thyroid-stimulating hormone (TSH) and serum thyroglobulin assays are only useful in postoperative follow-up; they are not useful in making the diagnosis of thyroid malignancy, as most nodules are hypoactive regardless of presence or absence of malignancy. Calcitonin levels, however, should be checked at presentation and at follow-up exams for patients with MTC, as calcitonin serves as a sensitive tumor marker. In addition, those with MTC need to be evaluated for the *RET* proto-oncogene mutation, and a 24-hour urine for vanillylmandelic acid, catecholamines, and metanephrines is needed to evaluate for possible pheochromocytoma as part of MEN II syndrome.

Imaging

Once a diagnosis of malignancy is made, all individuals should have a **chest x-ray** to evaluate for metastases to the lung. An extensive staging workup is necessary only in anaplastic thyroid cancers, as they are often metastatic at presentation. Patients with anaplastic tumors should receive complete imaging of the neck with ultrasound or MRI and have a contrast-enhanced CT scan of the chest. Consideration should also be given to abdominal imaging with CT or MRI.

Staging

The staging of thyroid cancer is different from other malignancies. In addition to tumor size, it also depends on tumor histology and the patient's age at presentation. For example, in patients <45 years old, well-differentiated papillary or follicular cell carcinomas are never classified higher than stage II. On the other hand, all anaplastic tumors are classified as stage IV regardless of anatomic extent due to their aggressive nature and high potential for metastasizing. In MTC, staging information comes from evaluation of the total thyroidectomy and cervical lymph node dissection.

TREATMENT

Treatment of the three main types of thyroid cancer varies significantly. Radioactive iodine, external-beam radiation, surgery, and systemic chemotherapy each have their role in comprehensive therapeutic regimens.

- **Well-differentiated thyroid carcinoma (i.e., papillary, follicular, and Hürthle)** is mainly treated by surgical resection in all stages. Patients younger than 40 years have an excellent prognosis with thyroidectomy alone. Factors increasing the chance of recurrence include advanced age and tumor size >1 cm. For these patients, a total thyroidectomy is recommended; otherwise, unilateral lobectomy can be considered for smaller tumors. Recurrent laryngeal nerve damage resulting in hoarseness is an uncommon complication of thyroid lobectomy. A total thyroidectomy carries the additional risk of hypocalcemia from hypoparathyroidism. In more advanced disease, dissection of the central and lateral cervical lymph nodes should be considered.
    - **Radioiodine therapy** with ^{131}I induces cytotoxicity and is the key adjuvant therapeutic agent. External-beam radiation therapy, on the other hand, rarely has a role in differentiated thyroid carcinomas. There are two main indications

for use of ^{131}I. The first is to ablate residual normal thyroid tissue post–total thyroidectomy to improve the sensitivity of subsequent diagnostic ^{131}I scans in detecting recurrence. The second is to treat metastatic disease and destroy microscopic malignant foci. Follow-up imaging with ^{131}I determines treatment efficacy by revealing residual normal tissue as well as carcinoma. Treatment ends when there is no further radioactive iodine uptake present.

  - **Adjuvant hormonal therapy** with exogenous thyroid hormone is also routinely used in well-differentiated thyroid carcinomas to suppress TSH, since both normal and neoplastic thyroid tissue depend on TSH for growth. In addition, thyroid hormone is also necessary to prevent symptoms of hypothyroidism. One should keep in mind, however, the potential side effects of higher rates of bone loss and an increased incidence of atrial fibrillation. Suppression of TSH to undetectable levels for the initial 5 to 10 years is reasonable. After this time, if there is no evidence of recurrent disease, exogenous thyroid hormone supplementation may be decreased, such that the TSH levels rise to the lower limits of normal.
  - **Chemotherapeutic agents** are rarely administered because they are typically less effective and have a worse side-effect profile than radioactive iodine.
- **MTC** is sporadic in most cases, but ~20% of cases are part of inherited tumor syndromes (MEN IIA and IIB and familial MTC). This possibility makes ruling out a *RET* proto-oncogene mutation, hyperparathyroidism, and pheochromocytoma essential to the initial preoperative management, along with calcitonin measurement. Total thyroidectomy with bilateral central neck dissection is the mainstay of therapy for MTC because of the high frequency of bilateral disease. Although MTC is somewhat indolent in its progression, no effective systemic chemotherapy regimens exist, and MTC cells take up radioactive iodine poorly. For this reason, patients with genetic predisposition to the disease (i.e., *RET* mutations) should be highly encouraged to undergo prophylactic total thyroidectomy with central lymph node dissection. Complications of local MTC invasion mirror those of anaplastic tumors, yet progression is less rapid. Doxorubicin is the most effective cytotoxic chemotherapeutic agent, but an objective response is <40%, with no patients having a complete response.
- **Anaplastic thyroid carcinoma** is poorly responsive to therapy and is often locally invasive, if not metastatic, at the time of presentation. These poor prognostic features mean that this histology is always classified as stage IV at diagnosis regardless of size, grade, node involvement, or metastasis. The invasive nature makes tumor resection difficult or even impossible. At initial presentation, the tumor may encompass the carotid arteries, esophagus, and/or trachea. Recurrent or superior laryngeal nerve damage may also occur. The complications of local invasion account for the major morbidity of this cancer, often leading patients to require gastrostomy tubes or a tracheostomy.
  - **Resection.** If imaging reveals limited disease, resection should be pursued for improved local control and delay of complications, although survival is not altered.
  - **Radiation/Chemotherapy.** Radioactive iodine is rarely taken up by anaplastic carcinoma cells, so external-beam radiation therapy is a necessary component of treatment. Administration should be undertaken concurrently with systemic radiosensitizing chemotherapy. Doxorubicin is the most commonly used agent.
  - End-stage care typically includes managing local complications, with ~50% of patients dying from airway obstruction.

FOLLOW-UP

For routine follow-up of well-differentiated thyroid carcinoma, physical exam, TSH, thyroglobulin level measurement, and chest x-ray are recommended twice yearly for 4 years, then once yearly for 10 years. Thyroglobulin levels are expected to be <5 ng/mL if complete thyroid ablation has been successful. For MTC, serum calcitonin and carcinoembryonic antigen levels should initially be followed at 2 to 3 months postoperatively, and then yearly. Abnormal serum markers should trigger diagnostic imaging evaluation.

PROGNOSIS

Well-differentiated thyroid carcinomas have an excellent prognosis. Cure rates reach nearly 100% at 10 years, even with capsular invasion, as long as there is no vascular involvement. The two most important predictors of mortality are age (>45) and tumor stage at the time of initial therapy. Relative survival at 10 years for papillary, follicular, and Hürthle cell carcinomas is 93%, 85%, and 76%, respectively. Anaplastic tumors carry a grim prognosis, often leading rapidly to death within the first few years after diagnosis regardless of treatment. MTCs have 5-year survival rates >80% in stage I and II disease but <40% in stage III or IV disease.

Thirty percent of patients will have a recurrence, the majority locally, with distant recurrence mainly involving the lungs.

PARATHYROID CARCINOMA

GENERAL PRINCIPLES

Although adenomas of the parathyroid glands are a common endocrine abnormality, parathyroid carcinoma is quite rare. Primary hyperparathyroidism is categorized pathologically into three groups: single parathyroid adenoma (83% to 85%), multiglandular hyperplasia (15%), and parathyroid carcinoma (0.5% to 3%). Unlike benign hyperparathyroidism, which is found primarily in the postmenopausal female population, parathyroid carcinoma is found equally in both genders at younger ages. With an incidence of only 0.015 in 100,000, parathyroid cancer is classified as one of the rarest human cancers. Although no etiologic causes are known, parathyroid cancer is seen in the autosomal dominant disease of MEN I.

DIAGNOSIS

Patients with parathyroid carcinoma often present with either **hypercalcemia** or a **neck mass.** On physical exam, 30% to 50% of patients with parathyroid carcinoma have palpable masses in the central neck region. A hyperfunctional parathyroid tumor leads to excessive production of parathyroid hormone and, ultimately, the clinical syndrome of primary hyperparathyroidism. Clinical signs and symptoms include fatigue, renal stones, bone disease, and neuromuscular/neuropsychiatric disturbances related to hypercalcemia. Grossly elevated calcium levels lead to nausea, vomiting, polyuria, and dehydration. Cytologic examination of a needle aspirate is considered an unreliable criterion for diagnosis of malignancy. Definitive diagnosis of parathyroid carcinoma is made in the operating room, where local invasion and metastasis can be assessed.

TREATMENT

- The mainstay of treatment is **surgical exploration of the neck and complete en bloc resection of the tumor along with the ipsilateral thyroid lobe and central cervical lymph nodes.**[1] There is no proven role for adjuvant chemotherapy or radiation therapy. Likewise, the only effective therapy for recurrent or metastatic disease is complete resection.
- The management of severe hypercalcemia includes saline hydration, furosemide diuresis, and bisphosphonates. Octreotide and calcimimetic agents are occasionally used to lower calcium in patients refractory to other therapeutic interventions.

PROGNOSIS

Hypercalcemia is the major cause of morbidity and mortality. The prognosis for parathyroid carcinoma depends on the adequacy of the initial en bloc resection. The most common site of recurrence is local followed by lung, liver, and bone, in order of decreasing incidence. Early recurrence correlates with death from the disease. The overall survival is ~85% at 5 years and 50% to 70% at 10 years.[2]

PITUITARY NEOPLASMS

GENERAL PRINCIPLES

Pituitary neoplasms are rare endocrine malignancies that arise from epithelial origin in the adenohypophysis. Pituitary adenomas account for 10% to 15% of intracranial tumors. Previously classified by histopathology (acidophilic, basophilic, chromophobic), pituitary adenomas are now classified by the hormones they secrete, that is, prolactin, growth hormone, adrenal corticotropin hormone (ACTH), gonadotropins, and TSH. Tumors that do not secrete hormones above physiologic levels are termed nonfunctional adenomas.

Epidemiology

Incidence peaks in the third and fourth decades of life. In general, males and females are affected equally, with the exception of some subtypes, such as ACTH and prolactin-secreting adenomas, which are more common in females.

DIAGNOSIS

Clinical Presentation

Initial symptoms include headache, visual disturbance, and increased intracranial pressure, as well as syndromes related to the type of hormone secreted (Cushing's syndrome, acromegaly, hirsutism, hyperprolactinemia, or hyperthyroidism).

Diagnostic Testing

Initial evaluation involves a dedicated **gadolinium-enhanced MRI of the pituitary** and **laboratory evaluation** for active adenomas with a panel consisting of growth hormone (GH), insulin-like growth factor 1 (IGF-1), prolactin (PRL), TSH, free T4, T3, ACTH, cortisol, luteinizing hormone (LH), follicle-stimulating hormone (FSH), and testosterone. Diagnosis is made on imaging, substantiated by hormone levels in active adenomas, and, when appropriate, confirmed pathologically by transsphenoidal biopsy or resection. No TNM staging classification exists for these rare tumors, and prognostic markers include levels of hormone secreted, size of tumor, and extent of suprasellar extension.

TREATMENT

Management of pituitary adenomas depends on the type, but in general, transsphenoidal surgical resection is the favored curative approach. The exceptions are prolactin-secreting microadenomas, which are managed by dopamine agonists, or inactive adenomas, which remain stable in size on serial imaging. The goals of surgery are to alleviate mass effect while preserving pituitary function and abating endocrine hyperactivity. Postoperative management depends on the type of pituitary adenoma.

Prolactin-Secreting Adenomas

- Prolactin-secreting adenomas are the most commonly diagnosed pituitary tumor, representing ~30% of cases. Symptoms of hyperprolactinemia include galactorrhea and hypogonadism (oligomenorrhea or amenorrhea, dry vaginal mucosa, sterility, decreased libido, and impotence).[3] Prolactinomas are usually slow-growing microadenomas in premenopausal women, but can grow to a larger size (macroadenomas) in men and postmenopausal females. Macroadenomas can cause mass effect, classically manifested by visual disturbances (bitemporal hemianopsia) and headaches.
- The **differential diagnosis** of hyperprolactinemia includes pregnancy, prolactin-stimulating drugs, hypothyroidism, and renal failure. The definitive diagnosis requires radiographic evidence of an adenoma and a persistently elevated prolactin level (>200 ng/mL in females and >100 ng/mL in males), with the other etiologies of hyperprolactinemia having been ruled out.
- **Treatment** of prolactinomas is dependent on size. Microadenomas are treated medically, since most do not increase in size and surgery is rarely curative. Medical treatment is achieved with dopamine agonists (e.g., bromocriptine), where the response rates are 70% to 80% for tumor shrinkage and 80% to 90% for restoration of ovulation. In cases where dopamine agonist therapy is not tolerated (~30% of cases) or fertility is not a concern, oral contraceptives containing estrogen and progesterone can be used to treat the symptoms of hypogonadism. In cases of macroadenomas with significant suprasellar involvement or in pregnancy (which stimulates growth of adenomas), surgery or radiation therapy can be used, often in combination with dopamine agonists.
- **Follow-up** should include yearly prolactin levels. If prolactin increases to >250 ng/mL or neurological symptoms develop, repeat MRI is indicated. For patients with macroadenomas, visual field testing and MRI at 6 months after commencement of therapy should be performed. When prolactin levels are normalized for 2 years and at least 50% tumor reduction is observed, a trial of tapering the dopamine agonist may be considered.

Growth Hormone–Secreting Adenomas

- Growth hormone–secreting adenomas account for 30% of pituitary adenomas. Growth hormone excess results in acromegaly (coarse facial features, macroglossia, and acral growth). Growth hormone leads to an increase in IGF-1, which affects bone and tissue growth and can ultimately lead to organomegaly, hypertension, cardiomyopathy, arthropathies, and restrictive lung diseases. Symptoms include arthralgias, oily skin, hyperhidrosis, headaches, and fatigue.
- The **diagnosis** is suggested by a physical exam showing acromegaly, elevated IGF-1 levels (preferred over fasting GH because the levels are more stable), oral glucose suppression test failing to suppress IGF-1, elevated GH, and a pituitary adenoma evident on MRI.
- The **treatment** of choice is a transsphenoidal resection. In patients not eligible for surgery, external-beam radiation may be used. Medical treatment with dopamine agonists or somatostatin analogs such as octreotide are not curative, but may be used for symptomatic control of acromegaly.
- **Follow-up** should include monitoring GH and IGF-1 levels. Monitoring for hypopituitarism after radiation is also essential.

Adrenal Corticotropin Hormone–Secreting Adenomas

- These less common pituitary adenomas result in Cushing's disease. Cushing's disease is more common in women. The clinical presentation is most often a result of an endocrinopathy and less commonly secondary to a mass effect. Increased ACTH results in adrenal hyperplasia and hypercortisolism. Hypercortisolism results in centripetal obesity, moon facies, buffalo hump, hirsutism, abdominal striae, and acne (i.e., Cushing's syndrome). Clinical signs include hypertension, bone loss, myopathies, diabetes, and psychiatric disorders.
- **Diagnosis** is made by confirming hypercortisolism with 24-hour urinary cortisol. The pituitary origin of cortisol is demonstrated by failure of the low-dose dexamethasone suppression test to suppress serum cortisol to <10 μg/dL. Finally, serum ACTH should be elevated to rule out an adrenal adenoma. Ectopic ACTH syndrome is excluded if the high-dose dexamethasone suppression test results in reduction of cortisol levels to <50% of baseline. If the above laboratory testing is inconclusive, inferior petrosal sinus sampling for ACTH can be performed to confirm the pituitary etiology. Imaging studies are less reliable, as 50% of ACTH-secreting adenomas may not be detectable by MRI; nonetheless, MRI remains essential to guiding therapy and is performed in all cases.
- **Treatment** of choice is transsphenoidal resection, with cure rates ranging from 76% to 94%. External-beam radiation can be used for poor surgical candidates or as adjuvant therapy to surgery. Medical therapy with ketoconazole or mitotane can be used for symptom control in those unable to tolerate surgery or in relapsed cases.
- **Follow-up** requires replacement hormonal therapy for up to 1 year after surgery and monitoring for hypopituitarism after radiation.

Gonadotropin-Secreting Adenomas and Nonsecreting Pituitary Adenomas

- These adenomas account for 30% of pituitary tumors. They are associated with an older population. Most are nonsecretory, but demonstrate secretory granules containing FSH and LH. **Clinical presentation** typically presents secondary to a mass effect, with symptoms of headaches, visual changes, and hypopituitarism.

- **Diagnosis** is suggested by increased LH and FSH and by MRI findings of a macroadenoma. Postmenopausal women may have naturally elevated FSH and LH, and diagnosis relies on final surgical pathology.
- The **treatment** is primarily transsphenoidal resection. Adjuvant external-beam radiation therapy may be considered in patients with residual tumor on imaging postoperatively. **Follow-up** several months postoperatively with repeat MRI is essential since most tumors are nonsecretory.

TSH-Secreting Adenomas

- TSH-secreting adenomas are the least common pituitary tumor, comprising ~1% of pituitary adenomas. Clinical presentation is typically with symptoms of hyperthyroidism (heat intolerance, diarrhea, weight loss, or exophthalmos) or mass effect.
- **Diagnosis** is made by demonstrating increased TSH despite elevated T4 and T3. MRI may confirm the presence of an adenoma.
- **Treatment** is primarily transsphenoidal resection. Adjuvant external-beam radiation is used in refractory cases. Palliative medical therapy with octreotide has been used in refractory cases, with response rates of 90%. **Follow-up** requires monitoring of TSH, T4, and T3 levels.

ADRENAL CORTICAL TUMORS

GENERAL PRINCIPLES

The majority are benign, nonfunctioning adenomas found incidentally on imaging. Others are benign hormone-secreting adenomas causing diseases such as Cushing's. Only 50% of adrenal tumors are endocrinologically active. The third type of adrenal tumor is an adrenal cortical carcinoma that is a very rare and extremely aggressive tumor type.

DIAGNOSIS

Clinical Presentation

- Adrenal "incidentalomas" can be found on 1% to 3% of CT scans of the abdomen. The differential diagnosis includes benign adenomas and metastases. The chance of malignancy is directly related to the size of the mass (<3 cm, benign; >6 cm, malignant), with most carcinomas presenting as large masses.
- Adrenal adenomas can secrete cortisol, sex hormones, or aldosterone, or can be inactive. The clinical presentation is dependent on the predominant hormone secreted. The most common clinical presentation is Cushing's syndrome, which results from a cortisol excess. Sex hormone excess can lead to acne, oligomenorrhea, and virilization/hirsutism in women and feminization in men. Rarely, these carcinomas may produce aldosterone, resulting in hypertension and hypokalemia.

Diagnostic Testing

- Initial evaluation involves staging with imaging with a **CT of the abdomen and pelvis,** and determination of hormone levels, which are used to monitor for recurrence and progression.

- The definitive diagnosis is obtained by surgical pathology. High urinary free cortisol and serum cortisol, low ACTH, and lack of suppression in a high-dose dexamethasone suppression test occur in the instance of cortisol-secreting carcinoma. Virilizing sex hormone–secreting carcinomas demonstrate high levels of testosterone, androstenedione, and dehydroepiandrosterone sulfate (DHEA-S) while feminizing tumors demonstrate high estradiol levels. Some tumors are nonsecretory, and definitive diagnosis relies on pathologic diagnosis.
- The staging of adrenal carcinoma depends on tumor size, nodal involvement, and presence of distant metastasis. Tumors <5 cm with no nodal involvement are stage I; those >5 cm without nodal involvement, stage II; those with nodal involvement, stage III; and those with distant metastasis, stage IV.

TREATMENT

- **Surgical resection** is the treatment of choice, even in advanced disease. Debulking of the tumor and metastectomy are often considered. Adjuvant chemotherapy can be considered in advanced disease, but it is thought to be minimally effective, as there is not enough evidence to support any single regimen.
- In patients ineligible for surgery, most chemotherapeutic regimens will include **mitotane,** which selectively targets the adrenal cortex and results in selective chemical ablation.[4] Overall response rate to mitotane is ~33%, but its effect on overall and disease-free survival has not been conclusively determined. Other medical therapies aimed at palliating symptoms include ketoconazole and aminoglutethimide.
- Finally, adjuvant external-beam radiation therapy may also be effective for local control after resection or for symptomatic metastasis.

PROGNOSIS

The prognosis of adrenal carcinoma depends on initial stage and resectability. For surgically resectable tumors, the median overall survival is almost 6 years, but with medical therapy alone <10% of patients live to 6 years. Follow-up with repeat CT scans and hormone levels at 6 month intervals is recommended.

DIFFUSE ENDOCRINE SYSTEM TUMORS

Some endocrinologically active tumors are not localized to any one organ, but share the common embryonic origin of the neural crest and neuroectoderm. These include gastroenteropancreatic neuroendocrine tumors, pheochromocytomas, and the MEN syndromes.

GASTROENTEROPANCREATIC NEUROENDOCRINE TUMORS

GENERAL PRINCIPLES

Tumors of the gastroenteropancreatic axis are classified according to their secretory products: insulinoma, gastrinoma, somatostatinoma, glucagonoma, vasoactive intestinal

TABLE 25-2 HORMONE STUDIES AND CLINICAL SYMPTOMS IN NEUROENDOCRINE TUMORS

	Laboratory Test(s)	Clinical Symptom(s)
Carcinoid	5-HIAA 24-h urine Chromogranin A	Carcinoid syndrome: flushing/diarrhea/wheezing
Gastrinoma	Gastrin	Ulcer disease
Insulinoma	Proinsulin Insulin/glucose ratio >0.3 C-peptide	Hypoglycemia
VIPoma	VIP	Watery diarrhea and hypokalemia
Glucagonoma	Glucagon Serum glucose CBC	Dermatitis/diabetes/deep vein thrombosis
Other pancreatic islet cell tumors	Chromogranin A Somatostatin Pancreatic polypeptide	Diabetes/steatorrhea/gallbladder disease
	Calcitonin	Hypercalcemia
	Parathyroid hormone-related peptide	Hypocalcemia
Pheochromocytoma	Metanephrines (plasma and urine) Urine catecholamines	Cyclic hypertension

5-HIAA, 5-hydroxyindolacetic acid.

Adapted from Clark OH, et al. Neuroendocrine tumors. *J Natl Compr Canc Netw.* 2006;4(2):102–138.

peptide-oma (VIPoma), and carcinoid. Some are nonsecretory and classified as extrapulmonary small-cell carcinomas. Half of neuroendocrine tumors are of the carcinoid variant, followed by gastrinomas, insulinomas, VIPomas, and glucagonomas, in order of decreasing incidence.

DIAGNOSIS

Most neuroendocrine tumors are malignant and are commonly identified at the time of metastatic disease, with the exception of insulinomas, which are slow growing. Clinical presentation depends on the hormones secreted and the site of disease. The initial laboratory analysis should focus on specific hormones associated with those clinical symptoms as outlined in Table 25-2.

TREATMENT

Tumor localization is essential for successful management of limited disease. CT and MRI may detect larger tumors, but often scintigraphy or angiography with venous hormone sampling may be required to localize tumors. Therapy varies from surgical resection for localized tumors, to medical therapies and dietary changes to palliate symptoms, to chemotherapy and arterial embolization. Chemotherapy has variable activity depending on the type of gastroenteropancreatic tumor. Typical agents used include 5-FU, streptozotocin, doxorubicin, and dacarbazine. **Octreotide** is commonly used in the treatment of gastroenteropancreatic malignancies for symptom relief (e.g., flushing, wheezing, and diarrhea); it also has a direct inhibitory effect on tumor growth and is used in the perioperative setting as suppressive therapy.

CARCINOID TUMORS

GENERAL PRINCIPLES

Carcinoid tumors are the most common neuroendocrine tumors, with a yearly incidence of 1.5 in 100,000 in the United States. Benign and malignant tumors occur at approximately equal frequency, and either type may be symptomatic. They can secrete various vasoactive substances, including histamine, serotonin, catecholamines, and prostaglandins. The small bowel is the most common location for these tumors, but they may occur in the appendix, colon, rectum, lung, stomach, or ovary as well.[5] Symptomatic carcinoid tumors usually result from small bowel tumors with metastases to the liver and do not occur with rectal carcinoid. Carcinoid syndrome is due to excessive production of serotonin and other bioactive compounds that then have direct access to the systemic circulation.

DIAGNOSIS

Clinical Presentation

- Appendiceal and small (<1 cm) rectal tumors rarely metastasize, cause symptoms, or affect survival. Small bowel tumors are more likely to be problematic. One-third of small intestine tumors are multicentric, and the chance of metastases increases with increased tumor size (tumors >2 cm have a high rate of metastasis). In general, the progression of small intestinal carcinoid tumors is indolent. However, once metastasis of tumor cells occurs, prognosis is considerably worse. Five-year survival with localized disease, with only nodal involvement, and, finally, with liver metastases is ~95%, 65%, and 20%, respectively. Urinary 5-hydroxyindoleacetic acid levels inversely correlate with survival.
- Approximately 40% of carcinoid tumors found in living patients are hormonally active, leading to **carcinoid syndrome** in 10% of cases. This syndrome rarely occurs without liver metastasis. Symptoms may include facial flushing and edema, abdominal cramping and diarrhea, bronchospasm, hypotension, and cardiac valvular lesions (typically on the tricuspid and/or pulmonic valve if the tumor secretions originate in the bowel). Alcohol, stress, or exercise may precipitate symptoms. Tumors that are not endocrinologically active can also cause devastating effects such as bowel obstruction, appendicitis, or painful liver metastases.

Diagnostic Testing

- An elevated **24-hour urinary 5-hydroxyindoleacetic acid level** is often used for diagnosis, but it is not useful for detecting carcinoid at the early stages when it is curable. Levels >25 mg/d are the typical finding (normal value of excretion is <9 mg/d). Patients should avoid excessive intake of nuts, bananas, avocados, and pineapples for ~2 days before testing, as these may result in erroneously high levels.
- **Plasma chromogranin A level** may also be a useful test with a high sensitivity and without significant variability or need for a 24-hour urine collection.
- Routine blood tests, with attention to liver function tests, hepatic and upper gastrointestinal system imaging, a chest x-ray, and eventual tissue acquisition should all be part of the workup. If available, somatostatin receptor scintigraphy is a useful imaging test. There is no accepted staging system for carcinoid.
- Finally, pathologic diagnosis is confirmed with positive stains for chromogranin, synaptophysin, and neuron-specific enolase.

TREATMENT

- For localized disease, surgical resection is the standard curative modality, with a 5-year overall survival of 70% to 90%. In metastatic disease, overall survival is ~2 years, with the focus of therapy on palliating symptoms both surgically and medically. As survival with untreated carcinoid tumors can exceed 10 years, therapy is usually focused on controlling symptoms. Dietary tryptophan restriction, along with serotonin antagonists and other symptom-controlling drugs, is the initial mainstay of therapy.
- The somatostatin analog **octreotide,** used at doses of 100 to 600 mcg SC/d in two to four divided doses, is effective at symptom alleviation in nearly 90% of patients. A depot formulation of octreotide available as monthly dosing has become standardized. Histamine blockers, prochlorperazine, and cyproheptadine may decrease flushing. Atropine, diphenoxylate, and cyproheptadine can be used for diarrhea. Monoamine oxidase inhibitors (MAOIs) are contraindicated.
- **Surgery** can be risky, as anesthesia often precipitates attacks. However, resection is indicated and highly successful in localized carcinoid tumors. Preoperative administration of octreotide is necessary to prevent carcinoid crisis.
- **Radiation** and various **chemotherapy** regimens are typically reserved for symptomatic control of metastases in advanced disease.

PHEOCHROMOCYTOMA

GENERAL PRINCIPLES

- Pheochromocytomas arise from chromaffin cells primarily in the adrenal medulla (90%), although they can also arise along the aorta, within the carotid body, intracardiac, and even within the urinary bladder. The "rule of 10" is also useful in recognizing general features of pheochromocytomas: 10% are malignant, 10% are extra-adrenal, and 10% are bilateral. This widespread distribution reflects the location of chromaffin cells associated with the sympathetic ganglia. Pheochromocytoma is present in only 0.1% of hypertensive patients who undergo urinary catecholamine quantification.

- The incidence of malignancy in pheochromocytomas ranges from 5% to 45% in several series. Extra-adrenal tumors are more commonly malignant. Pheochromocytomas are associated with several inherited disorders. Bilateral adrenal medullary pheochromocytomas are elements of the inherited MEN IIA and MEN IIB neuroendocrine syndromes. Although ~25% of patients with von Hippel–Lindau disease develop pheochromocytomas, <1% of patients with neurofibromatosis and Von Recklinghausen disease are found to have the tumor.

DIAGNOSIS

Clinical Presentation

The most common presenting complaint is severe hypertension unrelated to physical or emotional stress. The production of catecholamines results in the clinical symptoms of episodic or sustained hypertension and anxiety attacks. Pheochromocytomas have been known to produce other hormones, including ACTH, somatostatin, calcitonin, oxytocin, and vasopressin. Classically, patients describe spells of hypertension, palpitations, headaches, and diaphoresis. Other presenting findings include lactic acidosis, hypovolemia, and unexplained fever. Clinically, the cluster of symptoms can be recalled by remembering the **five Ps: pain, pressure, palpitation, perspiration, and pallor.** However, it should be appreciated that many patients do not exhibit these "classic" episodes and may have persistent hypertension, rather than episodic.

Diagnostic Testing

- Traditionally, diagnosis has been based on a **24-hour measurement of catecholamines and metabolites** in the urine, including vanillylmandelic acid and metanephrines. New data suggest that a **random plasma metanephrine level** is extremely sensitive (~99%) in diagnosing pheochromocytoma and is an excellent choice for initial screening. Although rarely used in clinical practice today, the clonidine suppression test has been used in the past. Normally, clonidine suppresses plasma levels of epinephrine and norepinephrine. In the presence of pheochromocytomas, no such suppression is observed.
- Localization of a pheochromocytoma is accomplished by **chest and abdominal imaging with CT or MRI.** Nuclear scanning after the administration of labeled metaiodobenzylguanidine can be done if the tumor is not localized by CT or MRI. Metaiodobenzylguanidine is structurally similar to norepinephrine and is selectively taken up by adrenergic tissue.

TREATMENT

- After diagnosis, tumor localization and operative preparation are indicated, as **surgical resection** represents the mainstay of curative therapy.
- **Preoperative alpha-adrenergic blockade** is necessary for patients with pheochromocytomas. Traditionally, phenoxybenzamine has been used to control hypertension. Propranolol may be used to control tachycardia, but must always follow alpha-adrenergic blockade to avoid hypertensive exacerbation due to

unopposed vasoconstriction. Intraoperative hypertensive episodes are controlled with alpha-adrenergic blockers or sodium nitroprusside.

- **Malignant pheochromocytomas** are difficult to distinguish from benign pheochromocytomas by pathology alone. Natural history, secondary tumor sites, and recurrence help determine the nature of the pheochromocytoma. Aggressive disease may require combination chemotherapy with cyclophosphamide, vincristine, and dacarbazine. Routine follow-up consists of blood pressure measurements and urinary catecholamines in addition to regularly scheduled CT, MRI, or metaiodobenzylguanidine scanning to monitor for recurrence.

MULTIPLE ENDOCRINE NEOPLASIA SYNDROMES

MEN syndromes are a group of rare genetic disorders that confer an increased risk of malignancy of endocrine tissues. These disorders are grouped by the major cell type of malignancy that the affected patients are at risk for developing (Table 25-3). They share a common cell of origin (amine precursor uptake and decarboxylation [APUD] neuroendocrine cells) and are inherited in an autosomal dominant pattern.

- **Multiple endocrine neoplasia I (Werner syndrome)**
  This syndrome has high penetrance, with **parathyroid glands** most frequently involved. One-third of gastrinomas are associated with MEN I, and pituitary adenomas can also be discovered. The MEN I gene locus has been mapped to 11q13 and codes for a tumor suppressor gene. Inheritance of the mutation is autosomal dominant. Morbidity and mortality are predominately related to duodenopancreatic malignancies. Treatment is directed by sites of tumor involvement. Patients require close follow-up for evidence of additional sites of involvement in the pituitary, parathyroid, pancreas, duodenum, adrenals, thymus, and lungs.

TABLE 25-3 FEATURES OF MULTIPLE ENDOCRINE NEOPLASIA (MEN) SYNDROMES

Syndrome	Associated Tumors and Abnormalities
MEN I	Pituitary adenomas Pancreatic islet cell tumors or duodenal (35%–75%) Parathyroid hyperplasia (90%)
MEN IIA	Medullary carcinoma of thyroid Pheochromocytoma (bilateral) Parathyroid hyperplasia
MEN IIB	Medullary carcinoma of thyroid Pheochromocytoma (bilateral) Multiple mucosal ganglioneuromas Colonic and skeletal abnormalities with marfanoid body habitus
FMTC	Medullary carcinoma of thyroid

FMTC, familial non-MEN medullary thyroid carcinoma.

- **Multiple endocrine neoplasia IIA (Sipple syndrome) and IIB**
  MEN II syndromes demonstrate an autosomal dominant inheritance of an activating mutation of the *RET* proto-oncogene, located on chromosome 10. Nearly all patients develop medullary thyroid carcinoma (MTC), which is typically multifocal and bilateral and occurs at a young age. Other features of these syndromes are expressed variably and are reported in Table 25-3. Treatment is directed by sites of tumor involvement. All patients presenting with MTC should be considered for genetic screening for *RET* proto-oncogene mutations. Furthermore, **all patients with MTC should be evaluated for possible pheochromocytoma** before undergoing thyroidectomy to avoid a life-threatening hypertensive crisis.
- **Familial non-multiple endocrine neoplasia medullary thyroid carcinoma (FMTC)**
  This disease is also associated with an autosomal dominant inheritance of the *RET* proto-oncogene; however, these patients develop MTC without other abnormalities associated with MEN II syndromes. **Patients with MEN IIA and FMTC almost invariably develop MTC at an early age, and therefore, prophylactic thyroidectomy should be considered in patients with a known mutation.**

REFERENCES

1. Kearns AE, Thompson GB. Medical and surgical management of hyperparathyroidism. *Mayo Clin Proc.* 2002;77(1):87–91.
2. Lee PK, Jarosek SL, Virnig BA, et al. Trends in the incidence and treatment of parathyroid cancer in the United States. *Cancer.* 2007;109(9):1736–1741.
3. Schlechte JA. Clinical practice. Prolactinoma. *N Engl J Med.* 2003;349(21):2035–2041.
4. Terzolo M, Angeli A, Fassnacht M, et al. Adjuvant mitotane treatment for adrenocortical carcinoma. *N Engl J Med.* 2007;356(23):2372–2380.
5. Kulke MH. Clinical presentation and management of carcinoid tumors. *Hematol Oncol Clin North Am.* 2007;21(3):433–455.

Urological Malignancies 26

Parvin F. Peddi

PROSTATE CANCER

GENERAL PRINCIPLES

Prostate cancer is the most common non-cutaneous cancer among men in the United States and is the second leading cause of cancer death in men after lung cancer. The American Cancer Society estimated that there would be 217,730 new cases and 32,050 deaths from prostate cancer in 2010. One man in 6 would get prostate cancer during his lifetime and one in 36 die of this disease. The course is often indolent and the average age at presentation is late in life. As a result of widespread screening, most patients today are diagnosed with asymptomatic, prostate-confined disease.

Risk Factors

Age is the most significant risk factor, and 2 out of every 3 prostate cancers are found in men older than 65 years, as per the American Cancer Society. Increased risk is also conferred to patients with a **positive family history** and those of **African American descent. High-fat and red meat diets** appear to correlate positively with prostate cancer development. **Benign prostatic hypertrophy is not a risk factor.**

Prevention

No method of prevention has been found to be effective in clinical trials. 5-Alpha-reductase enzyme inhibitors, finasteride[1] and dutasteride[2], have been found to temporarily shrink tumors that probably would not have been fatal, without being able to prevent cancer from development. Furthermore, they suppress levels of prostate-specific antigen (PSA) and may provide a false sense of security that may have contributed to finding of higher grade tumors found in patients treated with finasteride compared with placebo.

DIAGNOSIS

- **Screening for prostate cancer in asymptomatic patients remains controversial.** US death rates from prostate cancer have been falling since introduction of PSA testing. However, it's unclear whether the harms of testing outweigh the benefits for the general asymptomatic population. Preliminary results from the US Prostate, Lung, Colorectal, and Ovarian (PLCO) Cancer Screening Trial showed no mortality benefit from combined screening with PSA testing and digital rectal exam during a medical follow-up of 11 years.[3] Meanwhile, preliminary results from the European Randomized Study of Screening for Prostate Cancer (ERSPC) Trial noted that 1410 men needed to be screened and 48 needed to be treated to prevent one prostate cancer–related death in a 10-year period.[4] These trials as well as several others, such as Prostate Cancer Intervention Versus Observation Trial (PIVOT) in the United States, are ongoing and the final results are pending.

- The American Cancer Society does not currently recommend routine PSA testing and recommends individualized discussion between the patient and his physician. US Preventive Services Task Force most recent recommendations from 2008 recommend against screening for men older than 75 years and conclude there is insufficient data to recommend for or against routine testing for younger men. As of November 2009, the American Urological Association continues to recommend PSA testing starting at age 40 years.

Clinical Presentation

Often patients with prostate cancer are asymptomatic. However, obstructive symptoms as well as dysuria, back pain, and hematuria can be initial presenting symptoms. In some cases, disease may become evident only after investigation of metastatic symptoms such as spinal cord compression or bone pain, which is the favored site of metastasis.

Physical Exam

Carcinoma of the prostate can develop within the posterior surfaces of the lateral lobes, which are palpable during the **digital rectal exam** (DRE). Sensation of hard irregular nodules on the DRE is characteristic. Deeper or more anterior lesions, however, are not detectable on routine DRE. One should also recognize that detection sensitivity also varies significantly between examiners owing to differences in experience and technique. Trials for detecting early disease suggest that the physical exam, or even an ultrasonography (U/S) exam, is less sensitive than measurement of PSA.[5] On occasion, disease disseminates to the lymph nodes, causing evidence of scrotal or lower-extremity lymphedema on physical exam.

Diagnostic Testing

Laboratories

Because signs and symptoms are often nonspecific or nonexistent, diagnosis is often suggested by use of serum markers. The relatively high sensitivity (70% to 80%) and noninvasive nature of the **total serum PSA assay** have made it the most often used test. Although PSA levels fall on a continuum, a normal level is considered to be <4 ng/mL. Of note, levels typically elevate with age and following prostatic massage, and they can also be elevated in patients with benign prostatic hypertrophy and prostatitis. On the other hand, men with high Gleason score tumors may have tumors so undifferentiated that they do not synthesize large amounts of PSA. In the general population, sensitivity of PSA >4 has been estimated at 70% to 80%, while the specificity is estimated to be about 60% to 70%.[6] Perhaps the most important feature of PSA testing is the ability to follow its change over time (PSA velocity).

Imaging

Although **transrectal ultrasound** has been used for screening and staging in some situations, its greatest use is to guide prostatic biopsies. **Bone scan** is useful in identifying bone metastasis and is recommended for men with PSA >20. **CT** can supplement clinical evaluation and should also be used with PSA >20 or T3/T4 stage tumors to evaluate for lymph node involvement. Role of PET and MRI is not yet clear.

Diagnostic Procedures

Biopsy is essential for diagnosis. The sensitivity can also be increased when more needle cores are obtained. A minimum of 6 cores is standard, although many patients routinely have 8 to 12 cores/biopsy sessions. **Histologic grade** is an important determinant of disease course and patient survival. Adenocarcinomas represent >95% of prostate cancers and are graded histologically using the **Gleason scoring system.** This system takes the two most predominant histologic patterns in the area of the tumor and assigns each a number from 1 to 5. These numbers are then added together to give the total score. *Higher scores* correlate with more poorly differentiated tumors and worse prognosis. Squamous and transitional cell tumors make up the majority of the remaining prostate tumors, with another important subset being the high-grade neuroendocrine or small-cell tumors.

TREATMENT

The key determinants in considering the optimal treatment of prostate cancer are estimates of life expectancy and risk of cancer progression. The risk of cancer progression can be estimated using the **pathologic stage,** which is determined by the clinical stage (based on DRE), preoperative PSA, and biopsy Gleason score. The National Comprehensive Cancer Network publishes a staging monogram based on these three features in their Clinical Practice Guidelines in Oncology. It is freely accessible at http://www.nccn.org/. Patients with prostate cancer can be divided for the purposes of treatment into three groups to guide treatment: localized prostate cancer, locally advanced prostate cancer, or advanced prostate cancer.

- **Localized prostate cancer.** By definition, cancer is confined to the prostate. These patients are further subdivided into three risk categories:
  - **Low risk** (T1-T2a, Gleason score ≤6, PSA <10): Expectant management, radical prostatectomy (RP), external beam radiation therapy (EBRT), or brachytherapy are all reasonable options for treatment. If expectant management is chosen, PSA should be checked at least every 6 months and DRE at least once a year. Curative therapy is initiated at onset of disease progression. No clinical trials have compared expectant management with immediate treatment. Choice of therapy otherwise is based on patient preferences, as no clinical trials have found any treatment modality to be superior.
  - **Intermediate risk** (T2b-T2c or GS 7 or PSA 10 to 20): Unless expected survival is less than 10 years, expectant management is not acceptable in this category. Otherwise, RP, EBRT, or brachytherapy are equivalent management options.
  - **High risk** (T3a or GS 8 to 10 or PSA >20): These patients are treated with either RP with pelvic lymph node dissection or EBRT combined with at least 2 to 3 years of androgen deprivation therapy[7] (ADT; see below).
- **Locally advanced prostate cancer (T3b-T4).** Similar to patients with high-risk localized disease, these patients are treated with either RP with pelvic lymph

node dissection or EBRT combined with 2 to 3 years of ADT. It is also acceptable to treat this group with only ADT.

- **Metastatic prostate cancer.** Surgery is not usually used for these patients. Radiation or TURP can be used to palliate obstructive symptoms. Otherwise, initial choice is ADT followed by chemotherapy in castrate-resistant prostate cancer.
- **PSA only recurrence.** These patients have a "biochemical recurrence" that occurs after either radiation therapy or surgical resection, and no source of recurrence other than elevated PSA can be found clinically or through imaging. Treatment options include watchful waiting, radiation therapy if they had previously had RP, or in selected patients salvage RP if they were originally treated with radiation therapy.
- **Watchful waiting.** This refers to complete deferment of therapy and instead proceeding with palliative therapy. Prostate cancer is often indolent in nature, which allows for watchful waiting as a reasonable approach in selected patients. In general, this option is reserved for patients whose life expectancy is <10 years and/or who have other comorbidities limiting treatment options.
- **Androgen deprivation therapy.** Prostate cancer is testosterone dependent, and androgen deprivation often aids in controlling the disease. ADT can be achieved either surgically through orchiectomy or through hormonal suppression. Most men opt for hormonal therapy instead of orchiectomy for psychological reasons. GnRH agonists are first-line therapy for ADT and are as efficacious as bilateral orchiectomy. Continuous treatment with GnRH agonists induces suppression of LH synthesis and, therefore, testosterone production. Due to being agonists, however, they cause a temporary flare in symptoms on initiation. Therefore, GnRH agonists should be coupled with androgen receptor antagonists when first initiated and continued for at least 7 days. There are several GnRH agonists available, such as leuprolide and goserelin. If patients progress through GnRH agonists, an androgen receptor antagonist (e.g., flutamide, bicalutamide, nilutamide) can be added to the regimen to achieve complete androgen blockade.
- Another option for androgen deprivation is suppression of adrenal androgen synthesis with high dose **Ketoconazole.** Corticosteroids are also effective for suppressing the adrenal androgen synthesis by reducing the production of pituitary ACTH.
- The main **adverse effects** of ADT include hot flashes, decreases in libido, and loss of muscle mass. Osteoporosis also occurs at a higher rate with long-term androgen deprivation. A baseline bone density screen is therefore recommended prior to initiation of ADT. Patients should be supplemented with calcium and vitamin D and bisphosphonate therapy should also be offered to men who are found to be osteopenic or osteoporotic.
- **Chemotherapy.** Many men receiving ADT will eventually develop increasing PSA values despite continued therapy. This progression of disease is termed androgen-independent or castrate-resistant prostate cancer. This resistance is due to adaptations at the cellular level that allows the prostate cancer cell to grow despite a low-androgen environment. A **docetaxel**-based regimen with prednisone is the current standard-of-care therapy for patients with androgen-independent prostate cancer, based on a demonstrated survival benefit of 2 to 3 months over mitoxantrone- and corticosteroid-based regimens in two phase III trials (Southwest Oncology Group [SWOG] 9916[8] and TAX 327[9]).

RENAL CELL CARCINOMA

GENERAL PRINCIPLES

Primary cancers of the kidney can be divided into cancers of the renal parenchyma and cancers of the renal pelvis that are generally transitional cell tumors. This section focuses on cancers of the renal parenchyma, which are generally adenocarcinomas (renal cell carcinoma [RCC]). Histologically RCC comprises of four main subtypes. Clear cell is the most common and accounts for ~80% of the cases. Papillary or chromophilic RCC accounts for 10%, followed by chromophobic RCC and collecting duct RCC.

Epidemiology

The American Cancer Society estimates 58,240 new cases of RCC and 13,040 cancer deaths in 2010. The overall incidence of RCC is rising for unclear reasons. It is more common in men currently and slightly more common in blacks. The higher incidence in males may change as smoking rates equalize between men and women.

Risk Factors

As with prostate cancer, age is the major risk factor for RCC. Accordingly, disease predominantly presents in the sixth to eighth decades of life. Other risk factors include cigarette smoking, obesity, hypertension, acquired cystic kidney disease associated with dialysis, polycystic kidney disease, and occupational exposure to heavy metal, asbestos, or petroleum products. Although not common, there are several hereditary forms of renal cancer as well. A well-known example is von Hipple–Lindau syndrome in which approximately two-thirds of patients develop RCC.

DIAGNOSIS

Clinical Presentation

- Unfortunately many patients are asymptomatic until advanced stages of disease. Hematuria, abdominal pain, and a palpable flank or abdominal mass are the classic triad of RCC diagnosis, but occur in combination only 10% of the time.[10]
- **Hematuria** is the most common finding in RCC. Other symptoms include fever, night sweats, malaise, and weight loss. One interesting potential presenting symptom in men is a left-sided varicocele, secondary to obstruction of the left testicular vein. Paraneoplastic syndromes are rare, but include erythrocytosis and hypercalcemia from overproduction of erythropoietin or parathyroid hormone-related protein, respectively. Stauffer's syndrome is another RCC paraneoplastic syndrome to keep in mind, which consists of hepatic dysfunction in absence of liver metastasis. This dysfunction may be due to production of tumor cytokines.

Diagnostic Testing

Imaging

The best initial imaging modality for a suspected RCC is an **ultrasound.** It is inexpensive, is without radiation, and has a high sensitivity. It is also very useful for distinguishing simple cysts from complex and malignant masses. If a suspicious mass is found, ultrasound is typically followed by **abdominal CT or MR** to further characterize lymph node and regional involvement. Role of **PET** in initial diagnosis is unclear. Bone scan is indicated if patients have bone pain or unexplained elevated alkaline phosphatase that could be due to Stauffer's syndrome (see "Clinical presentation").

Diagnostic Procedures

Despite the sensitivity of imaging studies, **biopsy** of suspected metastatic lesions or nephrectomy is needed to definitely establish RCC diagnosis, as well as to delineate histologic subtype. Needle biopsy of the renal mass is not recommended due to concern for seeding of the peritoneum, as well as sampling errors that result in a negative biopsy.

TREATMENT

Table 26-1 lists a simplified staging of RCCs and their associated prognosis based on contemporary studies.[11] RCC is one of the most resistant tumors to therapy, so **surgery remains the gold standard.** Treatment decision and prognosis is based mostly on feasibility of surgical resection, and it is controversial whether histological subtype affects management.

- **Resectable disease.** Surgical resection can be curative and is the treatment of choice in patients with stage I, II, and III disease. This includes even patients with tumor thrombus involving the inferior vena cava (IVC). Patients with a solitary metastasis should also be considered for resection of primary renal mass and site of metastasis. Either radical nephrectomy or partial nephrectomy are performed depending on the size of mass and the patient's reliance on the affected kidney for total renal function.
  - **Adjuvant therapy.** There is no role for either chemotherapy or radiation in the adjuvant setting currently, even though a portion of these patients will have recurrence of disease.
  - After surgical resection, patients should be followed with repeat imaging for evidence of recurrence. A repeat surgical resection can be considered in suitable patients with recurrence.

TABLE 26-1 STAGING OF RENAL CELL CARCINOMA AND 5-YEAR SURVIVAL

Description of Disease Extent	Stage	5-Year Survival (%)
Confined to renal capsule		
≤7 cm	I	90%–100%
>7 cm	II	75%–95%
Extends through renal capsule but not through Gerota's fascia	III	60%–70%
Renal vein, IVC, or regional nodal involvement	III	
Extends through Gerota's fascia or with distant metastases	IV	15–30%

- **Unresectable disease.** Until 2005, only high dose interleukin-2 had been approved by the FDA for treatment of advanced RCC. Although toxic, this treatment was effective in a very small minority of patients. Studies on pathophysiology of RCC have now revealed reliance of a majority of the tumors on von Hipple–Lindau protein inactivation and subsequent activation of hypoxia-induced vascular endothelial growth factor (VEGF) overexpression for tumor angiogenesis. Two oral, small-molecule kinase inhibitors, sunitinib and sorafenib, which inhibit VEGF, are now approved on two phase III trials.[12,13] Both drugs were found to improve progression-free survival in patients with metastatic clear-cell renal carcinoma. Other treatments based on the same rationale include bevacizumab (anti-VEGF antibody)[14] and temsirolimus (an inhibitor of the mammalian target of rapamycin [mTOR])[15] can be used. Both drugs improved survival in patients with metastatic RCC and are currently approved by the FDA for metastatic RCC.

TESTICULAR CANCER

GENERAL PRINCIPLES

Due to remarkable advances in treatment, testicular cancer is now one of more curable solid organ cancers. This is especially important since it affects a much younger population than most neoplasms. Five-year survival rate is now over 95%.

Classification

Testicular tumors are divided into **seminoma** and **nonseminoma tumors.** The nonseminoma tumors include embryonal carcinomas, teratomas, choriocarcinomas, and mixed germ cell types. Leydig, granulosa, and Sertoli cell tumors occur rarely. Nonseminomas are clinically more aggressive tumors. If elements of both seminoma and nonseminoma are found on biopsy, management follows that of nonseminoma, which is the more aggressive tumor type.

Epidemiology

As per the American Cancer Society, ~8500 new cases of testicular cancer were diagnosed in 2010 with 350 dying of the disease. It remains the most common cancer among men aged 15 to 35 years.

Risk Factors

Although it can affect men of any age, 9 out of 10 cases are in men between 20 and 54 years. White men have five times the risk of black men and three times the risk of Asian Americans for unclear reasons. Other risk factors include cryptorchidism, Klinefelter syndrome, and family history.

DIAGNOSIS

Clinical Presentation

A **painless testicular mass** is the classic presenting symptom. Testicular pain or swelling can be present, but typically suggests epididymitis or orchitis, and an initial course of antibiotics may be appropriate in this situation. **Gynecomastia** as the first sign of testicular cancer is seen in ~10% of patients. It is due to tumor production of human chorionic gonadotropin (hCG).

Physical Exam

A thorough physical exam is essential in patients with suspected testicular cancer. Exam should focus on the testicles, lymphadenopathy (particularly supraclavicular), scrotal edema, and evaluation for gynecomastia. Early metastases to bone are rare but possible, and back pain can also result from bulky retroperitoneal lymphadenopathy.

Laboratories

Three serum markers have roles in testicular cancer: **alpha fetoprotein** (AFP), **β-hCG,** and **lactate dehydrogenase** (LDH). These tumor markers are useful for diagnosis, prognosis, and assessment of treatment. Although nondiagnostic by themselves, it is important to know that pure seminomas do not produce AFP, and β-hCG is elevated in only 15% to 20% of these cancers. By contrast, AFP and/or β-hCG are elevated in more than 80% of non-seminomas.

Imaging

Testicular ultrasound is the initial test of choice in suspected testicular cancer. Subsequent tests include a **chest x-ray** to rule out pulmonary metastasis and **abdominal and pelvic CT** exam with oral and intravenous contrast to assess nodal enlargement and staging. **Chest CT** should be included if any retroperitoneal lymphadenopathy is present or if there is high suspicion of pulmonary metastasis. Other imaging options, such as bone scan or brain imaging, are guided by the patient's symptoms.

Diagnostic Procedures

Biopsy of a testicular mass should be avoided due to a concern for seeding and dissemination of an otherwise curable cancer. A radical inguinal orchiectomy is therefore recommended when workup, including imaging and labs, indicates testicular cancer. Trans-scrotal orchiectomy has an increased risk of seeding. In addition, retroperitoneal lymph node dissection is frequently used in patients with low-stage nonseminomas for staging and curative purposes, and to remove remaining viable tumor tissue in the lymph nodes.

TREATMENT

Treatment is **based on histology type and stage.** In general, stage I disease is localized to the testis, stage II disease has spread to retroperitoneal lymph nodes, and stage III disease is metastatic or has spread to non-regional lymph nodes. Prognosis is generally very favorable with >90% of patients being cured with therapy, including 70% to 80% of patients with advanced tumors. Sperm banking should be discussed before initiation of any therapy.

- **Seminomas** are very radiation and chemo sensitive. Stage I tumors are treated with either adjuvant radiation therapy or single-agent carboplatin for one to two cycles. Active surveillance is also an acceptable option in motivated patients due to low risk of spread. Stage II seminomas are treated with radiation therapy in non-bulky disease and cisplatin-based combination chemotherapy, such as BEP (bleomycin, etoposide, cisplatin) in bulky disease. Stage III seminomas are treated similarly to bulky stage II with chemotherapy.
- **Nonseminomas** are less radiosensitive, and patients often require additional surgical therapies following orchiectomy. Most of these patients will undergo retroperitoneal lymph node dissection for either diagnostic or therapeutic

purposes. The major morbidity of this surgery is retrograde ejaculation with resulting infertility, which occurs in ~10% of cases using an open nerve dissection technique. Adjuvant chemotherapy is often recommended if the surgical resection reveals lymph node involvement. Etoposide and cisplatin ± bleomycin is the chemotherapeutic regimen of choice.

MONITORING/FOLLOW-UP

Patients with testicular cancer should have close follow-up after diagnosis and treatment. This includes serial chest x-rays, CT scanning of the abdomen and pelvis, and blood work for relevant tumor markers, in addition to a detailed clinical exam. The National Comprehensive Cancer Network recommends tumor markers and chest x-ray monthly for the first year and every 2 months for the second year, and specific guidelines for follow-up is found on its Web site (www.nccn.org). It also recommends abdominal and pelvic CT every 3 months in the first 2 years. PET scan may have a role in surveillance, but this has yet to be fully determined. Screening for **late effects** of platinum-based chemotherapy, most commonly dyslipidemias, cardiovascular disease, and cerebrovascular diseases, should be included in follow-up as well.

BLADDER CANCER

GENERAL PRINCIPLES

Bladder cancer is primarily a malignancy of the epithelium. Urothelial (transitional cell) carcinomas are the most common histological subtype and account for >97% of bladder tumors. Other histologic subtypes include squamous cell carcinoma, adenocarcinoma, and small-cell tumor.

Epidemiology

The American Cancer Society estimates that over 70,000 new cases of bladder cancer were diagnosed in 2010 with 14,680 deaths. Similar to prostate cancer, the median age at presentation is late in life (65 years). Medical comorbidities and life expectancy play key roles in management decisions.

Risk Factors

Bladder cancer affects more men than women almost threefold. The most important risk factor is **cigarette smoking**, with smokers twice as likely to get bladder cancer as nonsmokers. Other known risk factors include occupational exposure to aromatic amines in the dye industry, and work in certain other industries such as rubber, leather, textile, paint, printing, and hairdressing industries. Although uncommon in the United States, squamous cell carcinoma is a prevalent subtype in areas endemic for *Schistosoma haematobium*.

DIAGNOSIS

Clinical Presentation

Symptoms are not always appreciated by patients, but **hematuria** is present in ~90% of individuals with bladder cancer. This may be intermittent or constant, frank or microscopic, and is occasionally associated with symptoms of urinary frequency or urgency. Otherwise unexplained hematuria in an individual older than 40 years denotes bladder or renal cancer unless proven otherwise.

Diagnostic Testing

Laboratories

Urinalysis, including microscopic and gross examination, should be performed to detect presence and degree of hematuria. **Urine cytology** has low sensitivity, but it is usually sent as noninvasive adjunctive test that may yield the diagnosis.

Imaging

Imaging studies are performed to determine extent of disease involvement usually after bladder cancer is already confirmed by cystoscopy. **Abdominal and pelvic CT,** with and without IV contrast, is the test of choice. MRI is also efficacious but is more expensive. Ultrasound has no role in evaluation of bladder cancer. The role of PET is being studied.

Diagnostic Procedures

Cystoscopy is the diagnostic test of choice for evaluation and initial staging of suspected bladder cancer. If a suspicious lesion is found, cystoscopy is usually repeated under anesthesia to obtain biopsy.

TREATMENT

For purposes of treatment, bladder cancer is divided into three categories: superficial, muscle invasive, or metastatic.

- **Superficial bladder cancer.** Up to 75% of bladder cancers are superficial at presentation. Most can be completely resected by transurethral resection of the bladder tumor (TURBT). Most patients with superficial bladder cancer will have recurrence within 5 years, even with seemingly complete initial resection. Therefore, it is recommended that patients undergo cystoscopy every 3 months after initial resection and, depending on level of progression, be considered for intravesical therapy. Bacillus Calmette-Guérin (BCG) is the most common and effective intravesicular agent used. Other agents, including mitomycin, interferon, and anthracyclins, are also used. None has been shown to be superior to BCG.
- **Muscle invasive bladder cancer.** The standard treatment is radical cystectomy with pelvic node dissection. In males this also includes removal of prostate and seminal vesicles, and in females the uterus, ovaries, and fallopian tubes. Neoadjuvant chemotherapy has been found to improve outcome in patients with muscle invasive bladder cancer. MVAC (methotrexate, vinblastin, doxorubicin, cisplatin) is one of the commonly used regimens, as a trial demonstrated a doubling of median survival with this approach.[16] A cisplatin-based adjuvant chemotherapy regimen can be used in patients who did not receive neoadjuvant therapy.
- **Metastatic bladder cancer.** Cisplatin-based combination therapy is the treatment of choice. MVAC is the most commonly used regimen. Sometimes TURBT or radiation is used palliatively for symptoms of obstruction. Unfortunately, median survival remains in the range of 12 months.

REFERENCES

1. Thompson IM, Goodman PJ, Tangen CM, et al. The influence of finasteride on the development of prostate cancer. *N Engl J Med.* 2003;349:215–224.
2. Andriole GL, Bostwick DG, Brawley OW, et al. Effect of dutasteride on the risk of prostate cancer. *N Engl J Med.* 2010;362:1192–1202.
3. Andriole GL, Crawford ED, Grubb RL III, et al. Mortality results from a randomized prostate-cancer screening trial. *N Engl J Med.* 2009;360:1310–1319.
4. Schröder FH, Hugosson J, Roobol MJ, et al. Screening and prostate-cancer mortality in a randomized European study. *N Engl J Med.* 2009;360:1320–1328.
5. Catalona WJ, Richie JP, Ahmann FR, et al. Comparison of digital rectal examination and serum prostate specific antigen in the early detection of prostate cancer: results of a multicenter clinical trial of 6,630 men. *J Urol.* 1994;151:1283–1290.
6. Brawer MK. Prostate-specific antigen: current status. *Cancer J Clin.* 1999;49:264–281.
7. Bolla M, de Reijke TM, Tienhoven GV, et al. Duration of androgen suppression in the treatment of prostate cancer. *N Engl J Med.* 2009;360:2516–2527.
8. Petrylak DP, Tangen CM, Hussain MH, et al. Docetaxel and estramustine compared with mitoxantrone and prednisone for advanced refractory prostate cancer. *N Engl J Med.* 2004; 351:1513–1520.
9. Tannock IF, de Wit R, Berry WR, et al. Docetaxel plus prednisone or mitoxantrone plus prednisone for advanced prostate cancer. *N Engl J Med.* 2004;351:1502–1512.
10. Skinner DG, Colvin RB, Vermillion CD, et al. Diagnosis and management of renal cell carcinoma. A clinical and pathologic study of 309 cases. *Cancer.* 1971;28:1165–1177.
11. Pantuck AJ, Zisman A, Belldegrun AS. The changing natural history of renal cell carcinoma. *J Urol.* 2001;166:1611–1623.
12. Motzer RJ, Hutson TE, Tomczak P, et al. Sunitinib versus interferon alfa in metastatic renal-cell carcinoma. *N Engl J Med.* 2007;356:115–124.
13. Escudier B, Eisen T, Stadler WM, et al. Sorafenib in advanced clear-cell renal-cell carcinoma. *N Engl J Med.* 2007;356:125–134.
14. Escudier B, Bellmunt J, Négrier S, et al. Phase III trial of bevacizumab plus interferon alfa-2a in patients with metastatic renal cell carcinoma (AVOREN): final analysis of overall survival. *J Clin Oncol.* 2010;28:2144–2150.
15. Hudes G, Carducci M, Tomczak P, et al. Temsirolimus, interferon alfa, or both for advanced renal-cell carcinoma. *N Engl J Med.* 2007;356:2271–2281.
16. Grossman HB, Natale RB, Tangen CM, et al. Neoadjuvant chemotherapy plus cystectomy compared with cystectomy alone for locally advanced bladder cancer. *N Engl J Med.* 2003; 349:859–866.

Gynecologic Oncology

27

Andrea R. Hagemann and
Israel Zighelboim

Tumors of the female reproductive tract are often diagnosed and managed by the combined efforts of the primary care physician, gynecologist, gynecologic oncologist, medical oncologist and radiation oncologist. This chapter describes the approach to common gynecologic oncology evaluations and briefly discusses selected gynecologic tumors.

VAGINAL BLEEDING

GENERAL PRINCIPLES

Vaginal bleeding can be caused by exogenous hormones, endocrine imbalances including hyper- or hypothyroidism and diabetes mellitus; anatomic causes such as fibroids, polyps, or cervical lesions; hematologic causes such as coagulopathy; infectious causes such as cervicitis from *Chlamydia trachomatis;* and neoplasia. Organic causes are either related to genital tract pathology or secondary to a systemic disease. Cervical and endometrial cancers are the most common malignancies that result in vaginal bleeding. Dysfunctional uterine bleeding (DUB) is considered a diagnosis of exclusion and is the term used to describe abnormal bleeding for which no specific structural cause can be identified.

DIAGNOSIS

Clinical Presentation

History

A thorough medical and gynecologic history, with careful attention to last menstrual period and amount and duration of bleeding, should be obtained.

Physical Examination

A careful gynecologic exam, including a **speculum exam and pelvic exam,** should be performed. A **Papanicolaou (Pap) smear** should be obtained, and any suspicious cervical or vulvar lesions should be biopsied. A **rectal exam with stool guaiac** should also be performed.

Diagnostic Testing

Laboratories

Appropriate laboratory studies include a **complete blood count** to detect anemia or thrombocytopenia and a pregnancy test in reproductive-age women. In certain individuals, **thyroid-stimulating hormone** and screening **coagulation studies** may be appropriate to rule out thyroid dysfunction and a primary coagulation problem, respectively. Von Willebrand disease is a common cause of heavy menses, especially in adolescent women (see Chap. 7).

Diagnostic Procedures

Women with chronic anovulation, women with obesity, and those older than 35 years of age require further evaluation. A **transvaginal ultrasound** can be helpful in evaluating for anatomic abnormalities, and assessment of endometrial stripe thickness may prove useful in postmenopausal women. **Endometrial sampling,** accomplished in the office using disposable plastic cannulae, should be performed in these women, as they are at risk for polyps, hyperplasia, or carcinoma of the endometrium.

TREATMENT

Medications

In most cases, abnormal bleeding can be managed medically. Acute, profound vaginal bleeding should first be managed by assessing for a primary coagulation disorder. If anovulatory bleeding is established as the working diagnosis, **hormonal therapy** with oral or intravenous estrogen will usually control bleeding. If hormonal management fails, a structural cause of bleeding is more likely. Hormonal management, including oral contraceptives, can be used to significantly reduce blood flow. When estrogen is contraindicated, progestins can be used, including cyclic oral medroxyprogesterone acetate, depot forms of medroxyprogesterone acetate, and the levonorgestrel-containing intrauterine device, which has been shown to decrease menstrual blood loss by 80% to 90%.

Surgical Management

Options range from dilatation and curettage, endometrial ablation, hysteroscopy with resection of uterine polyps or leiomyomas, myomectomy, uterine artery embolization, magnetic resonance-guided focused ultrasonography ablation, and, most definitively, hysterectomy.

PELVIC MASSES

A variety of entities may result in the development of a pelvic mass. These may be gynecologic in origin or, alternatively, may arise from the urinary or gastrointestinal (GI) tracts. Gynecologic causes of a pelvic mass may be uterine, adnexal, or, more specifically, ovarian. Age is an important determinant of the likelihood of malignancy.

- **Ovarian masses**

  These can be functional or neoplastic; neoplastic masses can be either benign or malignant.

  - **Ovarian cysts.** Functional ovarian cysts include follicular cysts, corpus luteum cysts, and theca lutein cysts. Women with endometriosis can develop ovarian endometriomas. Follicular cysts, defined by a diameter >3 cm, are most common, and are most often <8 cm. They usually resolve spontaneously and only require expectant management. Corpus luteum cysts can rupture, leading to hemoperitoneum, which may occasionally require surgical management. Theca lutein cysts are usually bilateral and occur with pregnancy due to ovarian stimulation by human chorionic gonadotropin (hCG).

These cysts may be prominent in certain conditions such as multiple and molar pregnancies. Combination monophasic oral contraceptives can reduce the incidence of these functional cysts.

 - **Neoplastic masses.** The most common benign ovarian neoplasm is the mucinous cystadenoma. Eighty percent of cystic teratomas (dermoid cysts) occur during the reproductive years. Epithelial tumors of the ovary increase with age, and benign tumors of this type include serous and mucinous cystadenomas, fibromas, and Brenner tumors. Malignant ovarian neoplasms are discussed in the following section.
 - **Other masses.** Adnexal masses arising from the fallopian tube are primarily related to inflammatory causes in the reproductive age group. Examples of masses in this category include ectopic pregnancy, tubo-ovarian abscesses, and paraovarian or paratubal cysts.

- **Uterine masses**

  Uterine leiomyomas, commonly referred to as fibroids, are the most common benign uterine tumors. Asymptomatic fibroids are present in up to 50% of women older than age 35 years. Degenerative changes can occur in these tumors. Smooth muscle tumors of the uterus rather represent a continuum that ranges from benign lesions (leiomyoma or fibroid) to malignant neoplasms (uterine leiomyosarcoma). Smooth muscle tumors of uncertain malignant potential have 5 to 9 mitoses per 10 high-power fields (hpf) and do not demonstrate nuclear atypia or giant cells. Leiomyosarcomas typically have ≥10 or more mitoses/hpf and demonstrate nuclear atypia.

DIAGNOSIS

Clinical Presentation

History

History should include any history of urinary or GI symptoms, pelvic pain, or vaginal bleeding.

Physical Exam

A complete pelvic exam, including a rectovaginal exam and Pap test, should be performed. Evidence of ascites or a pleural effusion heightens the suspicion for a malignant ovarian tumor.

Diagnostic Testing

Laboratory and Diagnostic Procedures

Workup usually includes **cervical cytology, complete blood count,** testing of **stool for occult blood,** and a **pregnancy test** in reproductive-age women. **CA-125** is a nonspecific tumor marker that may be obtained, but be aware that a number of benign conditions, including leiomyomas, pelvic inflammatory disease, pregnancy, and endometriosis, *to name a few,* can cause elevations of this marker. **Endometrial sampling** with an endometrial biopsy or dilatation and curettage is necessary if both a pelvic mass and abnormal bleeding are present.

Imaging

Pelvic ultrasonography, usually done transvaginally, will help to clarify the origin and characteristics of gynecologic masses. Additional imaging by means of computed tomography and/or magnetic resonance can be used in selected cases to further delineate the anatomy or evaluate concurrently other anatomic sites. A barium enema or endoscopic study of the lower GI tract may be indicated to exclude a GI etiology.

TREATMENT

- Once a nongynecologic problem is excluded, **management depends on the location and size of the mass as well as the age of the patient.** Premenopausal women with an adnexal mass <8 cm, with predominantly cystic features, can be followed with close observation and/or hormonal suppression. Women with a mass >8 cm, those with complex, solid, or suspicious features on ultrasound, and those whose masses persist or progress with close follow-up should be managed surgically by a gynecologist or a gynecologic oncologist.
- Recently, the American College of Obstetrics and Gynecologists, along with the Society of Gynecologic Oncologists, released guidelines for referral to a gynecologic oncologist for a pelvic mass. In these guidelines, they state that premenopausal women with any of the following should be referred: CA-125 >200 U/mL, ascites, evidence of abdominal or distant metastasis (by imaging or exam), or family history of breast or ovarian cancer in a first-degree relative. The criteria for referral for postmenopausal women are slightly different: CA-125 >35 U/mL, ascites, evidence of abdominal or distant metastasis (by imaging or exam), and family history of breast or ovarian cancer in a first-degree relative. Surgery can be done laparoscopically or by laparotomy depending on the size of the mass and concern for malignancy.
- Most postmenopausal women with an adnexal mass should undergo surgery to rule out an ovarian malignancy.

CERVICAL CANCER

GENERAL PRINCIPLES

Classification

The most common histologic types identified in cases of invasive cervical cancer are squamous cell carcinoma (85%) and adenocarcinoma (5%). Less common histologies include neuroendocrine carcinoma, melanoma, and sarcomas (embryonal rhabdomyosarcoma in children and young adults).

Epidemiology

It was estimated that in 2010, there would be 12,200 new cases of invasive cervical cancer in the United States, resulting in more than 4210 deaths. Worldwide, ~370,000 cases are identified each year. Despite the fact that screening programs are becoming more established, cervical cancer is still the leading cause of death from cancer among women in developing countries and second only to breast cancer worldwide.

Risk Factors

Invasive cancer of the cervix is considered a preventable disease. There is a long preinvasive state (cervical dysplasia), and cytologic screening programs as well as effective treatments are readily available. Cervical intraepithelial neoplasia is a precancerous lesion of the cervix.

Several risk factors for cervical cancer have been identified. These include young age at first intercourse (<16 years), multiple sexual partners, cigarette smoking, immunosuppression, African American or Hispanic ethnicity, high parity, and lower socioeconomic status. **Human papilloma virus** (HPV) **infection** is considered to play a causal role and can be detected in up to 99% of women with cervical cancer.

Prevention

- Cervical cancer can be prevented by detecting and treating cervical dysplasia, thus avoiding progression from the preinvasive into the invasive state. The **Pap smear** is the standard screening test for cervical cancer.
- Annual cervical cytology screening should begin ~3 years after the initiation of sexual intercourse but probably not earlier than age 21 years. Women younger than 30 years should undergo annual cervical cytology screening. Women aged 30 years and older who have had three consecutive negative cervical cytology screening test results, with no history of high-grade dysplasia, are not immunocompromised, and were not exposed to diethylstilbestrol in utero may extend the interval between cytology examinations to 2 to 3 years. The combination of cytology and screening for high-risk subtypes of human papilloma virus can be appropriate for women older than age 30 years. If such combined screening results are negative, they should be screened no more often than every 3 years.
- A quadrivalent **vaccine** against human papilloma virus types 6, 11, 16, and 18 (Gardasil®), is now approved for girls aged 9 to 26 years. A bivalent vaccine (types 16 and 18) has also been recently approved (Cervarix®) for girls 10 to 25 years of age. Cytologic screening is still recommended for those receiving the vaccine.

DIAGNOSIS

Clinical Presentation

The most common symptom in women with cancer of the cervix is **vaginal bleeding,** which can often be postcoital. Asymptomatic women are usually diagnosed on the basis of abnormal cytology. Advanced disease may present with symptoms of malodorous discharge, weight loss, or obstructive uropathy. Physical exam may reveal a palpable cervical mass, and palpation of the inguinal and supraclavicular nodes may reveal lymphadenopathy.

Diagnostic Testing

If a gross lesion is present, **cervical biopsy** should be performed. Abnormal cytologic screening should be evaluated as indicated with colposcopy and directed biopsies, along with endocervical curettage. Cervical cancer is a clinically staged disease, often via an exam under anesthesia to yield the most accurate assessment. Cystoscopy, proctoscopy, chest radiographs, and intravenous pyelograms may be used for staging purposes. CT, MRI, and PET scan are commonly used in the evaluation of disease extension and for treatment planning. However, such imaging modalities should not alter the clinical stage.

TREATMENT

The treatment of cervical cancer is **determined by the clinical stage of disease,** with the underlying principle that therapy should ideally consist of either radiation or surgery alone in order to prevent increased morbidity that results when the two are combined. Stage by stage, these modalities are equivalent in terms of survival outcomes.

Radiation Therapy

Radiation therapy can be classified as either primary or adjuvant therapy. **Primary therapy** combines external radiotherapy to treat parametria and regional lymph nodes and to lessen tumor volume with brachytherapy to target the central tumor. Brachytherapy is delivered by intracavitary or interstitial implants. Intensity-modulated radiotherapy utilizes computer algorithms to distinguish between normal and diseased tissues in order to optimize the delivery of radiation to the affected area while minimizing radiation complications. **Adjuvant radiotherapy** is often used postoperatively for patients with metastases to pelvic lymph nodes or channels, invasion of paracervical tissue, deep cervical invasion, or positive surgical margins. Adjuvant radiotherapy has been shown to decrease pelvic recurrence, but not necessarily to improve 5-year survival rates. Complications of radiation therapy include vasculitis and fibrosis of the bowel and bladder, as well as bowel and bladder fistulas.

Chemotherapy

Randomized trials have shown that the addition of chemotherapy to radiation therapy (known as chemoradiation) improves survival in patients with locally advanced cervical cancer. Chemotherapy allows for systemic treatment as well as sensitization of cancer cells to radiation therapy to improve local and regional control. **Cisplatin-based adjuvant chemotherapy** is the treatment of choice for patients with locally advanced cervical cancer. Single-agent platinum or multiagent chemotherapy with platinum in combination with topotecan or paclitaxel are usually prescribed in cases of advanced or recurrent cervical cancer. Multiagent chemotherapy may offer improved response rates and modest survival benefits at the expense of increased toxicity.[1]

Surgical Management

Surgical management is **generally limited to patients with disease limited to the cervix or with limited involvement of the upper vagina.** Depending on the clinical stage, fertility goals, and physical condition of the patient, surgical treatment ranges from cone excision of the cervix, to simple hysterectomy, to radical trachelectomy (where the cervix and parametria are removed with preservation of the uterine corpus), to radical hysterectomy. The removal of the fallopian tubes and ovaries is not part of the surgical therapy and should be considered on an individual basis. In fact, surgery, when feasible, represents an attractive option for younger women as it has the potential to preserve ovarian function and maximize quality of life.

Treatment for Recurrent Disease

Pelvic recurrences in patients initially treated by surgery are usually treated with radiation therapy. Cases of isolated central recurrences after radiation may be salvaged by radical or ultraradical (exenterative) surgical procedures. Systemic recurrences are most often treated with platinum-based chemotherapy.

MONITORING/FOLLOW-UP

Patients treated for cervical cancer require careful follow-up with clinical exams, Pap smears, and various imaging modalities, as indicated. Positron emission tomography at the completion of treatment appears to have important prognostic potential. Similarly, this modality is also capable of identifying localized and potentially salvageable recurrences.

OUTCOME/PROGNOSIS

The 5-year survival rate for early stage cervical cancer is ~85% with either radiation therapy or radical hysterectomy. For patients with locoregional extension, 5-year survival falls to ≤40%.

OVARIAN CANCER

GENERAL PRINCIPLES

Classification

Malignant ovarian tumors can arise from the germinal epithelium, the germ cells, or the sex-cord stroma. The World Health Organization has developed and maintained a complex classification schema for ovarian tumors. The following discussion concentrates in epithelial ovarian cancer. Most malignant epithelial tumors are high-grade serous adenocarcinomas. Other histologies include the mucinous, endometrioid, clear cell, and transitional cell types. Mixed varieties and other rare variants also exist (squamous cell, undifferentiated, and neuroendocrine).

Epidemiology

In the United States, 1 in 70 women will develop ovarian cancer in their lifetime (lifetime risk, ~1.4%). In 2010, it was estimated that 21,880 new cases of ovarian cancer would be diagnosed in the United States, and 13,850 deaths were expected to occur as a result of ovarian cancer. Epithelial ovarian cancer, which accounts for ~90% of all ovarian cancers, is the leading cause of death from gynecologic cancer in the United States. This type of cancer is often diagnosed at an advanced stage, as patients usually remain asymptomatic until metastasis occurs. The peak incidence of invasive epithelial ovarian cancer is 56 to 60 years of age. Germ cell and sex-cord stromal tumors are less common and typically occur in adolescents and younger women.

Risk Factors

Ovarian cancer has been associated with low parity and infertility; risk factors include early menarche and late menopause. Oral contraceptive use for ≥5 years has been shown to reduce the likelihood of ovarian cancer by 50%. Mutations in BRCA1 and BRCA2, along with Lynch or hereditary nonpolyposis colorectal cancer syndrome (HNPCC), are important genetic susceptibility factors for developing ovarian cancer. In some patients, prophylactic oophorectomy may be a reasonable approach, but this decision must be highly individualized.

Prevention

There is considerable public controversy regarding ovarian cancer screening, but unfortunately, the value of tumor markers and ultrasonography to screen for epithelial ovarian cancer has not been clearly established by prospective studies. The tumor marker CA-125 has played an important role in the diagnosis, management, and follow-up of patients with ovarian cancer. Particularly in premenopausal women, **CA-125 testing and transvaginal ultrasonography have not been shown to be cost effective and should not be used routinely to screen for ovarian cancer in the general population.** Different screening strategies are an active area of study in ovarian cancer research.

DIAGNOSIS

Clinical Presentation

- Symptoms from ovarian cancer can be vague and nonspecific, and many women remain asymptomatic for long periods of time. Abdominal distention, nausea, vomiting, early satiety, and increased abdominal girth may be reported.
- In premenopausal women, irregular or heavy menses may be noted. The Society of Gynecologic Oncologists has presented the Ovarian Cancer Symptoms Consensus Statement in an attempt to educate the general public about the signs and symptoms of ovarian cancer. The document states that women who have certain symptoms (bloating, pelvic and abdominal pain, difficulty eating, and early satiety as well as urinary urgency or frequency) on a daily basis for more than a few weeks should be specifically evaluated to rule out the possibility of ovarian cancer by means of a skillful pelvic exam, ultrasound examination, and CA-125 determination, as indicated. However, the value of screening for symptoms to diagnose ovarian cancer remains highly controversial.
- The most important sign on physical exam is the presence of a pelvic mass, abdominal mass, or ascites. Pleural effusions are not uncommon.

Diagnostic Testing

The diagnosis of ovarian cancer is most often made by surgical exploration and pathologic confirmation. Prior to exploratory laparotomy, a **CA-125 level** should be drawn, and other primary cancers metastatic to the ovaries should be excluded, specifically colon, gastric, or breast (via barium enema or colonoscopy, upper GI, and mammogram, respectively). Preoperative evaluation may also include a **CT of the chest, abdomen, and pelvis** to assess for extra-abdominal disease and parenchymal liver lesions. In certain circumstances, a preoperative pathologic diagnosis can be obtained by **cytologic study of pleural/ascitic fluid** or percutaneous biopsy.

TREATMENT

Surgical Management

Treatment of ovarian cancer has historically begun with surgical staging and cytoreduction. Thorough surgical staging is essential, as subsequent treatment will be based directly on the surgical stage. Cytoreduction, or debulking, refers to removing as much gross tumor as technically feasible. "Optimal cytoreduction" (now defined as

<0.5 cm largest residual tumor, or even better no gross visible residual disease) confers a significant survival advantage.

Chemotherapy and Biologics

After cytoreductive surgery, adjuvant chemotherapy with a taxane- and platinum-containing compound is used unless precluded by toxicity. Multiple studies have evaluated the role of intraperitoneal chemotherapy in patients with ovarian cancer. A randomized prospective Gynecologic Oncology Group (GOG172) study has shown that intraperitoneal cisplatin with intravenous paclitaxel improves disease-free and overall survival compared to intravenous cisplatin and paclitaxel in patients with optimally cytoreduced ovarian cancer. In general, the administration of intraperitoneal chemotherapy involves significant toxicity. However, quality of life 1 year after treatment is comparable in patients treated intravenously versus intraperitoneally. Multiple modifications to this intraperitoneal regimen are currently being evaluated.[2]

A recent Gynecologic Oncology Group (GOG218) study suggested that the addition of bevacizumab to intravenous carboplatinum and paclitaxel followed by bevacizumab maintenance might be associated with an improvement in progression-free survival.[3]

Neoadjuvant and Maintenance Chemotherapy

- A multinational Phase III study recently demonstrated non-inferiority of neoadjuvant chemotherapy followed by interval cytoreduction compared to up-front surgery followed by intravenous chemotherapy. Neoadjuvant chemotherapy must be considered in patients with obvious unresectable disease and medical comorbidities precluding up-front surgical cytoreduction.[4]
- There is some evidence that single-agent taxane maintenance may delay recurrences in patients who demonstrate complete response to up-front treatment. However, a survival benefit has not yet been documented. This modality should be reserved for patients participating in clinical trials.

Treatment for Recurrent Disease

Treatment in the recurrent setting usually consists of chemotherapy. Selected patients will undergo secondary cytoreductive surgery. In general, patients who present with recurrence or progression more than 6 months after platinum-based chemotherapy are "**platinum sensitive**" and therefore treated with combination chemotherapy including platinum compounds. Those who have recurrences within 6 months of platinum-based therapy are considered **platinum resistant.** These patients are treated with second-line chemotherapy agents such as pegylated liposomal doxorubicin, topotecan, and gemcitabine, among others. Biologic and/or hormonal agents are used in selected cases, alone or in combination with cytotoxic chemotherapy.

MONITORING/FOLLOW-UP

After completion of adjuvant therapy, patients are typically followed with clinical exams, Ca-125 levels, and imaging studies if clinically or biochemically indicated. Recent randomized data have called into question the benefits derived from routine surveillance using Ca-125. There appears to be no survival benefit derived from biochemical screening followed by "earlier" therapeutic intervention when compared to clinical follow-up.

OUTCOME/PROGNOSIS

Surgical staging is the most important prognostic variable for patients with ovarian cancer. Five-year survival rates are estimated to be 75% to 95% for patients with disease limited to the ovaries and 10% to 25% for those with extensive peritoneal disease or extraperitoneal metastases at diagnosis. Other independent prognostic variables include extent of residual disease after primary surgery, histologic grade, volume of ascites, patient age, performance status, and platinum-free interval before recurrence. Interestingly, surgical management by a gynecologic oncologist experienced in the management of this disease has consistently been associated with better outcomes.

ENDOMETRIAL CANCER

GENERAL PRINCIPLES

Classification and Risk Factors

Patients with endometrial carcinomas can be generally classified into two groups. The largest group is represented by **estrogen-dependent or type I tumors.** These patients tend to be younger at diagnosis. Unopposed estrogenic stimulation of the endometrium in these cases is thought to cause endometrial hyperplasia and well- to moderately differentiated endometrioid carcinomas. Tumors of this type usually carry an overall better prognosis. Risk factors for type I endometrial cancer include iatrogenic unopposed stimulation of estrogenic receptors in the uterus (estrogens or selective estrogen receptor modulators such as tamoxifen), chronic anovulation, truncal obesity, diabetes mellitus, hypertension, nulliparity, and late menopause. **Type II** patients are on average older at diagnosis and lack evidence of sustained unopposed estrogenic endometrial exposure as their main risk factor. Tumors in this group tend to be poorly differentiated and include more uncommon and aggressive histologic subtypes such as clear cell, papillary serous carcinoma, and carcinosarcoma (malignant mixed mullerian tumor).

Epidemiology

Endometrial cancer is the most common gynecologic malignancy diagnosed in developed countries and accounts for more than 90% of malignancies affecting the uterine corpus. It was estimated that in 2010, 43,470 new cases of uterine cancer would be diagnosed and 7950 women would die of this disease in the United States. The median age at diagnosis is 63 years.

Prevention

- Since <50% of cases of endometrial cancer will have abnormalities on a Pap smear, evaluation of the endometrial cavity to rule out malignancy requires histologic evaluation. Several biopsy devices are currently available and allow for endometrial sampling to be performed in the office setting with a sensitivity >90%. However, screening for endometrial cancer at the general population level is currently not recommended.
- Biopsy of the endometrium for screening purposes should be reserved for women at high risk. This includes postmenopausal women who have been treated with unopposed estrogen replacement therapy, premenopausal women with prolonged untreated chronic anovulation, and patients with estrogen-producing tumors.

Tamoxifen use does not represent an indication for endometrial surveillance with ultrasound or biopsy in asymptomatic patients. Endometrial cancer is associated with Lynch syndrome (HNPCC) as well as other familial cancer syndromes.

- Women diagnosed with Lynch syndrome have a 40% lifetime risk of developing endometrial cancer. Prophylactic hysterectomy with bilateral salpingo-oophorectomy is an effective strategy for preventing endometrial and ovarian cancer in these women.

DIAGNOSIS

Clinical Presentation

- More than 90% of cases will initially present with **abnormal uterine bleeding.** Therefore, the presence of abnormal peri- or postmenopausal bleeding should prompt immediate and thorough evaluation to rule out the presence of a gynecologic malignancy. If cervical stenosis is present, pyometra or hematometra may develop. Physical exam is usually unremarkable. Slight uterine enlargement may occasionally be present.
- A detailed history and physical examination should be performed. Physical examination may offer evidence of chronic anovulation. Pelvic and rectal exams will allow complete evaluation of the genital tract and pelvic structures. This will assist in ruling out other diagnoses and assessing the presence of extrauterine extension.

Diagnostic Testing

Office **endometrial biopsy** is very accurate (>90% sensitive) in detecting endometrial carcinoma. Patients with a nondiagnostic office biopsy or negative biopsies in the context of high clinical suspicion should be further evaluated with hysteroscopy and dilatation and curettage (D&C).

Initial evaluation usually includes investigation of blood counts, liver and renal function, and radiologic imaging as needed to evaluate for suspected advanced disease. This should include, at a minimum, a chest radiograph. When elevated, CA-125 may suggest extrauterine disease and assist in evaluating response to treatment.

TREATMENT

Surgical Management

All patients who are medically fit should undergo surgical exploration with complete staging. The surgical staging procedure includes pelvic washings for cytologic evaluation, evaluation of peritoneal surfaces with directed biopsies as indicated, extrafascial hysterectomy with bilateral salpingo-oophorectomy, and pelvic and para-aortic lymph node dissection. Nodal dissection can be omitted in cases of well-differentiated adenocarcinoma without myometrial invasion. Minimally invasive procedures are becoming increasingly common for the initial surgical staging and treatment of endometrial cancer.

Radiation Therapy

- Adjuvant treatment with radiation and/or cytotoxic chemotherapy is indicated for extrauterine disease or those with high-risk clinicopathologic features (high grade, deep myometrial invasion, and/or lymph-vascular space invasion).

- The use of adjuvant radiotherapy in patients with early-stage endometrial cancer has not been proven to improve survival, but may play a role in preventing local recurrences that can have an important impact on the quality of life for these patients. Radiation modalities include the use of vaginal brachytherapy, external radiotherapy, and intensity-modulated radiotherapy.

Chemotherapy and Biologics

- Many cytotoxic chemotherapeutic agents have been evaluated in patients with endometrial cancer.[5] The objective response rates to several cytotoxic agents have varied widely. **Platinum compounds** (cisplatin and carboplatin), **taxanes** (paclitaxel), and **doxorubicin** are among the most active agents and are commonly used alone or in combination for the treatment of advanced cases, with response rates ranging from 20% to >40%. Other cytotoxic agents such as topotecan, pegylated liposomal doxorubicin, and gemcitabine are also used in the advanced and recurrent setting. More recently, there has been an increasing interest in the use of **biologic noncytotoxic agents** such as bevacizumab and tyrosine kinase inhibitors in this disease.
- **Hormonal manipulation with high-dose progestins** approaches response rates of 20% in the presence of estrogen and progesterone receptors. This approach is often used for patients with advanced or recurrent disease whose tumors tested positive for these receptors (most commonly well- or moderately differentiated tumors) or in those with contraindication for cytotoxic chemotherapy or radiation.

Treatment for Recurrent Disease

Vaginal recurrences can often be salvaged with radiation therapy. Single site recurrences may be amenable of surgical resection and/or radiation. Distant failures are typically treated with chemotherapy as previously discussed.

MONITORING/FOLLOW-UP

Patients are followed with periodic clinical exams, Pap smears, and imaging studies if clinically indicated.

OUTCOME/PROGNOSIS

Early diagnosis in patients presenting with early symptoms accounts for high cure rates in patients with endometrial cancer. In general, long-term survivorship exceeds 75%. Patients with localized disease and well-differentiated tumors are usually cured by hysterectomy and bilateral salpingo-oophorectomy alone.

Several factors are associated with prognosis in patients with endometrial cancer. These include histologic type, age at diagnosis, tumor grade and stage, depth of myometrial invasion, and presence of lymph-vascular invasion. Overall, the survival by Federation of Gynecology and Obstetrics (FIGO) stage in endometrial cancer approaches 85% for stage I, 75% for stage II, 45% for stage III, and 25% for stage IV disease. However, these figures can vary considerably depending on tumor grade, histologic type, and other clinicopathologic variables.

GESTATIONAL TROPHOBLASTIC DISEASE

This entity encompasses a spectrum of pathologic conditions derived from placental tissues.

HYDATIDIFORM MOLE

GENERAL PRINCIPLES

Classification

- **Complete moles** are tumors characterized by edematous chorionic villi with variable degrees of trophoblastic proliferation. No fetal tissue is identified. Most commonly, they have a 46,XX karyotype resulting from duplication of the paternal haploid chromosomal complement. Approximately 5% of cases have a Y chromosome (46,XY) derived from double sperm fertilization. The uterine size is typically greater than expected for gestational age. It is often possible to identify ovarian theca lutein cysts as a result of ovarian stimulation by large amounts of hCG. The risk of postmolar gestational trophoblastic neoplasia (GTN) in cases of complete moles is ~15% to 20%.
- **Partial or incomplete moles** have variable and usually just focal villous edema. Trophoblastic proliferation is mild and usually coexists with a fetus or fetal tissues. Most commonly they have a triploid (69,XXX or XXY) chromosomal complement derived from one maternal and two paternal haploid sets of chromosomes. Most cases present as a missed abortion, with uterine size less than that expected for gestational age. The risk of postmolar GTN in cases of partial moles is generally <5%.

Epidemiology

In the United States, these conditions are rare and diagnosed in ~1 in 1500 pregnancies.

DIAGNOSIS

Clinical Presentation

- Patients with **complete moles** usually present in early pregnancy with an **abnormally elevated hCG.** Clinical presentation also includes first-trimester bleeding (95%), excessive uterine enlargement (50%), and medical complications (10% to 25%) such as hyperemesis gravidarum, early-onset preeclampsia, and hyperthyroidism. These systemic manifestations are mainly seen in cases with uterine enlargement >14- to 16-week size.
- **Incomplete moles** often present as **missed or incomplete abortions,** and incidental diagnosis is made upon histologic evaluation of products of conception. With the increased use of ultrasound and measurement of hCG levels in early pregnancy, this condition is usually diagnosed in the first trimester.

Diagnostic Testing

Once the diagnosis of molar pregnancy is suspected, **pelvic ultrasound is the imaging test of choice.** The **classic "snow storm pattern" sonographic appearance** is highly suggestive of molar pregnancy. Patients should be thoroughly evaluated with complete blood counts, coagulation studies, renal and liver function tests, blood type and antibody screen, determination of serum hCG level, and chest radiograph.

TREATMENT

Treatment consists of evacuation of the uterine cavity in the operating room by means of dilatation and suction curettage. High dose uterotonics are usually administered after evacuation to prevent post-evacuation hemorrhage.

MONITORING/FOLLOW-UP

- After evacuation, patients should be monitored with **periodic determinations of serum quantitative hCG levels.** These should be obtained weekly while hCG is elevated and then monthly for 6 months. The objective of this surveillance program is to identify patients who will develop postmolar GTNs. The hCG curve in these patients will usually demonstrate rising or plateaued levels.
- A normal pregnancy during the surveillance period would make identification of GTN by means of hCG follow-up virtually impossible. Therefore, effective contraception should be prescribed to these patients during this surveillance period. Oral contraceptives represent a highly desirable method for the motivated patient. This method does not increase the incidence of postmolar GTN and is usually associated with a cyclic and predictable uterine bleeding pattern.

OUTCOME/PROGNOSIS

- In general, the prognosis associated with this disease is excellent. However, ~20% of patients with complete moles and 5% of those with incomplete moles will go on to develop the more complicated GTN.
- After a mole, the vast majority of patients will have subsequent normal pregnancies. However, there is a 10-fold increased risk of a second hydatidiform mole (1% to 2%). Therefore, early obstetric ultrasound should be recommended in all subsequent pregnancies.

GESTATIONAL TROPHOBLASTIC NEOPLASIA

GENERAL PRINCIPLES

Classification

The term gestational trophoblastic neoplasia (GTN) or gestational trophoblastic tumor (GTT) refers to various histologic entities that have the ability to invade locally and/or metastasize. These conditions include persistent or invasive hydatidiform moles, placental site trophoblastic tumors, and choriocarcinomas.[6] GTN may develop after a normal pregnancy, after a molar pregnancy, or after an abortion or, alternatively, may present primarily.

DIAGNOSIS

Clinical Presentation

Most cases will be diagnosed as a result of **routine hCG level surveillance** after uterine evacuation following a molar pregnancy or a missed/incomplete abortion (plateau or rise in hCG levels). Patients with locally invasive persistent or recurrent disease often report **vaginal bleeding.** Diagnosis in these cases is usually clinical. D&C is generally avoided to prevent potential uterine perforations. Most patients with metastatic disease will have pulmonary involvement (80%). Other relatively common metastatic sites include the vagina (30%), liver, brain, spleen, and/or kidneys (≤10%). Biopsy of metastatic lesions should be avoided to avoid risk of uncontrollable hemorrhage.

Diagnostic Testing

Evaluation should include complete blood counts, coagulation studies, renal and liver function tests, pretreatment determination of serum hCG level, and radiographic survey to assess for metastatic disease in the head, chest, abdomen, and pelvis (usually CT scan and/or MRI).

TREATMENT

After radiographic studies and clinical determination of risk category (based on age, type of antecedent pregnancy, time interval from index pregnancy, hCG levels, largest tumor size, site and number of metastases, and history of previous failed chemotherapy), patients are assigned a stage and a risk score.

Surgical Management

Almost all patients with nonmetastatic GTN can be cured without hysterectomy. These cases are usually treated with single-agent chemotherapy (methotrexate or, less commonly, actinomycin D). In patients without a desire for future fertility, pretreatment hysterectomy will reduce the amount of chemotherapy required to induce remission.

Chemotherapy

- Patients with **non-metastatic or low-risk metastatic GTN** can be treated with single-agent chemotherapy (methotrexate or actinomycin D). Approximately 40% of low-risk metastatic cases will fail single-agent treatment and require additional multiagent treatment to achieve remission.
- Patients with **high-risk metastatic disease** or those who have **failed single-agent treatment** will require multiagent chemotherapy. The most effective and frequently used multiagent regimen involves weekly administration of etoposide, methotrexate, and actinomycin D, alternating with cyclophosphamide and vincristine (EMA/CO). Therapy with methotrexate, actinomycin D, and chlorambucil or cyclophosphamide (MAC) was the standard of care for many years before widespread use of EMA/CO. Salvage regimens usually include combinations with etoposide, cisplatin, and other agents. Occasionally, patients with high-risk metastatic disease will require multimodal treatment, incorporating surgical excision of metastatic lesions and radiotherapy.
- Surveillance of hCG is required during treatment. Chemotherapy is usually continued until after normalization of hCG levels.

MONITORING/FOLLOW-UP

Once complete remission is achieved, contraception is recommended and periodic physical exams and hCG levels should be followed strictly for 12 to 24 months. Imaging tests are used as necessary.

OUTCOME/PROGNOSIS

GTN is exquisitely sensitive to chemotherapy, and even patients with widespread disease can be cured. Cure rates exceed 95% in patients with nonmetastatic disease. Even in high-risk metastatic cases, multimodal treatment results in cure rates up to 75%.

REFERENCES

1. Long HJ. Management of metastatic cervical cancer: review of the literature. *J Clin Oncol.* 2007;25:2966–2974.
2. Rao G, Crispens M, Rothenberg ML. Intraperitoneal chemotherapy for ovarian cancer: overview and perspective. *J Clin Oncol.* 2007;25:2867–2872.
3. Burger RA, Brady MF, Bookman MA, et al. Phase III trial of bevacizumab in the primary treatment of epithelial ovarian cancer, primary peritoneal cancer, or fallopian tube cancer: a Gynecologic Oncology Group study. *J Clin Oncol.* 2010;28:946s.
4. Vergote I, Tropé CG, Amant F, et al. Neoadjuvant chemotherapy or primary surgery in stage IIIC or IV ovarian cancer. *N Engl J Med.* 2010;363:943–953.
5. Fleming GF. Systemic chemotherapy for uterine carcinoma: metastatic and adjuvant. *J Clin Oncol.* 2007;25:2883–2990.
6. Garner EI, Goldstein DP, Feltmate CM, et al. Gestational trophoblastic disease. *Clin Obstet Gynecol.* 2007;50(1):112–122.

Brain Tumors

28

Xiaoyi Hu

GENERAL PRINCIPLES

Brain tumors are neoplasms that originate in different cells of the brain (primary brain tumors) or originate elsewhere in the body and metastasize to intracranial compartment (secondary brain tumor). Metastatic tumors are the most common type of brain tumors.[1]

Classification

Primary brain tumors are classified according to cell type. The majority of primary brain tumors in adults are gliomas (oligodendrogliomas and astrocytomas), ependymomas, meningiomas, and primary CNS lymphomas. The most common parenchymal metastases are from lung cancer, renal cell cancer, melanoma, breast cancer, and lymphoma. Dural metastases are seen most commonly with breast or prostate cancer.

Epidemiology

Brain tumors are rare malignancies—the 16th most common in frequency among tumors in adult patients. Primary intracranial tumors have an incidence of 7.1 per 100,000, with ~22,000 people diagnosed and 13,000 deaths in the United States each year.[2] Metastases to the brain are more common, with one estimate that >100,000 patients per year die from a systemic cancer that has metastasized to the brain.

Risk Factors

Ionizing radiation and genetic predisposition in identified syndromes are currently the only known unequivocal risk factors for developing brain neoplasms. Irradiation of the cranium, even at low doses, can increase the incidence of meningiomas by a factor of 10 and the incidence of glial tumors by a factor of 3 to 7. Other potential risks, such as use of cellular phones, exposure to high-tension power wires, head trauma, and exposure to nitrosourea compounds have provided conflicting and unconvincing data and, currently, are not considered to be risk factors.

Management

Management of these tumors often involves a multidisciplinary approach involving the neurosurgeon, neuro-oncologist, radiation oncologist, and neurologist, among others. Rehabilitation efforts may be multidisciplinary and involve rehabilitation specialists, physical and occupational therapists, and nurses.

ASTROCYTOMA

GENERAL PRINCIPLES

The epidemiology of astrocytic tumors depends on their histological grade. Low-grade (grades I and II) astrocytomas are typically found in children and young adults. The peak incidence in adults occurs in the third to fourth decade of life. High-grade astrocytomas (grade III and IV) typically present in the fourth or fifth decade, and glioblastoma multiforme (GBM) usually presents in the sixth or seventh decade. High-grade glial tumors are most common, with an annual incidence of 3 or 4 per 100,000 populations. Of these, 80% are GBMs. GBMs may be either primary or secondary (meaning the GBM has arisen from a tumor that was initially a low-grade astrocytoma). These secondary GBMs tend to occur in younger adults, typically ≤45 years. The male-to-female ratio of malignant astrocytic tumors is 3:2.[1]

Classification/Grading

These tumors are graded by the World Health Organization's four-tiered grading system.[3] The criteria used to grade these tumors include the following features: nuclear atypia, mitotic activity, endothelial proliferation, and necrosis.

- Grade I: absence of all features
- Grade II: any one feature
- Grade III: any two features (anaplastic astrocytoma)
- Grade IV: any three features (GBM)

Pathophysiology

Astrocytomas are composed of cells with elongated or irregular, hyperchromatic nuclei and eosinophilic, expressing glial fibrillary acidic protein in the cytoplasma. GMBs may arise de novo from neural progenitor cells or transition from low-grade astrocytomas. Molecular genetic abnormalities include inactivation of tumor suppressor genes *P53, PTEN, CDKNA, CDKN2B,* and *RB,* overexpression of growth factors PDGF and EGFR, and *isocitrate dehydrogenase* mutation.[4]

DIAGNOSIS

Clinical Presentation

Presentation of these tumors depends on their grade. Low-grade astrocytomas present with seizure in ~90% of cases. Typically, the seizures are focal, but they may become generalized and cause loss of consciousness. Headache is found in 40% of patients. In general, the headache is worse in the morning and improves in a few hours, usually without treatment. On occasion, headache can be unilateral and throbbing, mimicking a migraine or even a cluster headache. Symptoms such as hemiparesis and mental status changes are found in 15% and 10% of patients, respectively. These symptoms reflect the location of the tumor. Malignant astrocytic tumors, on the other hand, present with seizure 15% to 25% of the time and present with headache 50% of the time. These tumors are much more likely to present with focal neurologic deficits such as hemiparesis, seen in 30% to 50% of patients, and mental status abnormalities, seen in 40% to 60% of patients.

Diagnostic Testing

The diagnosis of the tumors is usually suggested by **MRI.** Low-grade astrocytoma is usually seen as a diffuse, nonenhancing mass that typically has a local mass effect and evidence of cortical infiltration with abnormal signal, reaching the surface of the brain. The radiologic borders of these tumors are usually distinct, with no surrounding edema. High-grade astrocytomas have an irregular contrast enhancement, which is often ringlike. These lesions are usually associated with edema, and the mass effect can be severe enough to cause herniation. Pathologic diagnosis of these tumors can be done by stereotactic biopsy or surgical excision of the lesion. A **stereotactic biopsy** can (and often does) provide adequate tissue for grading. However, in some instances it can underestimate the grade, especially in large tumors.

TREATMENT

- Therapy of **low-grade tumors** involves **surgical debulking** of the tumor and perhaps excision of the entire tumor if the tumor does not involve critical structures such as the language areas. With low-grade lesions, the next step in treatment is typically **radiation** if the tumor is not completely resected, has high MIB-1 index, or the patient is over 40 years of age. In younger patients with low-grade tumors that are completely resected, observation is also appropriate. Radiation may be done immediately after surgery or may be deferred until there is radiographic evidence of tumor progression. Studies at this time have not shown a difference in survival benefit between immediate and delayed irradiation. Many physicians will wait to start radiation to provide another treatment option at the time of progression. **Chemotherapy** is also a treatment option in the recurrent setting. Surveillance for recurrence with an MRI is performed every 3 to 6 months for 5 years and then at least annually.
- Therapy of **anaplastic astrocytoma and GBM** is identical. The initial step is to **surgically excise** the tumor. Every effort should be made to remove as much tumor as possible, as this is associated with longer survival and improved neurologic function. Subtotal resection is done if maximal safe resection is not feasible. During surgery, carmustine (BCNU) wafers may be placed for local chemotherapy. This is followed by 60 Gy in 30 fractions of **high-dose irradiation** of the involved field with concurrent daily oral temozolomide (75 mg/m^2).[5] **Bactrim should be used for PCP prophylaxis during radiation.** After completion of radiation, the temozolomide is continued with monthly treatments of 5-day duration for 6 cycles. MRI is performed 2 to 6 weeks after radiation therapy, and then 2 to 4 months for 2 to 3 years. At the time of recurrence, if the disease is localized, a second resection and BCNU wafer insertion should be done if possible. **Bevacizumab,** a vascular endothelial growth factor inhibitor, is FDA approved as a single agent for recurrent or relapsed anaplastic astrocytoma and GBM.[6] Nitrosourea, cyclophosphamide, procarbazine, lomustine, and vincristine (PCV regimen) or platinum-based regimens are also treatment options for recurrence.[7]
- **Brainstem gliomas are inoperable.** These tumors are treated with irradiation. If there is increased intracranial pressure, a shunt may be placed.

PROGNOSIS

Prognosis associated with astrocytomas is determined by their grade. The median survival for adult low-grade astrocytomas is 5 years. Most of these patients die from the progression of their disease to a higher grade. The median survival for malignant astrocytomas is typically ~3 years. The median survival for GBM is typically 1 year.

OLIGODENDROGLIOMAS

GENERAL PRINCIPLES

Epidemiology

Oligodendrogliomas are usually low-grade neoplasms and account for <5% of intracranial tumors and ~20% of glial neoplasms. Mean age at presentation is 38 to 45 years, with a slight male predominance.

Pathophysiology

Oligodendrogliomas arise from oligodendroglial cells, which are responsible for axonal myelination. More than one-third of these tumors have intermixed astrocytic or ependymal elements and are therefore considered "mixed gliomas." They are classified as low-grade and anaplastic oligodendrogliomas (high-grade). Classical oligodendrogliomas are highly associated with the 1p/19q codeletion.

DIAGNOSIS

Clinical Presentation

Patients may present with seizure, progressive hemiparesis, or cognitive impairment, depending on tumor location. These tumors are known to have delicate vasculature and hemorrhage easily, and the patient may present with an acute onset of hemiparesis, headache, and/or lethargy.

Diagnostic Testing

Diagnostic evaluation usually begins with an **MRI.** The radiologic hallmarks differentiating this tumor from an astrocytoma are lack of contrast enhancement and calcification of the tumor. **Biopsy,** as in astrocytoma, is necessary for definitive diagnosis, and excisional biopsy is preferred to stereotactic biopsy. Exam by light microscopy shows oligodendroglioma cells that may have regular and rounded nuclei, with some nuclei having a halolike appearance (sometimes termed fried egg appearance). There are currently no immunohistochemical stains or markers that definitively establish the diagnosis.

TREATMENT

As is seen with low-grade astrocytomas, therapy may not be necessary at initial presentation if the patient is asymptomatic and seizures are adequately controlled. Therapy of low-grade tumors usually begins with the **excisional biopsy** performed to diagnose these tumors. After surgery, observation or focal irradiation and chemotherapy are performed. **Adjuvant chemotherapy** includes temozolomide, PCV regimen, nitrosourea, or platinum-based regimen. Studies have shown that 66% of these tumors respond to therapy.[7] Chemotherapy is not curative, but it can induce sustained remissions. Management should be individualized, and there is some evidence that 1p and 19q loss in the tumor is associated with increased survival.

PROGNOSIS

The median survival for patients with low-grade oligodendroglioma is currently 10 years and that for anaplastic oligodendroglioma is 3 to 5 years. This long survival is attributed to earlier diagnosis of these tumors with MRI and to their chemosensitivity. Most oligodendrogliomas progress by becoming malignant.

EPENDYMOMAS

GENERAL PRINCIPLES

Definition

Histologically, ependymomas arise from the ependymal cells, which are normally lining the ventricular chambers and the central canal of the spinal cord. Most are histologically benign. Usually they are classified as either high or low grade. These tumors may metastasize via cerebrospinal fluid (CSF) pathways. Spinal cord metastases that arise from a brain lesion are known as **drop metastases.** The overall risk of seeding is ~10%, and the greatest risk occurs with high-grade infratentorial lesions.

Epidemiology

Ependymomas have a bimodal incidence, with an early major peak at 5 years and a late minor peak at the median age of 34 years. They account for 5% of intracranial tumors in the adult population. There is a 3:2 male predominance.

Pathophysiology/Molecular Genetics

Ependymomas are generally slow-growing tumors. Genetic changes include losses of chromosome areas 6q and 22q and the X chromosome, or gains of either 1q or 9q, with monosomy 22 being the most frequent change in sporadic ependymomas.

DIAGNOSIS

Clinical Presentation

Clinical presentation depends on the location of the tumor. Most adult tumors occur in supra- and infratentorial regions. They are also frequently seen in the spinal canal, especially the lumbosacral region. The supra- and infratentorial lesions may lead to symptoms of increased intracranial pressure or focal neurologic deficits and seizures. Ataxia, vertigo, and neck stiffness are common presenting symptoms with infratentorial lesions.

Diagnostic Testing

Extent of disease is assessed with an **MRI of the brain and spinal cord.** More than 50% of these tumors will have calcification. Histological confirmation is required for diagnosis, and open surgery is favored to stereotactic biopsy. CSF cytology is important for staging.

TREATMENT

- Therapy is **surgical excision followed by observation if completely resected** or **irradiation if not completely resected.** Gross total resection is the best determinant of outcome. **Steroids** may be given both before and after surgery to help decrease edema and other complications. Targeting only the local site with methods such as high-fractionation radiotherapy and stereotactic radiosurgery has shown promise in treating the tumor and limiting some of the complications seen. There is no definitive role for chemotherapy at this time.[7]

- Evidence of dissemination, as determined by MRI, positive CSF cytology, or myelographic findings, warrants additional radiation of the spinal axis. The dose and the extent of irradiation are also determined by the histological grade, with anaplastic lesions generally receiving more intensive regimens.

PROGNOSIS

Prognosis for these patients is excellent after treatment if the tumor is completely resected. The 5-year disease-free survival is >80%. Ten-year survival rates range from 40% to 60%. Age is the most important prognostic factor, with younger patients having a worse outcome. Poor prognosis includes high histological grade, incomplete surgical resection, and a poor performance status. Patients should be followed by MRI, as the recurrence rate is significant.

MENINGIOMA

GENERAL PRINCIPLES

Meningiomas are extra-axial primary brain tumors. They are of leptomeningeal origin, arising from arachnoid cap cells. They account for 33.8% of all primary brain and CNS tumors.

Classification

Meningiomas typically are classified as one of **four histological patterns:** meningothelial, transitional, fibrous, and angioblastic. The first three subtypes account for the majority of the meningiomas and have benign behavior. The angioblastic subtype is the least common but most aggressive form. Malignancy is determined by the amount of brain invasion, increased and atypical mitotic figures, increased cellularity, a papillary histological pattern, and distant metastases. Malignant meningiomas account for between 1% and 10% of cases. Metastatic disease is seen in <0.1% of cases. Radiation-induced meningiomas are more commonly atypical or malignant.

Epidemiology

The annual incidence of meningiomas is ~7.8 per 100,000, although most are asymptomatic and discovered incidentally at autopsy. The incidence of symptomatic tumors is ~2 in 100,000, and they occur more frequently in women than men. They are primarily adult tumors, with a peak occurrence at age 45 years. There is an association with breast cancer, neurofibromatosis, and a history of cranial irradiation.

Pathophysiology/Molecular Genetics

Deletion and inactivation of *NF2* on chromosome 22 is a predominant feature in sporadic meningiomas. Additional genes on chromosome 22 are likely involved as well. 14q, 1p, 6q, and 18q are also lost in meningiomas. Meningiomas are reported in families of several cancer predisposition syndromes involving the genes *NF1, PTCH, CREBBP, VHL, PTEN,* and *CDKNA.*[8]

DIAGNOSIS

Clinical Presentation

Meningiomas can arise virtually anywhere along the leptomeninges. Ninety percent are intracranial, and 90% of these are supratentorial. The three most common sites are adjacent to the superior sagittal sinus, over the cerebral convexities, and along the sphenoid ridge. These three sites account for 60% of intracranial meningiomas. Clinical presentation of meningiomas varies greatly depending on where they arise. **Focal neurologic deficits are common,** as are **symptoms of increased intracranial pressure. Seizures** are particularly common, occurring in >50% of patients. Many are found incidentally on CT or MRI.

Diagnostic Testing

Diagnosis of these tumors is suggested by **MRI.** They have a characteristic appearance of marginal dural thickening that tapers peripherally (the "tail" sign), as well as circumscribed, extra-axial, homogeneously enhancing, dural-based masses. Peritumoral edema and mass effect are common. Twenty percent of the tumors have calcification.

TREATMENT

Observation is preferred for tumor <3 cm and asymptomatic patients. Surgical resection is recommended for tumor >3 cm or symptomatic patients.[7] Total resection is curative for low-grade meningiomas. High-grade meningiomas require radiation therapy followed by surgical resection. Stereotactic radiosurgery is frequently used for tumors at the base of the skull, which are usually unresectable, because they are intertwined with vital structures. At the time of recurrence, a second resection should be performed, followed by external-beam irradiation.

PROGNOSIS

Meningiomas have an excellent prognosis. Disease-free survival at 10 years is 80% to 90% for all meningiomas. If the tumor is partially resected, the 10-year progression-free survival is 50% to 70%. Nearly 65% of malignant meningiomas will recur in 5 years, and nearly 80% will recur in 10 years. Patients who are younger, do not have CNS invasion, and are able to have more extensive resection do better overall. All patients should be followed closely for recurrence.

PRIMARY CENTRAL NERVOUS SYSTEM LYMPHOMA

GENERAL PRINCIPLES

Primary central nervous system lymphoma (PCL) is an uncommon variant of extranodal non-Hodgkin lymphoma that can affect the brain, leptomeninges, eyes, or spinal cord without evidence of systemic disease.

Classification

Ninety percent of non-HIV-associated PCLs are diffuse large B-cell type, with the remaining 10% being poorly characterized low-grade lymphomas, Burkitt lymphomas, or T-cell lymphomas.

Epidemiology

PCL accounts for approximately 3% of primary brain tumors. Patients with congenital or acquired immunosuppression have a markedly increased risk of PCL. The incidence of non-HIV-related PCL peaks in the sixth to seventh decades, with a male-to-female ratio of 2:1. There are no environmental or behavioral risk factors that are associated with the development of this disease. In immunocompromised patients, the risk increases 100- to 1000-fold. This increase is believed to most likely be secondary to infection with Epstein–Barr or other lymphatic viruses, which have been speculated to be possible transforming events.[9]

DIAGNOSIS

Clinical Presentation

PCLs are solitary in ~50% of patients on presentation, and patients most commonly present with behavioral or cognitive changes, seen in approximately two-thirds of patients. Hemiparesis, aphasia, and visual field deficits are seen in ~50% of patients and seizures in 15% to 20%. Approximately 15% will develop uveitis, sometimes preceding cerebral symptoms by months.

Diagnostic Testing

These tumors are typically diagnosed with the use of **MRI.** They usually are periventricular in location and have a homogeneous pattern of enhancement. Approximately 25% to 50% of patients will also have cells identified in the CSF. **Stereotactic biopsy** is necessary for tissue diagnosis. **Further workup** should also include a slit-lamp eye exam, CSF cytology with cell count and protein assessment, spinal MRI, chest x-ray, HIV test, blood cell count, and complete metabolic panel to assess for other sites of disease.

TREATMENT

- Unlike other intracranial tumors, there is **no role for surgery** other than a stereotactic biopsy in primary CNS lymphoma treatment.
- **Corticosteroids** can work rapidly to cause tumor regression and decrease peritumoral edema, but should be held prior to diagnostic biopsy in clinically stable patients. They have a direct lymphocytolytic effect that may disrupt cellular morphology and lead to diagnostic inaccuracy.
- **High-dose methotrexate** as a single agent is now the standard care.
- **Whole-brain radiation therapy** is used as salvage treatment of recurrence. The radiation ports should include the orbits if retinal or vitreous disease is present and also the spinal axis if CSF cytology findings suggest meningeal disease.
- **Intrathecal chemotherapy** is needed if CSF cytology or spinal MRI is positive.

PROGNOSIS

Prognosis is dependent on treatment regimen. Radiation alone usually results in a median survival of 12 to 18 months, but is not recommended for patients older than 60 years. When chemotherapy is used before radiation, the median survival improves to 42 months, with 25% of patients alive at 5 years. Important indicators of poor prognosis include age >60 years, ECOG performance status >1, elevated serum LDH, elevated CSF protein, and involvement of deep regions of the brain.[10]

METASTATIC TUMORS OF THE CENTRAL NERVOUS SYSTEM

GENERAL PRINCIPLES

- Metastatic lesions to the brain typically occur via hematogenous spread and are 10 times as common as primary CNS tumors. There typically is a predilection for the gray matter–white matter junction in which cerebral blood flow is greatest. Spinal involvement may be secondary to spread from the primary site to the vertebral body, with subsequent compression of the spinal cord, retrograde spread via the vertebral venous plexus, or direct invasion of the epidural space via the intervertebral foramen. Alternatively, multifocal spread to the meninges may occur. Twenty percent of cancer patients will develop brain metastases, and 10% will develop spinal metastases. Refer to Chapter 35 for more information regarding spinal cord compression.
- The lung is the most common origin of brain metastases. Other sources include breast (especially ductal carcinoma), melanoma, renal cell cancer, lymphoma, GI malignancies, germ cell tumors, and thyroid cancer.

DIAGNOSIS

Clinical Presentation

Metastatic tumors present with the *same clinical features* common to any intracranial mass but occur with a *much more rapid rate of progression.* Focal deficits, seizures, and symptoms of increased intracranial pressure are the usual presenting symptoms. The rapid progression is believed to be secondary to the development of cerebral edema, which is usually associated with metastatic lesions.

Diagnostic Testing

Diagnosis of these lesions is suggested by their appearance on **MRI or CT using contrast.** Ring-enhancing or diffusely enhancing lesions, typically surrounded by a zone of edema disproportionate to the size of the lesion, are most commonly seen. MRI is also useful and is more sensitive in identifying multiple lesions. Meningeal involvement requires both brain and spinal imaging, where hydrocephalus or more diffuse enhancement may be seen. **CSF with positive cytology is diagnostic,** and an elevated CSF protein level is suggestive of meningeal disease. These cancers are typically considered incurable with few exceptions.

TREATMENT

Therapy is palliative in nature. High-dose **glucocorticosteroids** will frequently provide a rapid improvement in symptoms as the surrounding edema decreases. Improvement occurs within 6 to 24 hours and is sustained with continuous therapy. There is no role for prophylactic anticonvulsants in patients with brain metastases. Whole-brain radiation therapy is the primary treatment mode for focal brain metastases. For those patients who have a single lesion in the brain, surgical excision or gamma-knife radiation may be used as a palliative measure. Surgical excision is typically followed by whole-brain irradiation. For leptomeningeal disease, radiation is limited to symptomatic sites and intrathecal chemotherapy is initially administered weekly, and then monthly after four treatments. Methotrexate is the most often used regimen, but cytarabine and thiotepa are other options. In primary cancers that are chemotherapy responsive, systemic chemotherapy may provide some improvement, although there is typically less of a response than seen in the primary tumor.

PROGNOSIS

Survival in untreated brain metastases is typically 1 month. Survival improves to a median of 3 to 6 months with the use of steroids and radiation. If the tumor is amenable to surgical excision, the survival may improve to a median of 40 weeks.

REFERENCES

1. McLendon R, Rosenblum MK, Bigner DD. *Russell and Rubinstein's Pathology of Tumors of the Nervous System.* London: Hodder Arnold; 2006.
2. Jemal A, Siegel R, Xu J, et al. Cancer statistics, 2010. *CA Cancer J Clin.* 2010;60:277–300.
3. Louis DN, Ohgaki H, Wiestler OD, et al. The 2007 WHO classification of tumours of the central nervous system. *Acta Neuropathol.* 2007;114:97–109.
4. Parsons DW, Jones S, Zhang X, et al. An integrated genomic analysis of human glioblastoma multiforme. *Science.* 2008;321:1807–1812.
5. Stupp R, Mason WP, van den Bent MJ, et al. Radiotherapy plus concomitant and adjuvant temozolomide for glioblastoma. *N Engl J Med.* 2005;352:987–996.
6. Vredenburgh JJ, Desjardins A, Herndon JE, 2nd, et al. Bevacizumab plus irinotecan in recurrent glioblastoma multiforme. *J Clin Oncol.* 2007;25:4722–4729.
7. National Comprehensive Cancer Network. Central Nervous System Cancers. Version I, 2011. Adult cancer pain. In: *National Comprehensive Cancer Network Practice Guidelines in Oncology, 2011:1.* Last accessed: 4/5/2011 <http://www.nccn.org/professionals/physician_gls/pdf/cns.pdf>.
8. Wiemels J, Wrensch M, Claus EB. Epidemiology and etiology of meningioma. *J Neurooncol.* 2010;99:307–314.
9. Gerstner ER, Batchelor TT. Primary central nervous system lymphoma. *Arch Neurol.* 2010;67:291–297.
10. Ferreri AJ, Blay JY, Reni M, et al. Prognostic scoring system for primary CNS lymphomas: the International Extranodal Lymphoma Study Group experience. *J Clin Oncol.* 2003;21: 266–272.

Leukemias

29

George Ansstas

GENERAL PRINCIPLES

Leukemia is the result of somatically acquired genetic mutations leading to the dysregulation and clonal expansion of myeloid and/or lymphoid progenitor cells. The accumulation of neoplastic cells, both in the bone marrow and in the peripheral tissues, manifests as cytopenias with associated complications, elevation of the total WBC count, and dysfunction of the various involved organs. The diagnosis is typically suspected based on an abnormal CBC and peripheral smear and then confirmed on bone marrow biopsy. The prognosis and treatment depend on the age of the patient, accurate determination of the type of the leukemia, and cytogenetics and molecular markers.

ACUTE MYELOGENOUS LEUKEMIA

GENERAL PRINCIPLES

Definition

The acute leukemias are the result of abnormal clonal proliferation of mutated progenitor cells. The mutations cause a block in the maturation process, leading to an accumulation of immature cells. The expansion of the abnormal clone leads to suppression of the other elements in the marrow, often producing clinical bone marrow failure and making the patient gravely ill. The clinical course of untreated acute leukemia is very brief, with patients succumbing in days to weeks from the complications of marrow failure. Therapy involves intensive chemotherapy regimens, prolonged hospitalizations, and, potentially, stem cell transplantation.

Classification

The French–American–British (FAB) group identifies nine subtypes of AML that are based on morphology and staining (Table 29-1). They indicate the myeloid lineage and the degree of differentiation. Cytogenetic evaluation is crucial, as it helps to determine treatment and prognosis (Table 29-2). For example, the M3 subtype (acute promyelocytic leukemia; APL) is associated with the translocation 15;17, a distinct clinical phenotype (DIC), a good prognosis, and tailored therapy. M7 is associated with a poor clinical outcome in the absence of transplantation. The World Health Organization (WHO) has developed a classification system of AML based not only on morphologic findings but also on genetic and clinical findings (Table 29-3).[1] In the WHO system, AML is defined by >20% myeloblasts in the bone marrow aspirate. Patients with clonal cytogenetic abnormalities such as t(8;21), inv(16), and t(15;17) have AML regardless of the blast percentage. Gene mutations are increasingly being recognized as important diagnostic and prognostic markers in myeloid neoplasms. These include, among others, *NPM1, CEBPA, FLT3, RUNX1, KIT,*

TABLE 29-1 ACUTE MYELOGENOUS LEUKEMIA, FAB CLASSIFICATION

Subtype	Name	Frequency (%)	Peroxidase/ SB/NP[a]
M0	Myeloblastic with minimal differentiation	<5	–/–/–
M1	Myeloblastic without maturation	20	+/+/–
M2	Myeloblastic with maturation	25	+/+/–
M3	Promyelocytic (APL)	10	+/+/–
M4	Myelomonocytic	20	+/+/+
M4Eo	Myelomonocytic with abnormal eosinophils	5–10	+/+/+
M5	Monocytic	20	–/–/+
M6	Erythroleukemia	5	+/+/–
M7	Megakaryoblastic	<5	–/–/+

+, positive; –, negative.

[a]Myeloperoxidase, Sudan black (SB), and nonspecific esterase (NE) stains.

Adapted from DeVita VT, Hellman S, Rosenberg S. *Cancer: Principles and Practice of Oncology.* 6th ed. Philadelphia: Lippincott Williams & Wilkins; 2001.

WT1, DNMT3A, and *MLL* in AML; and *GATA1* in myeloid proliferations associated with Down syndrome. Although over- and underexpression of genes has proved to affect the prognosis in some myeloid neoplasms, at the present time analysis of gene dosage by quantitative RT-PCR is not practical on a daily basis, nor have gene expression arrays been introduced into routine use.[2] There are four main groups of AML recognized in this classification system:

1. AML with recurrent genetic abnormalities
2. AML with myelodysplasia-related features

TABLE 29-2 CYTOGENETIC ABNORMALITIES IN ACUTE MYELOID LEUKEMIA AND ASSOCIATED PROGNOSIS

Risk Group	Cytogenetic Findings	Preferred Consolidation Strategy
Favorable	t(15;17), t(8;21), inv(16)	Chemotherapy
Intermediate	Normal or ≤2 nonspecific chromosomal aberrations	Chemotherapy OR allogeneic transplant
Unfavorable	Complex karyotype (defined as ≥3 abnormalities, excluding the favorable-risk cytogenetics) inv(3), t(6;9), t(6;11), t(11;19) del(5q) –5, –7, +8	Allogeneic transplant

Adapted from Mrozek K, Bloomfield CD. Chromosome aberrations, gene mutations and expression changes, and prognosis in adult acute myeloid leukemia. *Hematol Am Soc Hematol Educ Program.* 2006:169–177.

TABLE 29-3 ACUTE LYMPHOBLASTIC LEUKEMIA, IMMUNOTYPE, AND FAB CLASSIFICATION

Immunotype	Frequency (%)	FAB Subtype	Staining
Pre-B cell	75	L1, L2	+TdT, +CALLA, B-cell markers (CD19, CD20)
T cell	20	L1, L2	+TdT, –CALLA, +acid phosphatase, +T cell markers (CD2, CD7, CD5)
B cell	5	L3	–TdT, +surface IgG

TdT, terminal deoxynucleotidyl transferase; CALLA, common acute lymphoblastic leukemia antigen.

3. Therapy-related AML and MDS
4. AML, not otherwise specified

- **AML with recurrent genetic abnormalities.** This WHO category contains AML variants that contain genetic abnormalities of prognostic significance:
  - **AML with t(8;21)(q22;q22); RUNX1-RUNX1T1.** This leukemia is associated with a more favorable prognosis. The presence of c-KIT mutations is an adverse prognostic features in patients with t(8;21).
  - **AML with inv(16)(p13.1q22) or t(16;16)(p13.1;q22); CEFB-MYH11** (previously acute myelomonocytic leukemia, AMML, FAB M4Eo). This leukemia occurs in younger patients and can present as an extramedullary myeloid sarcoma. It is associated with a more favorable prognosis although cases with an additional c-KIT mutation may do more poorly.
  - **APL with t(15;17)(q22;q12); PML-RARA.** It is notable that the malignant cells in APL are promyelocytes, making this another AML where the presence of 20% blasts is not required. Outcomes in this variant of AML are generally favorable. It can present with disseminated intravascular coagulation (DIC).
  - **AML with t(9;11)(p22;q23); MLLT3-MLL.** This type of leukemia is usually monocytic and more common in children. It can present with DIC, and high white cell counts with gingival or skin infiltration. It has an intermediate prognosis.
  - **AML with t(6;9)(p23;q34); DEK-NUP214.** This is a rare type of leukemia that is associated with basophilia, pancytopenia, and dysplasia. It has a generally poor prognosis.
  - **AML with inv(3)(q21q26.2) or t(3;3)(q21;q26.2); RPN1-EVI1.** This leukemia is also rare, accounting for only 1% or 2% of cases. Patients are anemic but may have normal or elevated platelet counts. It is frequently associated with dysplasia and is associated with aggressive disease and a short survival time.
  - **AML (megakaryoblastic) with t(1;22)(p13;q13); RBM15-MKL1.** This type of leukemia is also rare, but is typically a megakaryoblastic process occurring in infants, although it is not seen in patients with Down Syndrome. Sometimes it can present as a mass and mimic sarcoma.

- Two provisional entities identified at the molecular level are
  - **AML with mutated NPM1.** The mutation is seen in about one-third of all cases of AML making it overlap other types. In almost all cases, the mutation is seen in AML with normal cytogenetics. The presence of the NPM1 mutation confers a better prognosis, but only if it is seen alone. When seen in conjunction with mutations in FLT3, it is associated with a poor prognosis.
  - **AML with mutated CEBPA.** Mutation in CEBPA is seen in ~6% to 15% of AML, commonly in cases with a normal karyotype. Cases with this mutation are associated with a good prognosis.
- **Mutation in FLT3** occurs in 30% to 40% of patients with AML and normal cytogenetics. Patients with this mutation often present with high WBC counts. Two variants exist: FLT3 mutation with internal tandem duplication and a less prevalent mutation affecting the tyrosine kinase domain of the enzyme. The presence of a FLT3 mutation can overcome the favorable effects of NPM1 and CEBPA mutations when they occur concurrently.

Epidemiology

AML is the most common acute leukemia in adults and accounts for ~80% of cases in this group. In the United States, the incidence has been stable at 3 to 5 cases per 100,000 population. In contrast, AML accounts for less than 10% of acute leukemias in children less than 10 years of age. In adults, the median age at diagnosis is ~65 years. The incidence increases with age with ~1.3 and 12.2 cases per 100,000 population for those under or over 65 years, respectively. The male-to-female ratio is ~5:3.

Risk Factors

Radiation, previous chemotherapy with alkylating agents or topoisomerase inhibitors, myelodysplasia, myeloproliferative disorders, aplastic anemia, and exposure to benzene are known risk factors for the development of AML. Higher risk for AML is seen in people with Down syndrome (particularly AML-M7), Turner, and Klinefelter syndromes. In most cases, no risk factors are clearly defined.

DIAGNOSIS

Clinical Presentation

Marked cytopenias from leukemic infiltration of the marrow result in diverse presentations, including fatigue, pallor, and dyspnea on exertion from anemia; hemorrhage from thrombocytopenia; and fevers and infection from neutropenia. Extramedullary tissue invasion by leukemic cells (most commonly with AML-M5) may result in hepatomegaly, splenomegaly, lymphadenopathy, rashes (leukemia cutis), gingival hypertrophy, CNS dysfunction and cranial neuropathies, intestinal involvement, lytic bony lesions, or even establishment of infiltrative masses (granulocytic sarcomas or chloromas). With myeloblast counts >50,000, **leukostasis** may occur, resulting in dyspnea from pulmonary infiltrates or CNS dysfunction (ranging from somnolence to cerebral ischemia). **Spontaneous tumor lysis syndrome** may cause hyperuricemia, hyperphosphatemia, hypocalcemia, or hyperkalemia and renal failure. Patients may also present with disseminated intravascular coagulation (DIC; with excessive bleeding), which is more commonly seen in the M3 and M5 subtypes.

Diagnostic Testing

Workup should include the following.

- **CBC.** Pancytopenia or leukocytosis may be present
- **Coagulation profile.** INR, prothrombin time, partial thromboplastin time, D-dimer, and fibrinogen to look for DIC.
- **Electrolytes.** Tumor lysis may cause hyperkalemia, hypocalcemia, hyperphosphatemia, or hyperuricemia.
- Lactate dehydrogenase (LDH)
- **Peripheral smear.** Leukemic myeloblasts on Wright–Giemsa stain of the peripheral blood and bone marrow aspirate demonstrate large nuclei with scant cytoplasm and may contain Auer rods (eosinophilic needlelike inclusions).
- **Lumbar puncture.** This should be done if neurologic symptoms are present.
- **Bone marrow aspirate and biopsy,** evaluated for the following:
  - Morphology and histochemical staining
  - Flow cytometry, to distinguish AMLs from lymphoid and to determine the subtype of AML
  - Cytogenetics, which is critical in the initial workup for AML since it provides a wealth of prognostic information and helps to guide therapy
  - Molecular studies, abnormalities in certain genes, such as mutations in FLT3, nucleophosmin (NPM1), KIT, or CEBPA, to confer prognostic significance in adult patients with AML

TREATMENT

Treatment is divided into two phases: **induction** and **consolidation.** The goal is to achieve remission, defined as <5% blasts in the bone marrow and recovery of peripheral blood counts.

- **Induction** chemotherapy consists of 7 days of cytarabine (Ara-C) and 3 days of an anthracycline (daunorubicin or idarubicin; "7+3" regimen). Complete remission can be obtained in ~70% to 80% of patients <60 years and in ~50% of older patients. In patients with AML who are older than 60 years of age, escalation of the dose of daunorubicin to twice the conventional dose effects a more rapid response and a higher response rate than does the conventional dose, without additional toxic effects.[3] Patients are generally admitted to the hospital during induction for nearly a month, require frequent blood and platelet transfusions, and often have febrile neutropenia.
- **Consolidation** therapy is essential to prevent relapse and is guided by cytogenetics, age, and patient comorbidities. Therapeutic options include allogeneic bone marrow transplantation or further chemotherapy with high-dose cytarabine (HiDAC) or other regimens. HiDAC is efficacious in younger patients and those with core binding factor leukemia. It is considered too toxic for general use in patients over 60 years with AML due to a higher incidence of cerebellar ataxia (>30% in patients ≥60 years), which is irreversible in some patients. Autologous transplants offer little to no benefit over chemotherapy.
- For **promyelocytic** (M3) **leukemia, all-trans retinoic acid** (ATRA) is given with induction chemotherapy. ATRA ameliorates the coagulopathy associated with M3 but is also associated with the potentially dangerous APL **differentiation syndrome.** Maintenance therapy with lower-dose ATRA is commonly used.

Recent data show that consolidation with **arsenic trioxide** (ATO) decreases risk of relapse and improves overall survival. Relapse occurs in 5% to 10% of patients with APL and in ~20% to 30% of those with **high-risk APL** as defined as those who present with a white blood cell count above 10,000 and a platelet count less than 40,000. ATO is the treatment of choice for most patients with **relapsed APL.** Second complete remission can be obtained in 85% to 88% of patients. It is unclear whether adding ATRA to ATO is better than ATO alone. ATO is able to penetrate the blood-brain barrier and so can be used in patients with CNS involvement. If a second remission is obtained and reverse transcription polymerase chain reaction (RT-PCR) testing is negative for the PML/RAR-alpha transcript, consolidation with either autologous hematopoietic cell transplantation (HCT), allogeneic HCT, or further ATO is recommended. If PCR negativity is not obtained, allogeneic HCT becomes the favored treatment.

- In the case of **relapse,** patients should be salvaged with intensive chemotherapy and then considered for allogeneic bone marrow transplantation. Patients who are not transplant candidates, due to age or comorbidities, should be considered for treatment on clinical trials.

COMPLICATIONS

Leukostasis may cause symptoms that require emergent cytoreduction with hydroxyurea and/or leukapheresis. Tumor lysis syndrome, fever, and neutropenia are all concerns as well (see Chap. 35). Cytopenias should be supported with transfusions, and coagulopathy should be corrected. Prospective trials have identified 10,000/μL as a relatively safe transfusion threshold for platelets during inpatient induction chemotherapy. If the patient has received a bone marrow transplant, he or she should be followed closely for symptoms of opportunistic infections and graft-versus-host disease (see Chap. 31).

PROGNOSIS

Leukemia can typically be divided into good, poor, and intermediate prognostic groups.

- **Good-prognosis** leukemias are those with favorable cytogenetics: translocation (15;17) (associated with M3 AML), translocation (8;21) (associated with M2 AML), and inversion 16 (associated with M4 AML with eosinophilia). These patients are typically offered induction therapy followed by chemotherapy-based consolidation, as they have a relatively high rate of cure by this strategy (~60% to 70%).
- **Poor prognostic indicators** include age >60 years; AML secondary to myelodysplastic syndrome or antecedent hematologic disorder; deletion of 5q, 7q, or trisomy 8; and lack of the favorable cytogenetics noted earlier. Patients with poor-prognosis leukemia have a high rate of relapse and should be considered for allogeneic bone marrow transplant in first remission.
- Patients with normal cytogenetics fall into an intermediate risk group, and management should be individualized after remission. New molecular prognostic markers such as mutations in the FLT-3, NPM, DNMT3A, and MLL genes may help guide therapy in this group. Clinical trials are always ongoing, and

whenever appropriate, patients in all groups should be considered for participation. Since 1970, the 5-year survival rate has increased from 15% to 40% with advances in antileukemic and supportive therapies (i.e., antibiotics, antifungals, improvement in transfusion medicine).

ACUTE LYMPHOBLASTIC LEUKEMIA

GENERAL PRINCIPLES

Definition

Acute lymphoblastic leukemia (ALL) results from the abnormal proliferation of a lymphoid hematopoietic progenitor cell. It accounts for 80% of childhood leukemias and 20% of adult acute leukemias. The median age at diagnosis is 13 years old, with 39% of cases diagnosed in patients older than 20 years. People with Down syndrome are at a higher risk for developing ALL. This section deals only with adult ALL, which has a worse prognosis than childhood ALL.

Classification

Classification is based on morphologic (FAB system) and immunophenotypic information (Table 29-3). Many different translocations have been reported in B ALL, three of which predict response to intensive chemotherapy.

- **The Philadelphia chromosome: t(9;22)(a34;q11); BCR/ABL** is the most frequent rearrangement in adult ALL and is associated with a poor prognosis. It is present in 25% of adult and 3% of childhood cases. The incidence of t(9;22) increases with age and is present in 40% to 50% of patients older than 60 years.
- **t(v;11q23); MLL rearranged:** associated with a poor prognosis, seen in infants <1 year and adults.
- **t(12;21)(p12;q22) TEL/AML1:** associated with a good prognosis and hyperdiploidy, this is the most common rearrangement seen in children.

The t(9;22) and t(v;11q23) are often associated with a pro-B immunophenotype and a poor prognosis, while the t(12;21) is associated with common pre-B ALL.

DIAGNOSIS

Clinical Presentation

The clinical phenotype of ALL is very similar to that of AML. Patients present with malaise, fatigue, dyspnea, and bone pain. Patients also typically have signs of marrow failure such as bleeding, bruising, fever, and infection. More commonly than in AML, in up to 10% of patients, the CNS may be involved at presentation, manifesting as headache and/or cranial nerve palsies. Leukostasis may also be present. Hepatosplenomegaly and lymphadenopathy can be seen. ALL can be associated with an anterior mediastinal mass (in T-cell subtypes) or large abdominal lymph nodes (in B-cell subtypes).

Diagnostic Testing

Basic workup is similar to that for AML. A **peripheral smear** will usually demonstrate the presence of circulating blasts. **Bone marrow** will be hypercellular, with >30% blasts. Cytoplasmic granules and Auer rods should be absent. However, it can be extremely difficult to diagnose ALL on clinical and morphologic grounds alone. Immunophenotyping is often necessary to distinguish ALL from AML. Thirty percent of adult ALL patients exhibit the Philadelphia chromosome t(9;22), as seen in chronic myelogenous leukemia (CML).

TREATMENT

Therapy for ALL consists of multiple phases.

- **Induction chemotherapy** typically consists of vincristine, a steroid, and an anthracycline. Most protocols include l-asparaginase as well. One regimen is hyper-CVAD (cyclophosphamide, vincristine, dexamethasone, and doxorubicin alternating with high-dose methotrexate and cytarabine with incorporated intrathecal therapy).[4] These multiagent protocols carry the burden of profound myelosuppression, and patients must be followed for infectious and cytopenic complications. Induction mortality rates range from 3% to 20% but these regimens boast complete remission rates of 65% to 90%. The BCR-ABL tyrosine kinase inhibitor imatinib has been incorporated into induction regimens in patients who harbor the Philadelphia chromosome (t(9;22)).
- **CNS prophylaxis** is an important component of therapy for ALL, as it has a high incidence of recurrence in the CNS. Regimens typically consist of intrathecal methotrexate and cytarabine.
- **Maintenance therapy** is typically continued for 2 years, often with mercaptopurine, prednisone, vincristine, and methotrexate (the so-called POMP regimen).
- **Relapse,** unfortunately, is common in adult ALL. Salvage chemotherapy regimens are able to induce a second complete remission in ~30% to 70% of persons, and when consolidated with allogeneic stem cell transplantation ~40% of patients will be alive at 4 years.

PROGNOSIS

Although 60% to 90% of patients can expect to undergo a complete remission with induction chemotherapy, the majority of patients will relapse. Patients who are younger and have good prognostic indicators have a cure rate of 50% to 70%. Those who are older and have poor prognostic indicators have a cure rate of only 10% to 30%. Adverse risk factors are summarized in Table 29-4.

TABLE 29-4 ADVERSE PROGNOSTIC FACTORS IN ADULT ACUTE LYMPHOBLASTIC LEUKEMIA (ALL)

Adverse Risk Factor	
Age	>60 y old
WBC at presentation	>50,000
Prolonged time to complete remission	>4–6 wk
Adverse cytogenetics	Hypodiploidy t(9;22) t(4;11) Trisomy 8

CHRONIC MYELOGENOUS LEUKEMIA

GENERAL PRINCIPLES

Epidemiology

CML accounts for 14% of all leukemias and 20% of adult leukemias, with an annual incidence of 1.6 cases per 100,000 adults. Since the advent of imatinib, the annual mortality has decreased to 1% to 2%. The median age at presentation is 65, and incidence increases with age.

Etiology

The etiology is unclear; no correlation with monozygotic twins, geography, ethnicity, or economic status has been observed. However, a significantly higher incidence of CML has been noted in survivors of the atomic disasters at Nagasaki and Hiroshima, in radiologists, and in patients treated with radiation to the spine for ankylosing spondylitis.

Pathophysiology

- CML is associated with the fusion of two genes: BCR (on chromosome 22) and ABL1 (on chromosome 9) resulting in the BCR-ABL1 fusion gene. This abnormal fusion typically results from a reciprocal translocation between chromosomes 9 and 22, t(9;22)(q34;q11), that gives rise to an abnormal chromosome 22 called the Philadelphia (Ph) chromosome. It is this derivative chromosome 22 which harbors the BCR-ABL1 fusion gene. The BCR-ABL1 fusion gene results in the formation of a unique gene product, the BCR-ABL1 fusion protein. This protein product includes an enzymatic domain from the normal ABL1 with tyrosine kinase catalytic activity, but relative to ABL1, whose kinase activity is tightly regulated, the kinase activity of BCR-ABL1 is elevated and constitutive due to fusion with a portion of BCR. It is this deregulated tyrosine kinase that is implicated in the pathogenesis of CML.[5]
- Blast-phase CML is characterized by **cytogenetic evolution** in ~70% of patients. The most common chromosomal abnormalities are trisomy 8, in 30% to 40% of patients, additional Ph chromosome, in 20% to 30%, and isochromosome 17, in 15% to 20%. Corresponding mutations in p53 are also seen in 20% to 30% of patients, amplification of c-myc in 20%, and, less commonly, mutations and deletions of ras, Rb, or p16. As with de novo AML, complex cytogenetics are associated with decreased response rates and survival.
- The natural history of CML is a **triphasic process.**
  - Most patients present in **chronic phase,** characterized by an asymptomatic accumulation of differentiated myeloid cells in the bone marrow, spleen, and peripheral blood. CML usually progresses through a transient **accelerated phase,** lasting 4 to 6 months, and then inevitably to **blast phase,** an incurable acute leukemia that is fatal within 3 to 6 months. In the 2 years after initial diagnosis of CML, 5% to 15% of untreated patients will enter blast crisis. In subsequent years, the annual rate of progression increases to 20% to 25%, with progression commonly occurring between 3 and 6 years after diagnosis.
  - The **definition of accelerated-phase CML** relies on several clinical and laboratory features and is characterized by increasing arrest of maturation. Current WHO criteria include at least one of the following: 10% to 19%

blasts in peripheral blood or bone marrow, ≥20% peripheral basophils, thrombocytopenia <100,000/μL and lack of response to therapy, increasing spleen size and increasing WBC unresponsive to therapy, and cytogenetic evidence of clonal evolution. Once either accelerated phase or blast crisis occurs, the success of any therapy declines dramatically.

DIAGNOSIS

Clinical Presentation

In most patients, CML is diagnosed incidentally. Symptoms can result from concurrent anemia and splenomegaly (fatigue, early satiety, and sensation of abdominal fullness) but may also include weight loss, bleeding, and bruising in advanced disease.

Diagnostic Testing

- **Blood smear** shows leukocytosis with a myeloid shift. In contrast to cases of acute leukemia, in which an arrest in maturation is the rule, **granulocytes at all stages of maturation** are observed. Anemia and thrombocytosis are common, while basophilia (>7%) occurs in only 10% to 15% of patients. Leukocyte alkaline phosphatase (LAP) activity is usually reduced but can be increased with infections, stress, on achievement of remission, or on progression to blast phase.
- The diagnosis is confirmed by the detection of the **Ph chromosome t(9;22) (q34.1;q11.21)**. In 5% of patients a BCR-ABL fusion can be detected without classic Ph chromosomal cytogenetics, and rarely translocations can involve three or more chromosomes. The bone marrow is typically hypercellular and devoid of fat. All stages of myeloid differentiation are present and megakaryocytes may be increased, suggesting that chronic-phase CML is a disease of discordant maturation, where a delay in myeloid maturation results in increased myeloid cell mass.

TREATMENT

Chronic-Phase Chronic Myelogenous Leukemia

The two main treatment options for patients with newly diagnosed CML in chronic phase are

- **BCR-ABL tyrosine kinase inhibitors** (TKIs), such as imatinib, dasatinib, and nilotinib
- **Allogeneic hematopoietic cell transplantation (HCT)**
  As the only treatment option with proven ability to cure CML, allogeneic HCT was the primary therapy for younger patients in chronic phase before the development of TKIs. However, now that TKIs have demonstrated long-term disease control and good tolerability, most patients are not referred for allogeneic transplantation as initial therapy. Instead, they are treated with TKIs and careful follow-up, with allogeneic HCT reserved for patients with refractory or progressive disease.
- **Imatinib mesylate** (Gleevec) is a targeted TKI, which antagonizes the activity of the ABL tyrosine kinase, as well as c-Kit and platelet-derived growth factors alpha and beta. At nanomolar concentrations, imatinib binds to the inactive conformation of the BCR-ABL ATP-binding pocket, resulting in

competitive inhibition of BCR-ABL and growth inhibition of BCR-ABL-positive bone marrow progenitor cells. In a large Phase III trial, patients randomized to imatinib 400 mg daily had complete hematologic and cytogenetic remission rates of 95% and 74%, respectively, which was clearly superior to the standard arm of interferon-alfa+low dose cytarabine.[6] Although a few case reports are emerging of patients with continued complete cytogenetic response after imatinib withdrawal, relapse is common, and lifelong maintenance therapy is recommended at this time. Side effects of imatinib mesylate are generally mild but include hematologic suppression (neutropenia, thrombocytopenia, and anemia), constitutional symptoms (diarrhea, edema, and rash), and rare organ damage (elevated transaminases, hypophosphatemia, and potentially cardiotoxicity). These can usually be managed with growth factors or dose reduction but occasionally require discontinuation, either briefly or permanently.

- Since the development of imatinib, more potent, **second-generation TKIs** have been developed. The three second-generation TKIs that have been studied most extensively are dasatinib, nilotinib, and bosutinib. Nilotinib and dasatinib are approved for the treatment of newly diagnosed CML. Phase III trials comparing dasatinib or nilotinib to imatinib as initial therapy for CML in chronic phase have demonstrated faster and deeper responses with these second-generation TKIs. At 12 months, the rates of major molecular response for nilotinib and dasatinib (~45%) were nearly twice that for imatinib. The rates of complete cytogenetic response by 12 months were significantly higher for nilotinib and dasatinib (~80%) than for imatinib (~65%).[7,8] Further follow-up is needed to confirm whether the substantial short term improvements will result in longer term benefits, such as improved survival.
    - The side effect profiles of dasatinib and nilotinib are different from each other and compare favorably to that of imatinib. A choice among agents should take into consideration these drug side effect profiles and the patient's comorbidities. For example, dasatinib might be preferred in a patient with a history of pancreatitis, elevated bilirubin, or hyperglycemia, while nilotinib might be chosen for a patient with a history of pleural or pericardial disease or effusions. Patients who are currently being treated successfully with imatinib who have achieved complete cytogenetic response with good tolerance of the side effects, should be continued on imatinib and should not be switched to dasatinib or nilotinib.
- Increased risk of progression to accelerated and blast phase has been demonstrated if patients do not achieve specific **clinical goals.** These currently include the following, from the time a patient starts TKI therapy:
    - 3 months: **complete hematologic response** with normal peripheral counts and a >1 log reduction in BCR-ABL transcripts by quantitative PCR (qPCR)
    - 6 months: **cytogenetic response** with <35% Ph chromosome-positive bone marrow cells
    - 12 months: **complete cytogenetic response** with undetectable Ph chromosome
    - 18 months: **major molecular remission** with a 3 log reduction by qPCR of peripheral BCR-ABL

    Failure to reach any of these goals warrants close follow-up, ABL tyrosine kinase domain mutation analysis, dose escalation, and/or change to second-line TKI and consideration of hematopoietic stem cell transplant.

- **Resistance to imatinib** has been noted in 2% to 4% of patients annually for the first 3 years of imatinib therapy and may decrease thereafter. Point mutations in the SH1 kinase domain are commonly associated with resistance. These mutations either decrease the affinity for imatinib binding in the ATP-binding pocket or shift the kinetics of BCR-ABL to prefer the active conformation, to which imatinib will not bind. Imatinib resistance can be overcome with either increasing doses or a second-line TKI, although the point mutation T315I confers a high degree of resistance to all available TKIs.
- While effective, **chemotherapy** is second-line to the well-tolerated TKIs. Hydroxyurea, busulfan, and interferon-alpha have been used with some success.
- **Allogeneic hematopoietic stem cell transplant** from either related or unrelated donors remains the only known curative therapy for CML. Transplantation from a matched sibling donor during chronic phase is associated with a 10-year survival of 50% to 70%, but this decreases to 20% to 40% and <20% in accelerated and blast phase, respectively.

Accelerated and Blast-Phase Chronic Myelogenous Leukemia

- As advances are made in the treatment of CML, fewer patients (~7% at 5 years) are progressing to accelerated phase or blast crisis. In addition, 10% to 15 % of patients will initially present in accelerated phase or blast crisis. In general, an attempt is made to return the patient to a chronic phase with plans to proceed to allogeneic hematopoietic cell transplantation after an initial response. Imatinib has been shown to improve survival in accelerated phase at higher doses (600 to 800 mg), but responses are often short lived.
- Treatment of BP-CML remains a challenge, with survival of only 2 to 4 months in nonresponders. Treatment is dictated by hematologic features. Myeloid features are seen in 50% of patients, lymphoid in 25%, and undifferentiated in 25%. Typical AML induction chemotherapy is used for BP-CML with myeloid features and ALL induction chemotherapy for lymphoid features. Each has a response rate of only 30%. Transplant during BP-CML remains the only curative options, but it is associated with a ~80% risk of relapse and a 5-year survival of only ~5%.

MONITORING/FOLLOW-UP

Follow-up during initial treatment requires CBC monthly, peripheral BCR-ABL qPCR every 3 months, and bone marrow biopsy every 6 months until major molecular remission is achieved. Once molecular remission is documented, BCR-ABL transcripts should still be followed every 3 months, with an annual bone marrow exam for cytogenetics. Rising BCR-ABL transcripts should be quickly reevaluated and treatment altered accordingly.

CHRONIC LYMPHOCYTIC LEUKEMIA

GENERAL PRINCIPLES

Chronic lymphocytic leukemia (CLL) is characterized by the progressive accumulation of monoclonal, functionally incompetent lymphocytes. Patients with CLL commonly

TABLE 29-5 CHRONIC LYMPHOCYTIC LEUKEMIA STAGING AND MOLECULAR PROGNOSTICS

Rai Stage 0: lymphocytosis Stage 1: lymphadenopathy Stage 2: splenomegaly Stage 3: Hgb <11 g/dL Stage 4: platelets <100,000/μL	Binet Stage A: lymphocytosis Stage B: lymphadenopathy in >3 areas Stage C: Hgb <10 g/dL or platelets <100,000/μL
High-risk molecular markers Elevated β2, LDH, sCD23 CD38+ in >30% lymphocytes ZAP70+ in >30% lymphocytes Germline IgVH	Good-risk cytogenetics Deletion 13q High-risk cytogenetics 14q rearrangement 11q rearrangement Deletion 17p Trisomy 12
Low risk: overall survival, 7–10 y Rai 0–1 Binet A Deletion 13q Doubling time >12 mo	High risk: overall survival, 2–5 y Rai 3–4 Binet C Molecular or cytogenetic changes noted Doubling time <12 mo

Hgb, hemoglobin; LDH, lactate dehydrogenase.

develop complications associated with the intrinsic immune dysfunction that results in immunodeficiency and the development of autoimmune disorders. CLL is considered to be identical to the mature (peripheral) B-cell neoplasm small lymphocytic lymphoma (SLL).

Classification

Classification of CLL is based on the extent of systemic infiltration of lymphocytes. This helps to determine the prognosis and initiation of treatment (Table 29-5). Molecular and cytogenetic markers have become increasingly useful for prognostication.

Epidemiology

CLL is the most common form of leukemia in adults, accounting for ~30% of adult leukemia in Western countries. According to the SEER cancer database, from 2000 to 2003 the median age at presentation was 72 years, and only 13% of patients were <55 years old at the time of diagnosis. Nearly 4% of elderly individuals have a monoclonal lymphocytosis, although most of these do not progress to CLL. The age-adjusted incidence rate for CLL was 3.8 per 100,000 per year, with a ~2:1 male:female ratio.

Pathophysiology

CLL is an accumulation of malignant, immunologically incompetent, but mature B-cell lymphocytes. The malignant cells of CLL express high levels of the antiapoptotic protein, bcl-2, and express common B-cell antigens CD19, CD20, and CD23. Of note, CD5 antigen, a T-cell antigen, is found in all cases of CLL. A Coombs-positive, warm antibody, hemolytic anemia occurs in 10% of patients, and an immune thrombocytopenia occurs in ~5% of patients. In 5% of patients, **Richter syndrome** develops, which is a malignant transformation to diffuse large B-cell lymphoma.

Risk Factors

Patients with a history of **immunodeficiency syndromes** have an increased risk of CLL. There are no clear environmental or occupational risk factors that predispose to CLL, and patients who are exposed to radiation do not appear to have an increased frequency of CLL.

DIAGNOSIS

Clinical Presentation

Many patients are discovered by routine CBC and are asymptomatic. However, chronic fatigue is a common initial complaints. With bone marrow involvement, patients may develop severe fatigue, anemia, bruising, weight loss, and fever. On physical exam, splenomegaly, hepatomegaly, and lymphadenopathy can be present. With advancing immunodeficiency, herpes zoster infections, *Pneumocystis jiroveci* pneumonia, and bacterial infections become more frequent.

Diagnostic Criteria

The essential diagnostic criteria for CLL identified by the CLL international working group include an absolute lymphocytosis of >5000/μL with a typical morphology, a bone marrow infiltrated with small lymphocytes accounting for >30% of nucleated cells, and a typical immunophenotype ($CD5^{+}$, $CD23^{+}$, $CD10^{-}$, $CD19^{+}$, $CD20^{+dim}$, $CyclinD1^{-}$, $CD43^{\pm}$) (Table 29-6).

Differential Diagnosis

It is important to consider benign causes of lymphocytosis, including Epstein–Barr virus mononucleosis, chronic infections, autoimmune diseases, drug and allergic reactions, thyrotoxicosis, adrenal insufficiency, and postsplenectomy. The other possible

TABLE 29-6 IMMUNOPHENOTYPIC FEATURES OF MALIGNANT CONDITIONS AFFECTING MATURE B LYMPHOCYTES

Disorder	Common Immunophenotype
CLL	DR+, CD19+, CD20+, CD5+, CD22–, CD23+, CD10–, weak sIg
Prolymphocytic leukemia	DR+, CD19+, CD20+, CD5–, CD22+, CD23–, CD10–, bright sIg
Mantle cell lymphoma	DR+, CD19+, CD20+, CD5+, CD22+, CD23–, CD10–, moderate sIg
Follicular lymphoma	DR+, CD19+, CD20+, CD5–, CD22+, CD23–, CD10+, bright sIg
Hairy cell leukemia	DR+, CD19+, CD20+, CD5–, CD22+, CD23–, CD10–, CD11c+, bright sIg

CLL, chronic lymphocytic leukemia; sIg, surface immunoglobulin.

malignancies to consider are hairy cell leukemia (HCL), cutaneous T-cell lymphoma, other indolent non-Hodgkin lymphomas (mantle cell, follicular, lymphoplasmacytic), and large granular lymphocytic leukemia.

Diagnostic Testing

A **CBC with differential** reveals an **absolute lymphocytosis,** with >95% small lymphocytes. A blood smear should show mature lymphocytes. The **classic smudge cell** is nonspecific, but more than 30% smudging has been suggested as a poor prognostic marker. Anemia and/or thrombocytopenia may be present from bone marrow infiltration or from an autoimmune phenomenon. It is important to assess renal and hepatic function, LDH, uric acid, beta-2-microglobulin, Coombs antiglobulin, serum protein electrophoresis, quantitative immunoglobulins, chest radiograph, and CT scan of the chest, abdomen, and pelvis. Patients with CLL typically have at least 30% lymphocytes in the bone marrow. A **bone marrow biopsy** should be obtained for cytogenetics. Cytogenetic markers have been noted to predict overall progression of disease and response to therapy. Important molecular markers include **ZAP70 and IgVH (immunoglobulin heavy chain variable region) gene rearrangements.**

TREATMENT

- It is not necessary to initiate therapy early in the course of CLL. However, CLL patients may be immunocompromised, and fever or any other signs of infection need to be evaluated promptly. **Indications for therapy** include eligibility for a clinical trial, symptoms (fevers, sweats, weight loss), obstructive or advancing lymphadenopathy, hepatosplenomegaly, stage III or IV disease, rapid elevation in lymphocyte count with a doubling time <6 months, and complications including immune hemolysis, thrombocytopenia, recurrent infections, threatened organ function, and transformation.
- There is no agreed upon standard treatment regimen for symptomatic CLL.[9] Treatment options include purine analogs (e.g., fludarabine, pentostatin), alkylating agents (e.g., chlorambucil, bendamustine), monoclonal antibodies (e.g., rituximab, alemtuzumab), or combinations of these agents. These treatment options have not been directly compared with each other. When prospective randomized trials have been performed, most of these regimens have been compared with chlorambucil, an alkylating agent that had been a standard of care for decades. While overall survival rates with these different regimens are similar, they differ in their rates of complete remission (CR), time to progression, and associated toxicities. For example, randomized clinical trials have established higher CR rates and progression-free survival intervals for fludarabine over alkylating agents, and for combination therapies such as FC (fludarabine, cyclophosphamide) over fludarabine alone; however, no difference in overall survival has been demonstrated. With elevated leukocyte counts, consideration of tumor lysis risk and prevention is important prior to therapeutic intervention. In addition, patients treated with purine analogs should be considered for prophylaxis against *Pneumocystis* and varicella zoster.
- Patients with del(17p) or del(11q) are at high risk of either not responding to initial treatment, or relapsing soon after achieving remission.[10] The appropriate treatment for these patients remains undefined at this time. Options include

- ○ Initial treatment with fludarabine combinations, followed by alemtuzumab, either after a number of cycles of initial debulking chemotherapy, or at the time of relapse.
- ○ Consideration of non-myeloablative allogeneic hematopoietic cell transplantation for younger patients with a matched related or matched unrelated donor.
- Alemtuzumab is the only FDA-approved agent that has demonstrated activity in cells lacking p53 function, as seen in patients with CLL and chromosome 17p deletion.
- **Refractory and relapsed disease** may be treated with retreatment of prior agents, if relapse is >12 months, or with further combination therapy.[11] FCR (fludarabine, cyclophosphamide, rituximab) and PCR (pentostatin, cyclophosphamide, rituximab) have both shown response rates of 30% to 60% in fludarabine-pretreated populations. Alemtuzumab is showing increasing promise as a single or combined agent in refractory disease.
- Autologous and allogeneic bone marrow transplantations are being explored as treatment options. Improved results have been noted with nonmyeloablative therapies. Young patients with high-risk disease should be considered for this therapy.

COMPLICATIONS

- **Autoimmune hemolytic anemia (AIHA) and autoimmune thrombocytopenia** occur more frequently in advanced-stage patients and those with unmutated IgVH. These complications should be evaluated with reticulocyte count, haptoglobin, LDH, and Coombs assay. The results should be interpreted in context of other features, as the reticulocyte count may be low due to bone marrow suppression or infiltration, the LDH may be elevated due to the disease, not hemolysis, and treatments such as fludarabine may induce AIHA by themselves. Treatment is typical of other AIHA and autoimmune thrombocytopenia processes with prednisone or equivalent glucocorticoid at a dose of 1 mg/kg/d, tapered after control of blood counts. Splenectomy may be needed if the blood counts do not improve on steroids. Local irradiation or splenectomy can control the effects of hypersplenism.
- **Infection** can result from hypogammaglobulinemia, T-cell dysfunction, and decreased phagocytic function. Hypogammaglobulinemic patients with recurrent infections should be treated with intravenous immunoglobulin, 400 mg/kg IV, every 3 to 4 weeks (goal IgG trough, ~500 mg/dL), which reduces serious bacterial infection rates without altering overall survival. Patients treated with fludarabine or alemtuzumab develop therapy-related T-cell immune defects and are at a significantly increased risk of cytomegalovirus (CMV) reactivation, *Pneumocystis,* varicella zoster, herpes viruses, *Listeria,* and other opportunistic infections. Prophylaxis against *Pneumocystis,* herpes simplex virus, and varicella zoster virus, as well as monitoring for CMV reactivation should be considered when treating CLL patients with these agents.

PROGNOSIS

Diffuse marrow involvement, rapidly increasing lymphocyte counts, and initial lymphocytosis of >50,000/μL indicate a poor prognosis for an individual patient with early-stage disease. Anemia and thrombocytopenia correspond with decreased median survival time. Overall, CLL is an indolent disease, and median survivals of >10 years are reported in stages 0, I, and II. Thus, patients may die of other conditions rather than from CLL. However, if a patient presents with advanced disease, the course may be rapid, with a median survival of months to years. It is unclear whether cytotoxic therapy improves survival, although it can effectively palliate disease-related symptoms. Advances in supportive care and infection therapy have improved survival and quality of life.

HAIRY CELL LEUKEMIA

GENERAL PRINCIPLES

Hairy cell leukemia (HCL) is an uncommon chronic B-cell lymphoproliferative disorder originally termed "leukemic reticuloendotheliosis" in the 1920s. It was described as a distinct clinical entity by Bouroncle and colleagues in 1958, and named HCL in the 1960s because of the prominent irregular cytoplasmic projections of the malignant cells. It accounts for 2% to 3% of all leukemias, usually affecting men >55 years old.

DIAGNOSIS

Clinical Presentation

Most patients present with malaise and fatigue. On physical exam, splenomegaly and hepatomegaly are evident in 95% and 40%, respectively. With more advanced disease, pancytopenia develops, and patients may present with bleeding or recurrent infections (bacterial, viral, fungal, or atypical mycobacterial).

Diagnostic Testing

A **peripheral smear** and **bone marrow** reveal the **pathognomonic mononuclear cells.** These cells have characteristic irregular hairlike projections around the border of the cytoplasm. CBC frequently shows anemia and thrombocytopenia and, less frequently, granulocytopenia. Although bone marrow aspiration is frequently unsuccessful, the biopsy may show the characteristic hairy cells. Hairy cells exhibit a mature B cell phenotype and typically express one or more heavy chains and monotypic light chains. Hairy cells strongly express pan-B cell antigens including CD19, CD20, CD22, and CD25, and usually lack expression of CD5, CD10, CD21, and CD23, and characteristically express CD11c, CD103, CD123, cyclin D1, and annexin A1. Also, hairy cells are TRAP (tartrate-resistant acid phosphatase) positive. Hairy cell leukemia is differentiated from CLL, lymphomas, and monocytic leukemia based on the characteristic cell morphology, TRAP test, and immune phenotype. There is no formal staging system.

TREATMENT

As with other chronic leukemias and lymphomas, early treatment does not improve overall outcome. The decision to treat is based on the development of cytopenias (hemoglobin, <10 g/dL, absolute neutrophil count, <1000/μL; platelets, <100,000/μL) and recurrent infections. Several treatment options are available (Table 29-7). Typically,

TABLE 29-7 THERAPEUTIC OPTIONS FOR HAIRY CELL LEUKEMIA

Therapy	Comment
Cladribine	First-line agent, 7-d IV infusion with >90% response rate. Alternative outpatient treatment schedules may be equally effective. Risk of myelosuppression
Interferon-alpha	Given for 1 y, >90% response rate
Pentostatin	Given for 3–6 mo, many patients have a complete response. Complicated by neurotoxicity and skin rash
Splenectomy	Achieves a 75% response rate

cladribine or pentostatin is used. However, both of these agents induce significant and prolonged immunosuppression. Prophylaxis for herpes simplex virus and *Pneumocystis,* especially if concurrent steroids are used, is advised.

OUTCOME/PROGNOSIS

Before treatment, median survival was between 5 and 10 years. Survival has markedly improved with current therapies, as most untreated and pretreated patients have excellent response rates to cladribine or pentostatin (85% to 97%), with 4-year survival rates of up to 96%.

REFERENCES

1. Vardiman JW, Harris NL, Brunning RD. The World Health Organization (WHO) classification of the myeloid neoplasms. *Blood.* 2002;100(7):2292–2302.
2. Vardiman JW, Thiele J, Arber DA, et al. The 2008 revision of the World Health Organization (WHO) classification of myeloid neoplasms and acute leukemia: rationale and important changes. *Blood.* 2009;114(5):937–951.
3. Löwenberg B, Ossenkoppele GJ, Van Putten W, et al. High-dose daunorubicin in older patients with acute myeloid leukemia. *N Engl J Med.* 2009;361(13):1235–1248.
4. Kantarjian HM, O'Brien S, Smith TL, et al. Results of treatment with Hyper-CVAD, a dose-intensive regimen, in adult acute lymphocytic leukemia. *J Clin Oncol.* 2000;18:547–561.
5. Faderl S, Talpaz M, Estrov Z, et al. The biology of chronic myeloid leukemia. *N Engl J Med.* 1999;341(3):164–172.
6. O'Brien SG, Guilhot F, Larson RA, et al. Imatinib compared with interferon and low-dose cytarabine for newly diagnosed chronic-phase chronic myeloid leukemia. *N Engl J Med.* 2003; 348:994–1004.
7. Saglio G, Kim DW, Issaragrisil S, et al. Nilotinib versus imatinib for newly diagnosed chronic myeloid leukemia. *N Engl J Med.* 2010;362(24):2251–2259.
8. Kantarjian H, Shah NP, Hochhaus A, et al. Dasatinib versus imatinib in newly diagnosed chronic-phase chronic myeloid leukemia. *N Engl J Med.* 2010;362(24):2260–2270.
9. Gribben JG. How I treat CLL up front. *Blood.* 2010;115(2):187–197.
10. Dohner H, Stilgenbauer S, Benner A, et al. Genomic aberrations and survival in chronic lymphocytic leukemia. *N Engl J Med.* 2000;343(26):1910–1916.
11. Byrd JC, Lin TS, Grever MR. Treatment of relapsed chronic lymphocytic leukemia: old and new therapies. *Semin Oncol.* 2006;33:210–219.

Lymphoma

30

Amie Jackson and Kristen M. Sanfilippo

INTRODUCTION

Lymphoma refers to a clonal tumor arising from the malignant transformation of mature or immature lymphocytes (B cells, T cells, or natural-killer (NK) cells). It represents the most common hematologic malignancy, and is a heterogeneous disease, comprised of over 30 subtypes as classified by the World Health Organization (WHO).[1] This diversity derives from the varied pathways leading to lymphoma, including the transformation of different lymphocyte types, at different developmental or differentiation stages, and through multiple molecular pathways. Lymphoma can be subdivided into two clinically distinct classes: Hodgkin lymphoma (HL) and non-Hodgkin lymphoma (NHL).

HODGKIN LYMPHOMA

GENERAL PRINCIPLES

HL is a clonal neoplasm derived from B lymphocytes. It accounts for 30% of lymphomas in the United States. It is defined by the presence of characteristic Hodgkin Reed–Sternberg (HRS) cells located in the appropriate cellular background.

Classification

The WHO classification groups nodular sclerosis, mixed cellularity, lymphocyte-deplete, and lymphocyte-rich subtypes together as **classical HL (cHL),** based on pathologic and clinical similarities. **Nodular lymphocyte-predominant** HL **(NLPHL)** represents a distinct clinical entity with unique pathologic characteristics and a more indolent clinical course[1] (Table 30-1).

Epidemiology

There are 160,000 patients living with HL in the United States, with an annual incidence rate of 2.8 per 100,000. cHL accounts for 95% of HL cases, and has a bimodal age distribution with a peak at 15 to 35 years and a second peak later in life. NLPHL accounts for 5% of HL, has a male predominance, and occurs most frequently in adults age 30 to 50.[1]

Pathophysiology

The malignant B cell in HL is the HRS cell, which is large, bi- or multinucleated, and expresses CD30 and CD15 cell surface antigens. NLPHL is characterized by a clonal B-cell population composed of lymphocytic and histiocytic cells (LHC) that express CD45, CD20, and CD79a.

TABLE 30-1 WHO CLASSIFICATION OF HODGKIN LYMPHOMA[1]
Classical Hodgkin lymphoma (cHL)
Nodular sclerosis cHL
Mixed cellularity cHL
Lymphocyte-rich cHL
Lymphocyte-deplete cHL
Nodular lymphocyte-predominant Hodgkin lymphoma (NLPHL)

Risk Factors

Epstein–Barr virus (EBV) is a clear risk factor for HL. Patients with a history of infectious mononucleosis have a higher incidence of HL, although the frequency of EBV positivity varies with geographic region. Human immunodeficiency virus (HIV) predisposes to the development of EBV-associated HL, likely through alterations in immune surveillance.

DIAGNOSIS

Clinical Presentation

HL typically presents as **asymptomatic enlarged lymph nodes**, with the disease originating in one lymph node group and spreading in a contiguous pattern. In older patients (>50 years), there may be a "skipped" lymph node segment. Sixty percent of patients present with localized (stage I-II) disease based on the modified Ann Arbor staging system. The most commonly involved lymph node groups are cervical (75%) and mediastinal (60%). Extranodal sites of involvement include the spleen (20%), bone marrow (5%), lung, and liver, and patients may present with symptoms specific to site of involvement. Systemic **B symptoms** of fever (>38.5°C), night sweats, and weight loss (>10% of body weight over 6 months) occur in up to 40% of patients. Patients with HIV associated HL usually present with advanced stage disease, extranodal site involvement, and B symptoms.

History

Painless lymphadenopathy is the hallmark of HL. Intense **pruritus** is reported in up to 25% of patients. Patients with mediastinal disease may report cough, chest pain, or shortness of breath. Other rare symptoms which may be elucidated from the history include pain in enlarged lymph nodes after alcohol ingestion and periodic fever. Performance status should be determined from the history.

Physical Examination

The physical examination should focus on the number, size, location, and character of palpable lymph nodes. The cervical nodes are most commonly involved, and the disease tends to spread in a contiguous pattern. The abdominal examination may reveal hepatosplenomegaly.

Differential Diagnosis

The differential diagnosis of suspected lymphoma typically includes other causes of lymphadenopathy. Infections, systemic rheumatologic disorders, or metastatic malignancies can also cause peripheral lymph node enlargement. For patients presenting with

TABLE 30-2 INTERNATIONAL PROGNOSTIC SCORE (IPS) FOR CLASSICAL HODGKIN LYMPHOMA[2]

IPS Factors

1. Serum albumin <4 g/dL
2. Hemoglobin <10.5 g/dL
3. Male gender
4. Stage IV
5. Age >45 y
6. WBC ≥15,000/μL
7. Lymphocytes <8% of WBC or <600/μL

Risk Factors	FFP at 5 y (%)	OS at 5 y (%)	Patients (%)
0	84	89	7
1	77	90	22
2	67	81	29
3	60	78	23
4	51	61	12
≥5	42	56	7

FFP, freedom from progression; OS, overall survival.

isolated splenomegaly, other etiologies include infection, portal hypertension, storage diseases, metastatic tumors, autoimmune disorders and myeloproliferative disorders.

Diagnostic Testing

A large **excisional lymph node biopsy** is preferred for the diagnosis of HL. In addition to morphologic evaluation, immunohistochemistry may be helpful in differentiating the CD15+, CD30+ HRS of cHL from the CD45+, CD20+ LHC cells of NLPHL. **Bone marrow biopsy** should be performed in advanced stage disease or in the presence of cytopenias or B symptoms.

Laboratories

Complete blood cell count (CBC) with differential, erythrocyte sedimentation rate (ESR), and a complete metabolic panel (CMP) should be obtained at diagnosis. ESR, white blood cell and lymphocyte counts, hemoglobin, and albumin are important for calculation of a patient's **international prognostic score (IPS)**, which can be used to estimate survival in cHL (Table 30-2).[2] Pregnancy testing in women of childbearing age and HIV testing in at risk patients is indicated.

Imaging

Positive emission tomography (PET) is preferred over computed tomography (CT) scan for initial imaging in HL. PET is more sensitive for detecting additional sites of disease and may improve the accuracy of the stage of disease as determined by the **modified Ann Arbor staging system** (Table 30-3). In some cases, serial PET imaging during therapy can be used to assess early response and prognosis, which can help guide clinicians in determining need for dose escalation and duration of therapy.[3] **Pulmonary function testing** should also be performed in patients who will receive chemotherapy containing bleomycin (see treatment, below).

TABLE 30-3 MODIFIED ANN ARBOR STAGING SYSTEM FOR LYMPHOMAS

Stage	
I	Single lymph node region or lymphoid structure
II	≥2 nodal regions on the same side of the diaphragm
III	Involvement of lymph nodes on both sides of the diaphragm
IV	Involvement of one or more extranodal sites
Modifiers	
A	No additional symptoms
B	Presence of fever, drenching sweats, or weight loss
X	Bulky disease (nodal mass >10 cm or more than one-third the width of the thorax)
E	Involvement of a single extranodal site contiguous or proximal to a nodal site
S	Splenic involvement

—
Adapted from Lister TA, Crowther D, Sutcliffe SB, et al. Report of a committee convened to discuss the evaluation and staging of patients with Hodgkin's disease: Cotswolds meeting. *J Clin Oncol.* 1989;7:1630–1636.

TREATMENT

- **Early stage cHL (stages I/II, no B symptoms, no bulky disease).** Early stage cHL has a good prognosis when treated with standard therapy, with high rates of complete remission (CR) and 5 year overall survival (OS) greater than 90%.[4] The focus of current clinical investigation is on maintaining excellent disease results while minimizing long-term complications of therapy. Standard treatment approaches (Table 30-4) include combined modality therapy with ABVD chemotherapy × 2 to 4 cycles plus involved field radiotherapy (IFRT) or chemotherapy alone with ABVD × 4 to 6 cycles. Recent evidence suggests that patients with early stage disease without adverse prognostic factors may receive reduced intensity radiotherapy with similar outcomes to full dose therapy. Patients at the highest risk for complications of IFRT (e.g., age <30 years, smokers, CAD risk factors, family history of early breast cancer) should be considered for treatment with chemotherapy alone.[5]
- **Advanced-stage cHL (stages III/IV, B symptoms, bulky stage II).** Standard treatment of advanced cHL includes systemic chemotherapy with **ABVD** × 6

TABLE 30-4 COMMONLY USED CHEMOTHERAPY REGIMENS IN CLASSICAL HODGKIN LYMPHOMA

ABVD	Doxorubicin, bleomycin, vinblastine, dacarbazine
Stanford V	Mechlorethamine, doxorubicin, vinblastine, vincristine, bleomycin, etoposide, prednisone
BEACOPP	Bleomycin, etoposide, doxorubicin, cyclophosphamide, vincristine, procarbazine, prednisone

to 8 cycles. Consolidative radiotherapy is typically recommended for all patients with bulky (>10 cm) disease. This approach results in 5- and 15-year failure-free survival rates of ~60% and ~45%, respectively, and 5- and 15-year OS rates of ~75% and ~60%. Alternative regimens include Stanford V and dose-escalated BEACOPP. These regimens are more intense with slightly higher CR rates, but increased toxicity, and may be utilized in patients with poor risk disease.[6–8]

- **Relapsed cHL.** The approach to patients with relapsed cHL takes into account the primary therapy and duration of remission. Historically, patients with early-stage HL were treated with radiation therapy alone; these patients are excellent candidates for standard systemic chemotherapy for cHL, which results in long-term DFS in 50% to 80%. Patients who received initial chemotherapy and relapse late (>1 year after remission) may be considered for standard dose chemotherapy, resulting in 30% to 50% long-term DFS. Patients who relapse early (<1 year after remission) or those with poor prognostic factors (e.g., stages III/IV at relapse, B symptoms) should be treated with aggressive salvage chemotherapy (e.g., ICE, ESHAP) and be considered for high-dose chemotherapy with autologous stem cell transplant (SCT). This can result in long-term DFS in 40%. Patients who relapse after autologous SCT should be considered for clinical and, in appropriate candidates, allogeneic SCT.[9]
- **NLPHL** is a distinct HL subtype best characterized as an indolent B-cell lymphoma with a good prognosis. Most patients present with stage I disease, for which IFRT alone should be considered. Trials with single agent rituximab have also shown promising results. For advanced-stage presentation, treatment with systemic chemotherapy in combination with rituximab has favorable results.[10]

COMPLICATIONS

Short-term adverse effects depend on the chemotherapy regimen used. The most common short-term complication of ABVD is myelosuppression, leading to cytopenias and an increased risk of infections. Lung injury due to bleomycin or radiotherapy may occur acutely, and the highest risk is in patients who are older, smokers, or have underlying lung disease. Long-term toxicities include secondary malignancies, which occur in 25% of patients and may be delayed by decades; patients treated with radiation therapy are at the highest risk. Hypothyroidism occurs in 50% of neck radiotherapy patients at 1 to 20 years after treatment. The risk of CAD is highest in patients irradiated when <30 years of age. The risk of infertility and secondary MDS/leukemia is low with standard ABVD chemotherapy but higher in patients who receive dose-intensive regimens.

FOLLOW-UP

During the first 2 years after obtaining a complete CR, routine follow-up includes history and physical examination, CBC, ESR, and CMP at 3-month intervals. Imaging is performed at 1 and 2 years post-remission and as clinically indicated. After 2 years, office visits and laboratories may be spaced out to every 6 months for the first 5 years. Additional surveillance is required for patients who received radiation therapy. Thyroid screening tests should be performed annually in patients who received radiation involving the neck. Surveillance for solid tumors (cancers of the skin, soft tissue, breast, and lung) should begin 5 to 10 years following therapy and continue for the lifetime of the patient.

NON-HODGKIN LYMPHOMA

GENERAL PRINCIPLES

NHL is an umbrella diagnosis that encompasses all lymphomas which do not meet HL criteria. It is composed of a diverse group of diseases that range from indolent to aggressive in nature. Given this heterogeneity, a detailed discussion of each NHL subtype is beyond the scope of this chapter. This section will review general information about NHL, focusing on **follicular lymphoma** (**FL**) and **diffuse large B-cell lymphoma** (**DLBCL**). Together these two entities account for two-thirds of NHL. Other specific NHL subtypes of interest are described at the end of this section under "Special Considerations."

Classification

The WHO classification subdivides NHL based on morphologic, immunophenotypic, genetic, and clinical features. Subtypes are grouped into precursor lymphoid neoplasms, mature B-cell neoplasms, or mature T- and NK-cell neoplasms based on their resemblance to normal stages of lymphocyte differentiation (Table 30-5). Precursor neoplasms are primarily diseases of childhood. Mature T- and NK-cell neoplasms are uncommon diseases accounting for only 12% of NHL. Mature B-cell neoplasms (including FL and DLBCL) account for greater than 90% of lymphoid neoplasms worldwide, and are by far the most common type of NHL in adults.[1]

Epidemiology

There are an estimated 430,000 patients in the United States with NHL. The incidence has been rising over the last 30 years, with an annual incidence of 30 per 100,000 and a death rate of 7 per 100,000 in the United States. Most mature B-cell NHLs have median ages in the 6th to 7th decades of life, although a few subtypes (e.g., primary mediastinal lymphoma) occur at younger ages.[1]

Pathophysiology

The genetic hallmark of FL is the translocation t(14;18)(q32;q21), present in over 90% of cases. This translocation places the anti-apoptotic BCL-2 gene under in the influence of the immunoglobulin (Ig) heavy chain gene enhancer, resulting in increased expression of BCL-2. Accumulation of additional karyotypic abnormalities is common in FL. Mutation of the BCL-6 gene on chromosome 3q27 is the most frequent genetic aberration in DLBCL, occurring in 40% of cases. BCL-6 is a transcription factor that regulates the genes involved in lymphocyte development and apoptosis.

Risk Factors

HIV infection, immunosuppressant therapy, and primary immune deficiency are associated with an increased risk of NHL. Certain autoimmune diseases (e.g., Hashimoto's thyroiditis) are also risk factors. Viral pathogens that have been linked to NHL subtypes include HIV, EBV, human herpresvirus-8, human T-cell leukemia virus type I, and hepatitis C virus. The most notable bacterial association is of *Helicobacter pylori* infection with gastric MALT lymphomas.

TABLE 30-5 WHO CLASSIFICATION OF NON-HODGKIN LYMPHOMA[1]

Precursor Lymphoid Neoplasms	Mature B-Cell Neoplasms	Mature T- and NK-Cell Neoplasms
Precursor B-cell lymphoblastic leukemia/lymphoma	Chronic lymphocytic leukemia/small lymphocytic lymphoma	T-cell prolymphocytic leukemia
Precursor T-cell lymphoblastic leukemia/lymphoma	B-cell prolymphocytic leukemia	T-cell large granular lymphocytic leukemia
	Splenic lymphoma/leukemia, unclassifiable	Chronic lymphoproliferative disorders of NK cells
	Lymphoplasmacytic lymphoma	Aggressive NK-cell leukemia
	Heavy chain disease	EBV+ lymphoproliferative disorders of childhood
	MALT lymphoma[a,b]	Adult T-cell leukemia/lymphoma[a]
	Follicular lymphoma	Mycosis fungoides
	Primary cutaneous follicle center lymphoma	Sèzary syndrome
	Mantle cell lymphoma	Primary cutaneous T-cell lymphoma[a]
	Diffuse large B-cell lymphoma[a]	Peripheral T-cell lymphoma, NOS
	Primary effusion lymphoma	Angioimmunoblastic T-cell lymphoma
	Primary mediastinal large B-cell lymphoma	Anaplastic large cell lymphoma[a]
	Plasmablastic lymphoma	
	T-cell/histiocyte rich large B-cell lymphoma	
	Burkitt lymphoma	
	B-cell lymphoma, unclassifiable	

[a]Variants of asterisked subtypes are omitted for clarity and space limitations.

[b]MALT: Extranodal marginal zone lymphoma of mucosa-associated lymphoid tissue. Diseases not included are reviewed in Chapters 13 and 29.

DIAGNOSIS

Clinical Presentation

Presenting symptoms in NHL vary with subtype and sites of involvement. Painless lymphadenopathy is the most common presentation. Systemic **B symptoms** are present in 33% of patients with DLBCL and 28% of patients with FL. **Extranodal involvement,** more common in DLBCL, may include bone marrow, skin, gastrointestinal tract, testes, salivary glands, liver, spleen, breast, adrenals, bone, sinuses, and CNS. Patients with bulky retroperitoneal disease may present with vague abdominal complaints.

Physical Examination

The physical examination should focus on the number, size, location, and character of palpable lymph nodes. Lymph node chains which should be examined include cervical, submental, supraclavicular, infraclavicular, axillary, epitrochlear, inguinal, and femoral as well as examination of Waldeyer ring (tonsils, oropharynx). The abdominal examination should include assessment for hepatic and splenic enlargement. Any patient with back pain or neurologic symptoms should have a complete neurologic examination to evaluate for cord compression or CNS involvement with lymphoma.

Differential Diagnosis

Other causes of peripheral lymphadenopathy include infection, rheumatologic disease, or other malignancy and may mimic NHL. See discussion in HL section.

Diagnostic Testing

When lymphoma is suspected, an **incisional** or **excisional biopsy** is preferred. An adequate biopsy specimen is critical for morphologic review and assessment of architecture by the pathologist. It also provides material for ancillary studies which may aid in subclassification, such as flow cytometry, immunohistochemistry, and genetic tests. Bilateral **bone marrow biopsy** and aspiration are required. If CNS involvement is suspected, **lumbar puncture** should be performed.

Laboratories

CBC may reveal cytopenias suggestive of bone marrow involvement. A **CMP** should be ordered to assess creatinine and calcium and to establish baseline liver function. **Lactate dehydrogenase** (LDH) is an important prognostic indicator. If tumor lysis syndrome is suspected, particularly in highly aggressive lymphomas (e.g., Burkitt lymphoma), serial assessment of uric acid, potassium, calcium, phosphorus and creatinine is important during initial treatment.

Imaging

CT of the chest, abdomen, and pelvis should be performed with contrast to complete staging. Sites of lymph node involvement are classified by the modified Ann Arbor staging system (Table 30-3). An initial **PET** is useful for aggressive, potentially curable NHL subtypes such as DLBCL, as it may detect additional sites of disease. PET is not routinely recommended for indolent or incurable lymphomas, such as FL.[3] If anthracycline-based chemotherapy is considered, assessment of left ventricular function with a multiple-gated acquisition (MUGA) scan or a transthoracic 2-D echocardiogram is warranted.

TREATMENT

- **Follicular lymphoma** (FL) is an indolent lymphoma with a median survival of 7 to 10 years in historical reports; survival is probably improving with modern therapy. Treatment with chemotherapy typically results in initial response followed by repeated relapses. Transformation to high-grade (large cell) NHL sometimes occurs. Given its indolent course, many patients with FL can be observed safely without treatment. Up to 20% of patients may never require

TABLE 30-6 COMMONLY USED CHEMOTHERAPY REGIMENS IN NON-HODGKIN LYMPHOMA

R	Rituximab (commonly combined with chemotherapy regimens, e.g., R-CHOP)
CHOP	Cyclophosphamide, doxorubicin, vincristine, prednisone
CVP	Cyclophosphamide, vincristine, prednisone
ESHAP	Etoposide, methylprednisolone, high-dose Ara-C, cisplatin
DHAP	Dexamethasone, high-dose Ara-C, cisplatin
ICE	Ifosfamide, carboplatin, etoposide
EPOCH	Etoposide, vincristine, doxorubicin, cyclophosphamide, prednisone
FND	Fludarabine, mitoxantrone, dexamethasone
FR	Fludarabine-rituximab
B	Bendamustine
hyper-CVAD	Hyperfractionated cyclophosphamide, vincristine, adriamycin, dexamethasone alternating with high-dose methotrexate and Ara-C

Ara-C, cytosine arabinoside.

therapy. The "watchful waiting" approach does not alter OS, but requires a reliable patient and clinical follow up every 3 to 6 months. Indications for treatment include symptomatic disease, bulky lymphadenopathy, threatened end-organ damage, cytopenias, and eligibility for clinical trials.

- **Early stage (I/II) FL** occurs in a minority of patients. It has a good prognosis when treated with IFRT alone, or in combination with immunochemotherapy such as R-CHOP (Table 30-6). Ten year OS ranges from 50% to 70%.[11]
- **Advanced stage FL (III, IV or bulky stage II).** Rituximab containing regimens improve PFS over chemotherapy alone in advanced stage FL. CHOP, CVP, FND, fludarabine or bendamustine plus rituximab are all effective, with three-year PFS ranging from 50% to 70%. Although there is no clear superiority of one regimen, R-CHOP and R-CVP are common initial choices, with high remission rates and long median PFS.[12,13] Recent data suggests that Bendamustine-R may have higher rates of PFS than R-CHOP. For elderly patients or those with poor performance status, single agent therapy with rituximab or chlorambucil may be used. Following induction chemotherapy, consolidation with radioimmunotherapy or maintenance rituximab may be considered.[14]
- **Relapsed FL.** Treatment of relapsed disease depends on prior therapies and the length of time since last treatment. Patients who initially receive R-chemotherapy and relapse less than one year from initial therapy are considered for aggressive salvage approaches. Alternative treatment regimens include other R-chemotherapy combinations, radioimmunotherapy, and autologous or allogeneic SCT.

- **Diffuse large B-cell lymphoma** (DLBCL) is an aggressive but potentially curable lymphoma. The majority of patients present with advanced disease, but a small number have limited disease on presentation.
  - **Advanced Stage (III/IV) DLBCL.** Standard initial therapy for advanced stage disease includes combination immunochemotherapy with R-CHOP, typically administered for 6 to 8 cycles, resulting in 5-year OS rates of 58%.[15] In contrast to FL, maintenance rituximab has no role in DLBCL. Patients with an increased risk of central nervous system relapse (involvement of testicular, paranasal sinus, epidural, bone marrow, or greater than two extranodal sites) should receive CNS prophylaxis.
  - **Limited Stage (I/II) DLBCL.** Twenty-five percent of patients have limited disease at presentation. These patients have a good prognosis, with 5-year OS estimates of 70% to 80% with standard therapy. Treatment options include combined modality therapy with three cycles of RCHOP followed by IFRT, or R-CHOP for 6 to 8 cycles with or without IFRT. Patients with bulky stage II disease (tumor size greater than 10 cm in greatest dimension) have a worse prognosis and are often treated as advanced stage disease.[16,17]
  - **Relapsed DLBCL.** Patients who relapse after CR should be considered for high dose chemotherapy and autologous SCT.[18] Common salvage chemotherapy regimens include DHAP, ESHAP, and ICE with or without rituximab.

SPECIAL CONSIDERATIONS

- **Transformation to aggressive lymphoma.** Indolent NHL patients have a 1% to 3% per year risk of transforming into aggressive NHL (most commonly DLBCL). Transformation may manifest as rapid enlargement of a single lymph node group, sudden rise in LDH, decline in performance status, hypercalcemia, or new extranodal involvement. Transformed NHL can occur regardless of treatment approach for the indolent NHL and has a poor prognosis. The optimal therapy is unclear and these patients are encouraged to enroll in a clinical trial. If a trial is not available, they are typically treated similarly to patients with high-risk, relapsed DLBCL.
- **Marginal zone lymphomas.** These commonly present with localized disease (approximately two-thirds) involving the GI tract, thyroid, orbit/conjunctiva, lung, breast, or salivary glands. Gastric MALT lymphomas are associated with *H. pylori,* and complete responses are seen after antibiotic therapy aimed at eradicating the infection. At other sites, early-stage disease has an excellent prognosis with IFRT alone. Advanced-stage MALT lymphomas are treated with chemotherapy, similarly to FL. Splenic marginal-zone lymphoma also has an excellent prognosis, and first-line therapy involves splenectomy or single-agent rituximab, both of which may result in a high rate of CR and long-term DFS. Nodal and extranodal marginal-zone lymphomas are treated in a similar fashion to FL.
- **Mantle cell lymphoma.** Mantle cell lymphoma is an aggressive NHL characterized by t(11;14), a translocation that results in the overexpression of cyclin D1, a protein involved in cell cycle regulation. Most patients present with advanced disease. Cure rates are low with standard aggressive NHL therapy, and in appropriate candidates, aggressive chemotherapy regimens are warranted, preferably as part of a clinical trial. Typical off-study approaches include rituximab plus hyper-CVAD or autologous stem cell transplant.

- **Burkitt lymphoma.** Burkitt lymphoma/leukemia is a highly aggressive NHL that may be endemic (e.g., equatorial Africa), associated with immunodeficiency (HIV), or sporadic (most common in the United States). The sporadic form is characterized by overexpression of the c-myc proto-oncogene, usually via the t(8;14) translocation. This NHL is rapidly life-threatening without therapy, has a poor prognosis, commonly involves the bone marrow and CNS, and is treated with aggressive combination chemotherapy (e.g., hyper-CVAD regimen) with CNS prophylaxis.
- **Lymphoblastic lymphoma.** Lymphoblastic lymphoma is another highly aggressive NHL. This disease is treated identically to ALL, with intensive chemotherapy, and also requires CNS prophylaxis. Prognosis is good for early-stage disease and intermediate for advanced-stage disease, with ~80% and ~50% chance of long-term DFS, respectively.
- **Small lymphocytic lymphoma.** This is considered to be part of the same disease process as chronic lymphocytic leukemia, and is treated as such. See Chapter 29.
- **Primary CNS lymphoma.** This is an aggressive NHL that presents with isolated CNS disease and, if untreated, has a rapidly fatal natural history. Compared to systemic DLBCL, its prognosis is worse, and treatment approaches include radiation therapy and/or chemotherapy that penetrates into the CNS (e.g., high-dose methotrexate).
- **Cutaneous T-cell lymphoma/mycosis fungoides.** Cutaneous T-cell lymphomas typically present as erythematous plaques or exfoliation of skin but may progress to involve lymph nodes. They are treated with topical medications (steroids, retinoids, chemotherapy), local radiation, PUVA therapy, oral methotrexate and retinoids, interferon, and, at advanced stages, combination chemotherapy.
- **Anaplastic large-cell lymphoma.** This aggressive NHL typically involves both nodal and extranodal sites (e.g., skin, lung, bone, soft tissues) and is characterized by overexpression of anaplastic lymphoma kinase (ALK)-1, usually via a t(2;5) translocation. The presence of ALK-1 confers a much more favorable prognosis, compared with ALK-1-negative cases. Standard treatment is anthracycline-containing combination chemotherapy similar to DLBCL (e.g., CHOP), with 70% long-term DFS).

FOLLOW-UP

Follow-up for DLBCL during the first 2 years after obtaining a remission includes H&P, CBC, LDH, and complete metabolic panel at 3-month intervals, with imaging typically repeated at 1 and 2 years and as clinically indicated. After 2 years, follow-up intervals may be lengthened, and after 5 to 10 years without relapse, patients may be followed by their primary care physician. For indolent NHL, follow-up is typically every 3 to 4 months, with imaging repeated annually and as clinically indicated.

PROGNOSIS

The prognosis of NHL is determined by multiple factors but starts with defining the subtype of NHL. In general, indolent NHLs are not considered curable, while aggressive NHL patients have a significant chance for long-term DFS after initial therapy. The **international prognostic index (IPI)** was developed to help predict CR and long-term survival in aggressive NHL such as DLBCL at a time when CHOP-like chemotherapy

TABLE 30-7 INTERNATIONAL PROGNOSTIC INDEX (IPI) FOR NHL

Risk Factors

1. Age >60 y
2. LDH >normal
3. ECOG PS 2–4
4. Stage III or IV
5. ≥2 extranodal sites

Standard IPI Score	Risk	CR (%)	OS at 5 y (%)
0–1	Low	87	73
2	Low-intermediate	67	51
3	High-intermediate	55	43
4–5	High	44	26

Revised IPI Score	Risk	PFS at 4 y (%)	OS at 4 y (%)
0	Very good	94	94
1–2	Good	80	79
3–5	Poor	53	55

LDH, lactate dehydrogenase; ECOG, Eastern Cooperative Oncology Group; PS, performance status; CR, complete remission; OS, overall survival; PFS, progression-free survival.

Data from: A predictive model for aggressive non-Hodgkin's lymphoma. The International Non-Hodgkin's Lymphoma Prognostic Factors Project. *N Engl J Med.* 1993;329(14):987–994 and Ref. 19.

was standard treatment. The IPI factors were used to develop a revised IPI to provide prognostic information with current front-line treatment approaches that combine rituximab with CHOP chemotherapy (Table 30-7).[19] The **follicular lymphoma IPI (FLIPI)** was developed to define overall prognosis in FL (Table 30-8), and results have shown that this index is useful in patients treated with current chemotherapy.[11]

TABLE 30-8 FOLLICULAR LYMPHOMA INTERNATIONAL PROGNOSTIC INDEX (FLIPI)[11]

FLIPI Factors

1. Age >60 y
2. Stage III or IV
3. >4 nodal areas
4. LDH >normal
5. Hemoglobin <12 g/dL

Risk	Factors	5-y OS (%)	10-y OS (%)	Patients (%)
Low	0–1	91	71	36
Intermediate	2	78	51	37
High	≥3	53	36	27

OS, overall survival.

REFERENCES

1. Swerdlow SH, Campo E, Harris NL, et al, eds. *WHO Classification of Tumours of Haematopoietic and Lymphoid Tissues.* Lyon, France: International Agency for Research on Cancer; 2008.
2. Hasenclever D, Dihl V. A prognostic score for advanced Hodgkin's disease. *N Engl J Med.* 1998;339:1506–1514.
3. Cheson BD, Pfistner B, Juweid ME, et al. Revised response criteria for malignant lymphoma. *J Clin Oncol.* 2007;25:579–586.
4. Armitage JO. Current concepts: early-stage Hodgkin's lymphoma. *N Engl J Med.* 2010; 363:653–662.
5. Engert A, Plütschow A, Eich HT, et al. Reduced treatment intensity in patients with early-stage Hodgkin's lymphoma. *N Engl J Med.* 2010;363:640–652.
6. Horning SJ, Hoppe RT, Breslin S, et al. Stanford V and radiotherapy for locally extensive and advanced Hodgkin's disease: mature results of a prospective clinical trial. *J Clin Oncol.* 2002;20:630–637.
7. Diehl V, Sieber M, Rüffer U, et al. BEACOPP: an intensified chemotherapy regimen in advanced Hodgkin's disease. The German Hodgkin's Lymphoma Study Group. *Ann Oncol.* 1997;8:143–148.
8. Diehl V, Franklin J, Pfreundschuh M, et al. Standard and increased-dose BEACOPP chemotherapy compared with COPP-ABVD for advanced Hodgkin's disease. *N Engl J Med.* 2003;348:2386–2395.
9. Schmitz N, Pfistner B, Sextro M, et al. Aggressive conventional chemotherapy compared with high-dose chemotherapy with autologous haemopoietic stem-cell transplantation for relapsed chemosensitive Hodgkin's disease: a randomized trial. *Lancet.* 2002;359:2065–2071.
10. Ekstrand BC, Lucas JB, Horwitz SM, et al. Rituximab in lymphocyte-predominant Hodgkin disease: results of a phase 2 trial. *Blood.* 2003;101:4285–4289.
11. Solol-Cèligny P, Roy P, Colombat P, et al. Follicular lymphoma international prognostic index. *Blood.* 2004;104:1258–1265.
12. Hiddemann W, Kneba M, Dreyling M, et al. Frontline therapy with rituximab added to the combination of cyclophosphamide, doxorubicin, vincristine and prednisone (CHOP) significantly improves the outcome for patients with advanced-stage follicular lymphoma compared with CHOP alone: results of a prospective randomized study of the German low-grade lymphoma study group. *Blood.* 2005;106:3725–3732.
13. Marcus R, Imrie K, Belch A, et al. CVP chemotherapy plus rituximab compared with CVP as first-line treatment for advanced follicular lymphoma. *Blood.* 2005;105:1417–1423.
14. Van Oers MH, Marcus RE, Wolf M, et al. Rituximab maintenance improves clinical outcome of relapsed/resistant follicular non-Hodgkin lymphoma in patients both with and without rituximab during induction: results of a prospective randomized phase 3 intergroup trial. *Blood.* 2006;108:3295–3301.
15. Coiffier B, Lepage E, Briere J, et al. CHOP chemotherapy plus rituximab compared with CHOP alone in elderly patients with diffuse large-B-cell lymphoma. *N Engl J Med.* 2002; 346:235–242.
16. Miller TP, Dahlberg S, Cassady JR, et al. Chemotherapy alone compared with chemotherapy plus radiotherapy for localized intermediate- and high-grade non-Hodgkin's lymphoma. *N Engl J Med.* 1998;339:21–26.
17. Persky DO, Unger JM, Spier CM, et al. Phase II study of rituximab plus three cycles of CHOP and involved-field radiotherapy for patients with limited-stage aggressive B-cell lymphoma: Southwest Oncology Group Study 0014. *J Clin Oncol.* 2008;26:2258–2263.
18. Philip T, Guglielmi C, Hagenbeek A, et al. Autologous bone marrow transplantation as compared with salvage chemotherapy in relapses of chemotherapy-sensitive non-Hodgkin lymphoma. *N Engl J Med.* 1995;333:1540–1545.
19. Sehn LH, Berry B, Chhanabhai M, et al. The revised international prognostic index (R-IPI) is a better predictor of outcome than the standard IPI for patients with diffuse large B-cell lymphoma treated with R-CHOP. *Blood.* 2007;109:1857–1861.

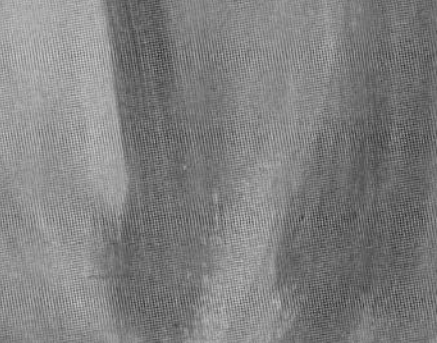

Introduction to Hematopoietic Stem Cell Transplantation

31

Armin Ghobadi

INTRODUCTION

Adult hematopoietic stem cells (HSCs) have two main characteristics: they are able to make identical copies of themselves for long periods of time (known as long-term self-renewal), and they can give rise to mature cells with specialized functions. Primitive stem cells create intermediate cells called precursor cells. Under specific signals these cells divide and become differentiated cells that finally mature to specialized blood cells.

More than 30,000 autologous transplantations and more than 25,000 allogeneic transplantations are performed annually worldwide.[1]

Sources of Hematopoietic Stem Cells

HSC transplant (HSCT) is a general term referring to the reconstitution of a patient's hematopoietic system by the administration of stored HSCs. The most common source of HSCs in adults is **peripheral blood,** accounting for ~70% of transplants. Cells are collected from peripheral blood through a process known as apheresis after mobilization of stem cells from the bone marrow into the peripheral circulation. **Bone marrow** is a source of HSCs in 20% of adult transplants. Cells are harvested directly from the bone marrow, usually from the iliac crests, under general anesthesia. **Umbilical cord blood** HSCs are currently used in 10% of transplants in adults, and the results are comparable to those achieved with adult unrelated donors (Fig. 31-1).[2]

Types of Hematopoietic Stem Cell Transplants

HSC transplants are divided into **allogeneic** and **autologous** transplants, depending on the relationship between the recipient and the donor.

- **Allogeneic transplant,** where the donor is different from the recipient, can be classified as **sibling-derived** or **matched unrelated donor.** The two main sources of matched unrelated donor transplants are **adult unrelated donors** and **umbilical cord blood.** In addition to the effect of the preparative high-dose chemotherapy, the antitumoral effect of allogeneic transplants is mediated by the **graft-versus-tumor effect** (GvT), which consists in the immune destruction of residual tumor cells by the donor's immune system. **Syngeneic transplant** is a sibling donor transplant from patient's identical twin. Because of absence of GvHD, transplant related mortality associated with syngeneic transplantation is significantly lower than matched unrelated donor transplant. However because of lower GVT effect, relapse rate is substantially higher than similar patients who receive HLA-identical sibling donor transplantation; as a result overall survival is similar in syngeneic and HLA identical sibling donor transplants. In general, sibling transplants suffer fewer problems with rejection and **graft-versus-host disease** (GvHD) than matched unrelated donor transplants, and thus, recipients

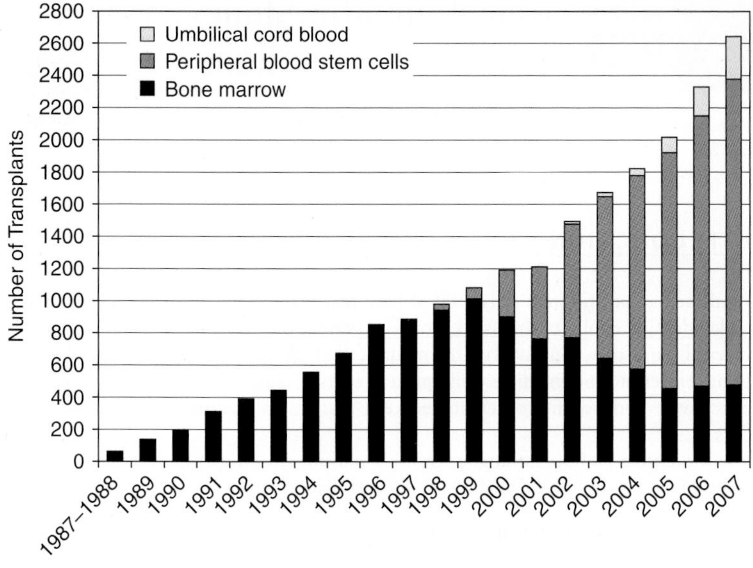

FIGURE 31-1. Number and source of adult transplants facilitated by national marrow donor program. (Ballen KK, King RJ, Chitphakdithai P, et al. The national marrow donor program 20 years of unrelated donor hematopoietic cell transplantation. *Biol Blood Marrow Transplant.* 2008;14:2–7.)

of the latter usually need more intensive immunosuppressive therapy in the posttransplant period (see Complications Related to Transplant, below).

- **Autologous transplant** refers to the infusion of a patient's own HSCs to reconstitute all of the hematopoietic lineages. This approach is used to allow very high doses of chemotherapy to be administered. Infusion of autologous HSCs rescues a patient's bone marrow function from the effects of the myeloablative doses of chemotherapy.

Indications

Indications for autologous stem cell transplantation include malignancies (multiple myeloma, non-Hodgkin's lymphoma, Hodgkin lymphoma, acute myeloid leukemia, neuroblastoma, germ-cell tumors) and nonmalignant disorders (autoimmune disorders and amyloidosis). Indications for allogeneic stem cell transplantation include malignancies (leukemia, non-Hodgkin's lymphoma, myelodysplastic syndromes) and nonmalignant disorders (aplastic anemia, paroxysmal nocturnal hemoglobinuria, fanconi's anemia, Blackfan–Diamond anemia, thalassemia major, sickle cell anemia, severe combined immunodeficiency, Wiskott–Aldrich syndrome, and inborn errors of metabolism).[3] More than 50% of allogeneic transplantations are performed for treatment of acute leukemias, followed by NHL (14%), and MDS (14%).

Transplant Immunology

- The major determinants of **histocompatibility** between donor and recipient, and thus risk for GvHD, are encoded by the **human leukocyte antigen** (HLA)

system on chromosome 6. These proteins normally function in antigen presentation in adaptive immunity. The HLA class I antigens are called A, B, and C and are found on all nucleated cells. Class II proteins, called DR, DQ, and DP, are found only on dendritic cells, B lymphocytes, and macrophages. Mismatches at HLA-DP are not associated with increased mortality. The perfect match is 10/10 HLA-A, HLA-B, HLA-C, HLA-DR, and HLA-DQ match. With high resolution DNA based HLA typing overall survival of patients undergoing 10/10 fully matched transplantations is similar to patients receiving 8/8 HLA-A, HLA-B, HLA-C, and HLA-DR matched transplantations.[4] According to NMDP guidelines, the minimal acceptable level of matching is 5 of 6 matches for HLA-A, HLA-B, and HLA-DRB.[5] Cord blood transplantations have a lower risk of GvHD. Optimal cord blood transplant is 6/6 matches for HLA-A, HLA-B, and HLA-DR.[6] The HLA locus can be considered a haplotype, so that all of the genes on one chromosome are inherited together (HLA A, B, and DR). Thus, for any given patient, the probability is one in four that a sibling will share the same two haplotypes and make a complete match.

- Other antigens called **minor histocompatibility antigens** (MHCs) are peptides also presented by HLA proteins but that elicit weaker responses compared to major antigens. These antigens are related to both GvHD and GvT effect. MHCs expressed only on the recipient HSCs will cause a GvT effect. MHCs expressed on both epithelial cells and HSCs will cause both GvHD and GvT.

THE TRANSPLANT PROCEDURE

Mobilization and Collection of Hematopoietic Stem Cells

In order to collect the necessary number of HSCs from the donor and to ensure rapid engraftment in the recipient's bone marrow, autologous and allogeneic HSCs are most commonly collected by leukapheresis from the peripheral blood after pretreatment with drugs that mobilize the HSCs from the bone marrow endosteal and vascular niches (**mobilization**). The most extensively studied mobilizing agent is granulocyte colony-stimulating factor (G-CSF). For G-CSF, the peak mobilization occurs after 4 to 6 days of daily treatment. Plerixafor, a small-molecule reversible CXC chemokine receptor 4 (CXCR4) inhibitor, can be added to G-CSF to improve stem cell collection. During the harvest procedure, called **apheresis**, stem cells are separated and removed from the other components of the blood by a cell-separator machine. The cells are then processed and stored for infusion into the patient.

Preparative Regimens

- In **allogeneic transplants**, the traditional preparative regimens are **ablative regimens**, consisting of very high doses of chemotherapy drug combinations intended primarily to eliminate the tumor cells and secondarily to suppress the donor immune system. Due to the high toxicity associated with this approach, and in order to extend transplants to older patients or patients with comorbidities, **reduced intensity** and **nonmyeloablative regimens** have been developed. The basic principle is to give drugs that are immunosuppressive to allow the GvT effect.
- In the **autologous** setting, the objective is to give high-dose chemotherapy to eliminate the tumor cells and then rescue the patient from aplasia with his or her own previously harvested and stored HSCs. In this case there is no GvT effect, and the disease control is exclusively due to the high-dose chemotherapy.

- Among the most commonly used drugs are cyclophosphamide, busulfan, fludarabine, melphalan, etoposide, and antithymocyte globulin. Total-body irradiation-based regimens combine high-dose chemotherapy with irradiation to the whole body.
- After the conditioning regimen is administered, patients will become profoundly pancytopenic (absolute neutrophil count, <100; platelet count, <10,000 cells/μL) for a period of between 12 and 24 days, depending on the source of HSCs (autologous or allogeneic) and preparative regimen used (ablative or nonablative).

Homing and Engraftment

- After infusion, HSCs migrate to specific sites in the bone marrow called niches, where they reside and undergo self-renewal and differentiation. The process of migration and adhesion is called **homing.** The interaction between HSC and their niches will result ultimately in **engraftment** and long-term durable repopulation.
- **Neutrophil engraftment** is defined as the first day of three consecutive days where the absolute neutrophil count is ≥500 cells/mm^3. **Platelet engraftment** is defined as an achievement of a platelet count of >50,000 platelets/mm^3 sustained for 3 consecutive days unsupported by a platelet transfusion. Median time to neutrophil engraftment after peripheral blood stem cell transplantation, bone marrow transplantation and cord blood transplantations is 14, 21, and 28 days, respectively. Median time to platelet engraftment after peripheral blood stem cell transplantation and bone marrow transplantation is 13, and 20 days, respectively. Median time to neutrophil engraftment after autologous stem cell transplantation is 11 days. Factors affecting time to recovery include the use of G-CSF during mobilization and harvest, degree of pretreatment chemotherapy, use of peripheral blood HSCs instead of bone marrow HSCs, and presence of infections.
- By days 18 to 21, natural killer cells are expanded and will provide antiviral responses. Within the first 30 days post transplant, natural-killer (NK) cells reach normal level and comprise the majority of lymphoid cells. Monocytes typically recover within a month after transplantation. B lymphocytes and CD8 T lymphocytes will reconstitute over months. CD4 T-lymphocyte recovery is usually prolonged over years (>5 years).[7]

Donor Lymphocyte Infusions (DLI)

Graft versus tumor mediated by donor T cells is a major component of the allogeneic HSCT anti tumor activity. DLI is defined as transfusion of nonmobilized lymphocyte concentrate or transfusion of mobilized peripheral blood stem cells without using immunosuppressant for GvHD prophylaxis. DLI can induce remissions in patients with relapse after allogeneic HSCT.[8]

SUPPORTIVE CARE

The posttransplant period is a critical time for patients who have undergone transplant. They become profoundly pancytopenic. During this time, there is significant potential morbidity and mortality from infectious agents, drug toxicity, and bleeding complications. Intensive care in a dedicated unit experienced in HSC transplant is required to support patients and provide optimal outcome.

Blood Products

All cytomegalovirus (CMV)-seronegative patients should receive CMV-negative blood and platelet products both prior to and during the transplant period. Blood products should also be irradiated or leukodepleted to avoid T-cell responses against host tissue (i.e., GvHD caused by the transfusion). Platelet products derived from a single donor are preferred to reduce alloantigen exposure.

Growth Factors

For both allogeneic and autologous transplants, **hematopoietic growth factors** have shown small reductions in the risk of documented infections, but with no effect on infection or treatment-related mortality. Specifically, in patients undergoing allogeneic HSC transplantation for myeloid leukemias, no long-term risk or benefit of using G-CSF after transplantation has been demonstrated. G-CSF shortens the post-transplantation neutropenic period by 4 to 5 days, without substantially affecting the hospitalization period or treatment-related mortality at days +30 and +100. Probabilities of acute and chronic GvHD, leukemia-free survival, and overall survival are similar whether or not G-CSF is given.

COMPLICATIONS RELATED TO TRANSPLANT

Graft-versus-Host Disease

- GvHD corresponds to an immune response of the donor T cells against the recipient. It is the main cause of morbidity and mortality after allogeneic HSC transplants. The exact cause and pathogenesis are still not completely understood, but it is believed to be caused by a reaction of donor T cells against the receptor HLA class I antigens. This inflammatory response is augmented by intestinal damage caused by the preparative regimens, which cause leakage of bacterial lipopolysaccharides into the bloodstream, increasing and maintaining the cytokine storm and tissue damage.
- GvHD has been divided into two phases, according to the timing of the symptoms. **Acute GvHD** occurs within 100 days after the transplant, and **chronic GvHD** occurs 100 days or more after the transplant, although the correlation between the two forms of GvHD is not very well understood. Moreover, not all cases of chronic GvHD are preceded by acute GvHD, although acute GvHD is the most important risk factor for chronic GvHD.
    - **Acute GvHD** occurs in 26% to 32% of recipients of sibling donor grafts, and 42% to 52% of recipients of unrelated donor grafts. It is graded as stages 0 to IV (most severe) according to the intensity of the symptoms. The usual organs compromised are the skin, mucous membranes, gastrointestinal tract, and liver. The risk factors for acute GvHD include HLA disparity, matched unrelated donors, older patients, gender-mismatched HLA, donors previously sensitized by transfusion or pregnancy, and CMV-positive donors.

    The most effective measure to prevent GvHD is an accurate HLA matching between donor and receptor. Other measures include posttransplant immunosuppressive drugs (methotrexate, cyclosporine, tacrolimus) and in vivo and ex vivo T cell depletion.

    Once GvHD is established, the first-line treatment remains corticosteroids. Topical corticosteroids and nonabsorbed steroid therapy are commonly used for skin GvHD and GI GvHD, respectively. There are a variety of second-line treatments, which generally have a low response rate.[9]

- **Chronic GvHD** develops in >50% of long-term survivors after HSC transplantation and affects both quality of life and survival. Manifestations resemble autoimmune diseases, suggesting T-cell immune deregulation, and include dermal, hepatic, ocular, oral, pulmonary, gastrointestinal, and neuromuscular manifestations.

  In contrast to acute GvHD, little is known about the causes and pathobiology of chronic GvHD. Presumably, MHCs are both responsible for and targets of this disease. It is also believed that chronic T-cell stimulation (as occurs in acute GvHD) could deregulate T cells, predisposing to chronic GvHD.

  - The most important risk factor for chronic GvHD is previous acute GvHD. Thirty percent of patients with grade 0 acute GvHD, versus 90% of grade IV acute GvHD patients, will develop chronic GvHD. Among patients with no or grade I acute GvHD, recipient age >20 years, use of non-T-cell-depleted bone marrow, and alloimmune female donors for male recipients predict a greater risk of chronic GvHD.
  - Prevention of chronic GvHD includes drugs such as cyclosporine, methotrexate, tacrolimus, corticosteroids, in vivo and ex vivo T cell depletion, and monoclonal and polyclonal antibodies. First line treatment of chronic GvHD includes a combination of corticosteroids and a calcineurin inhibitor (e.g., tacrolimus). Second-line therapies include ECP and mycophenolate mofetil.[10]

Sinusoidal Obstruction Syndrome (Veno-occlusive Disease)

- Sinusoidal obstruction syndrome (SOS) is a feared complication with a high mortality rate that can occur after either allogeneic or autologous transplant. The incidence ranges from 0% to 50%, depending on the preparative regimen. SOS can occur in up to 50% of patients receiving high dose cyclophosphamide plus total-body irradiation. Recently, the frequency and severity of SOS have decreased significantly because of lower doses of TBI and replacement of cyclophosphamide by fludarabine. Experimental studies have shown that the main damage occurs in the hepatic sinusoid.
- The major features accepted for diagnosis are jaundice, rising conjugated bilirubin, tender hepatomegaly, and ascites with fluid retention 10 to 20 days after the start of preparative regimen. There are no other specific lab tests to confirm this complication.[11]
- There is no satisfactory therapy for SOS. In 50% to 80% of patients, there is a gradual spontaneous resolution of the symptoms and signs in a 3-week period after onset of disease. During this period the focus of treatment should be management of fluid and electrolytes, and therapeutic paracentesis. **Defibrotide,** which has antithrombotic and profibrinolytic effects, is the best available treatment for sever SOS.

Pulmonary Complications

Pulmonary complications can occur in more than 60% of patients after HSCT. In the immediate post transplant period, **infections (viral, bacterial, and fungal)** are the most common causes of pulmonary complications. After engraftment, infections (viral, bacterial, and fungal), **interstitial pneumonia syndrome (IPS)** secondary to conditioning regimen and/or TBI, and **diffuse alveolar hemorrhage (DAH)** are the most common causes of pulmonary complications. **Bronchiolitis obliterans** is the most common late complication of HSCT, occurring more than 3 months after transplant.

- IPS is defined as diffuse noninfectious lung injury after transplantation. Corticosteroid is not beneficial in treatment of IPS. Treatment with etanercept is associated with a significant improvement in these patients.
- DAH is usually observed within the first month after HSCT, during peri-engraftment phase. High dose steroid is the treatment of choice for DAH, although its efficacy has not been proven in prospective clinical trials.
- Bronchiolitis obliterans occurs in 6% to 26% of allogeneic stem cell recipient. Patients with bronchiolitis obliterans present with gradually worsening dyspnea, nonproductive cough, and wheezing. Patients are usually afebrile. Pulmonary function test shows persistent obstructive pattern. High resolution CT scan shows evidence of air trapping. Immunosuppressive agents are the treatments of choice.[12]

Mucositis

Mucositis is extremely common during the neutropenic period and corresponds to the painful desquamation of the gastrointestinal epithelium. Almost 100% of patients will develop some grade of mucositis after the conditioning regimen, usually starting 3 to 5 days after the preparative regimen and lasting for 7 to 14 days.

The only demonstrated preventive treatment currently available is **Palifermin** (keratinocyte growth factor), which is able to reduce the frequency of severe mucositis from 60% to 20%. It was also associated with significant reduction in the duration of mucositis, from 9 to 3 days.[13] Others measures after mucositis is established include bland rinses, topical anesthetics, mucosal coating agents, and topical and systemic analgesics.

Engraftment Syndrome

Engraftment syndrome (ES) is characterized by a combination of noninfectious fever, erythematous rash, and noncardiogenic pulmonary edema occurring during neutrophil recovery phase following HSCT. It occurs most frequently after autologous HSCT. Treatment with a short course of corticosteroid is usually very effective especially in patients with significant pulmonary involvement.

Infections

Patients undergoing HSCT are at very high risk of infection due to the disease itself, previous chemotherapies, the preparative regimen, mucosal barrier breakdown, GvHD, and immunosuppressive drugs.

There are three periods of host defense recovery after HSC transplantation, and particular infections pose a threat in each period (Fig. 31-2).[14]

- The **phase I or preengraftment phase,** <30 days post posttransplant, is marked by **severe neutropenia** and mucosal barrier damage. As such, the patient is at risk of infection with skin and gastrointestinal organisms. Gram-negative bacilli, *Escherichia coli, Pseudomonas, Klebsiella,* and other enterics may cause local infection or sepsis. Enterococci or *viridans* streptococci may also cause bacteremia. Catheter-related bloodstream infection can be caused by staphylococci, particularly *Staphylococcus epidermidis.* Fungi, including *Candida*

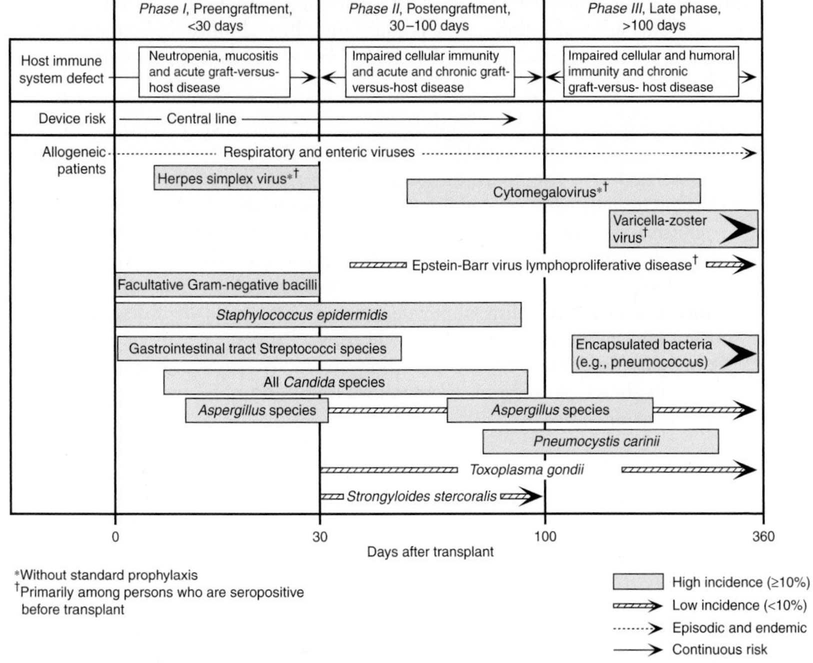

FIGURE 31-2. Phases of opportunistic infections among allogeneic HSCT recipients. Centers for Disease Control and Prevention. Guidelines for preventing opportunistic infections among hematopoietic stem cell transplant recipients: recommendations of CDC, the Infectious Disease Society of America, and the American Society of Blood and Marrow Transplantation. *MMWR Morb Mortal Wkly Rep.* 2000;49: 1–128. Available at: http://www.cdc.gov/mmwr/preview/mmwrhtml/rr4910a1.htm.

species and *Aspergillus,* may cause disseminated disease. Viral reactivation with herpes simplex virus (HSV) is common, as is varicella zoster virus (VZV), causing shingles. Human herpesvirus 6 commonly reactivates and is implicated in graft failure. BK virus is associated with encephalitis, hepatitis, and cystitis. Adenovirus and rotavirus may cause enteritis. Respiratory pathogens include adenovirus, influenza, parainfluenza, and respiratory syncytial virus.

Special consideration is given to nosocomial transmission of pathogens, including drug-resistant organisms. Thus, vigilance for methicillin-resistant *Staphylococcus aureus* is necessary, and broad coverage with vancomycin may be appropriate in the setting of neutropenic fevers without a known focus. Vancomycin-resistant enterococcus is commonly isolated from the stool but is often nonpathogenic; however, it requires treatment if isolated from the blood. *Clostridium difficile* causing colitis and diarrhea is problematic, as many patients receive broad antibiotics at some point during transplant. Contact isolation and strict adherence to routine hand washing are necessary to prevent outbreaks of nosocomial pathogens.

- The **phase II** or **postengraftment** is from day 30 to 100 posttransplant. It is characterized by intense cellular and humoral immunodeficiency, the appearance of GvHD, and increased risk of CMV reactivation.
- The **phase III** or **late phase** is after day 100 posttransplant. It is characterized by a T-cell-mediated immunodeficiency and the emergence of chronic GvHD. Several studies have demonstrated that although innate immunity recovers within several weeks, B cell and CD8 T cell counts take several months to normalize, and CD4 T cells can take several years or, indeed, may never recover in the presence of chronic GvHD.

  Among the most common infections in the later stages after transplantation is recurrent encapsulated bacterial infection, CMV reactivation, which can cause interstitial pneumonia and retinal compromise, and VZV reactivation. Patients are also at risk of *Pneumocystis jiroveci* (formerly *P. carinii*) and *Aspergillus* sp. pneumonia.[14,15]

Prevention of Infections

Strict adherence to hand-washing procedures and isolation precautions (visitor screening, HEPA filtered air, no fresh flowers) is mandatory in the care of the HSC transplant patient. Avoidance of unwashed fruits, vegetables, unroasted nuts, and raw food is recommended but its impact on infection prevention is not known. Also, good oral and body hygiene is recommended. Gut decontamination with antibiotics is no longer recommended.

Routine prophylaxis includes trimethoprim-sulfamethoxazole, dapsone, or pentamidine against *Pneumocystis;* acyclovir or valacyclovir against HSV and VZV; and fluconazole, itraconazole, or posaconazole against candidemia. Vaccination with inactivated vaccines can be started >12 months posttransplant, and patients will require a 23-valent pneumococcal vaccine as well as yearly influenza vaccinations (resuming 6 months posttransplant. Complete guidelines for preventing opportunistic infections among hematopoietic stem cell transplant recipients can be found at http://www.cdc.gov/mmwr/preview/mmwrhtml/rr4910a1.htm.

General Principles of Treatment of Infections

Workup should be directed at the most likely organisms based on time after HSC transplant. Under the minimal suspicion of infection, rapid labs and imaging, such as blood and urine cultures, CMV or aspergillus serologies, chest x-ray, and sinus or chest CTs, should be done. Treatment often requires broad-spectrum antibiotics and antifungals, which should be started as soon as possible and normally without knowing the causative agent. Acyclovir is used for HSV and VZV at therapeutic doses. For CMV, ganciclovir or foscarnet is required. Human herpesvirus 6 is responsive to ganciclovir or foscarnet. *Candida albicans* and *tropicalis* are sensitive to fluconazole but disseminated infection may require echinocandins (caspofungin, micafungin, or anidulafungin) voriconazole, or amphotericin. Other *Candida* species, such as *Candida glabrata* and *Candida krusei,* respond to itraconazole, voriconazole, echinocandins, or amphotericin. For aspergillosis, amphotericin is the standard; however, voriconazole and caspofungin are very effective, with fewer side effects. If IV amphotericin is required, lipid formulations may be used to reduce renal toxicity.

Blood Group Incompatibility

The inheritance of ABO and HLA are unrelated. ABO incompatibility occurs in 30% to 40% of allogeneic HSCT. It can be categorized into 3 subtypes. **Major mismatch** is characterized by presence of ABO antibody in recipient plasma against donor RBC antigens (recipient O, donor A, B, AB or recipient A or B, donor B, A, or AB). **Minor mismatch** is defined by presence of ABO antibody in donor plasma against recipient RBC antigens (recipient A, B, or AB, donor O or recipient AB, donor A or B). **Bidirectional mismatch** is the presence of both major and minor mismatches (donor A, recipient B or vice versa).[16]

- Major mismatch can lead to immediate hemolysis of RBCs in stem cell products, delayed hemolysis of donor RBCs or pure red cell aplasia (PRCA). Removal of RBCS from stem cell products can prevent immediate hemolysis. ABO antibodies are usually undetectable 2 months after major mismatch HSCT. Prolonged persistence of recipient B cells and plasma cells leading to persistence of ABO antibodies can occur for longer than 120 days after transplant. This can lead to delayed hemolysis or PRCA. Delayed hemolysis can be managed by transfusion of group O RBCs until anti-donor antibody has disappeared and recipient blood group has changed to donor blood group. PRCA can be managed by removal of recipient memory B cell and plasma cells by tapering immunosuppression permitting "graft versus plasma or B cell" or by using rituximab.
- Minor ABO mismatch can cause "passenger lymphocyte syndrome" that is attributed to rapid proliferation of lymphocytes transfused with stem cells. Hemolysis starts between days 3 and 15 posttransplant, lasts 5 to 10 days, and then gradually resolves as the patient incompatible RBCs are destroyed and replaced by transfused group O RBCs and/or donor RBC derived from engrafted stem cells. Passenger lymphocyte syndrome can be managed by transfusion of group O RBCs and in extreme cases plasma exchange.

HEMATOPOIETIC STEM CELL TRANSPLANT PROGNOSIS

Over the past decade, there have been substantial advances in the care of patients undergoing HSCT, resulting in significant improvements in transplant related mortality, relapse rate, and overall survival.[17] Despite significant advances in the knowledge of the biology and results of HSC transplantation, infections and other treatment-related complications are still a limiting factor in improving outcomes. Many complications are emergent and require admission to an ICU. Respiratory failure due to infections is common and may require mechanical ventilation. In addition, GvHD, infections and medication toxicities may contribute to multiple-organ dysfunction syndrome. The mortality rate is high in these situations, and overall prognosis should be discussed with the patient and family members promptly. Long-term survivors are at risk of complications such as chronic GvHD and secondary malignancies and should be closely followed. Factors such as age, comorbidities, and indication for and type of transplantation all contribute to the overall prognosis in each individual patient.

REFERENCES

1. Pasquini MC, Wang Z. Current use and outcome of hematopoietic stem cell transplantation. CIBMTR Summary Slides, 2010. Available at: http://www.cibmtr.org.
2. Ballen KK, King RJ, Chitphakdithai P, et al. The national marrow donor program 20 years of unrelated donor hematopoietic cell transplantation. *Biol Blood Marrow Transplant.* 2008; 14:2–7.

3. Copelan EA. Hematopoietic stem-cell transplantation. *N Engl J Med.* 2006;354:1813–1826.
4. Lee SJ, Klein J, Haagenson M, et al. High-resolution donor-recipient HLA matching contributes to the success of unrelated donor marrow transplantation. *Blood.* 2007;110: 4576–4583.
5. Bray RA, Hurley CK, Kamani NR, et al. National marrow donor program HLA matching guidelines for unrelated adult donor hematopoietic cell transplants. *Biol Blood Marrow Transplant.* 2008;14:45–53.
6. Scaradavou A. Unrelated umbilical cord blood unit selection. *Semin Hematol.* 2010;47: 13–21.
7. Geddes M, Storek J. Immune reconstitution following hematopoietic stem-cell transplantation. *Best Pract Res Clin Haematol.* 2007;20:329–348.
8. Huff CA, Fuchs EJ, Smith BD, et al. Graft-versus-host reactions and the effectiveness of donor lymphocyte infusions. *Biol Blood Marrow Transplant.* 2006;12(4):414–421.
9. Bacigalupo A. Management of acute graft-versus-host disease. *Br J Haematol.* 2007;137: 87–98.
10. Schlomchik WD, Lee SJ, Couriel D, et al. Transplantation's greatest challenges: advances in chronic graft-versus-host disease. *Biol Blood Marrow Transplant.* 2007;13:2–10.
11. McDonald GB. Hepatobiliary complications of hematopoietic cell transplantation, 40 years on. *Hepatology.* 2010;51:1450–1460.
12. Kotloff RM, Ahya VN, Crawford SW, et al. Pulmonary complications of solid organ and hematopoietic stem cell transplantation. *Am J Respiratory Crit Care Med.* 2004;170:22–48.
13. Spielberger R, Stiff P, Bensinger W, et al. Palifermin for oral mucositis after intensive therapy for hematologic cancers. *N Engl J Med.* 2004;351(25):2590–2598.
14. Centers for Disease Control and Prevention. Guidelines for preventing opportunistic infections among hematopoietic stem cell transplant recipients: recommendations of CDC, the Infectious Disease Society of America, and the American Society of Blood and Marrow Transplantation. *MMWR Morb Mortal Wkly Rep.* 2000;49:1–128. Available at: http://www.cdc.gov/mmwr/preview/mmwrhtml/rr4910a1.htm.
15. Hiemenz JW. Management of infections complicating allogeneic hematopoietic stem cell transplantation. *Semin Hematol.* 2009;46(3):289–312.
16. Petz LD. Immune hemolysis associated with transplantation. *Semin Hematol.* 2005;42: 145–155.
17. Gooley TA, Chien JW, Pergam SA, et al. Reduced mortality after allogeneic hematopoietic-cell transplantation. *N Engl J Med.* 2010;363:2091–2101.

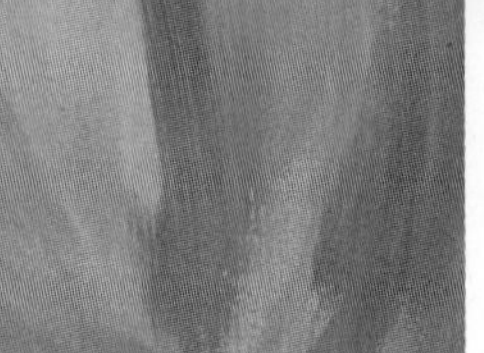

Human Immunodeficiency Virus–Related Malignancies

32

Xiaoyi Hu

INTRODUCTION

Patients infected with human immunodeficiency virus (HIV) are at significantly increased risk of developing a malignancy compared with the general population. HIV contributes to the development of cancer through immunosuppression promoting the tumorigenic effects of coinfecting oncogenic viruses. HIV infection also induces immune dysregulation causing chronic B-cell stimulation and cytokine activation that contributes to the initiation of malignancies. AIDS-defining malignancies include Kaposi sarcoma (KS), primary central nervous system lymphoma (PCNSL), non-Hodgkin lymphoma (NHL), and invasive cervical cancer. In addition, patients with HIV infection are also at increased risk of developing certain non-AIDS-defining malignancies.[1] Introduction of highly active antiretroviral therapy (HAART) has resulted in a significant change in the epidemiological and clinical profile of cancers in HIV-infected patients by decreasing the mortality associated with opportunistic infections and by improving the longevity of the patients. Although a significant decrease has been reported in certain AIDS-defining malignancies, such as KS, in the developed world, as patients live longer with chronic HIV infection, malignancy is becoming an important cause of morbidity and mortality.[2] Immune reconstitution following HAART and advances in chemotherapy and supportive care has resulted in improved outcomes of cancers in HIV infected patients compared to the pre-HAART era.[3]

KAPOSI SARCOMA

GENERAL PRINCIPLES

Epidemiology

KS is the **most common HIV-related malignancy.** The incidence of KS is approximately 15 times greater in men than in women. It is most common in homosexual or bisexual men. Since the introduction of HAART, the incidence of KS has declined markedly in HIV-infected patients. The standardized incidence ratio for KS compared to the general population fell from 22,100 to 3640. However, KS continues to be a problem of epidemic proportion in the parts of the world where HIV remains untreated.

Pathophysiology

KS-associated herpes virus, human herpes virus 8 (HHV-8), infection is found in all forms of KS. HHV-8 infection is transmitted by sexual contact, but it is also found in the saliva of infected patients. KS lesions are histologically characterized by neoangiogenesis and proliferating spindle-shaped cells admixed with an inflammatory infiltrate of lymphocytes, plasma cells, and macrophages. The malignant spindle-shaped cells are thought to be derived from HHV-8 infected circulating endothelial precursors.

HHV-8 and HIV infection act synergistically to produce cytokines, growth factors, anti-apoptotic signals, and angiogenic factors, which stimulate KS spindle cell growth and create an environment necessary to develop and sustain the tumor.[4]

DIAGNOSIS

Clinical Presentation

The clinical presentation of KS varies from minimal to fulminant disease. AIDS-related KS is generally an aggressive cancer resulting in serious morbidity and mortality. Although no organ is spared from involvement with KS, the most commonly involved sites are skin, mucous membranes, lymph nodes, gastrointestinal tract, and lungs.

- The **cutaneous lesions** are typically multifocal, plaque like or papular, and pinkish to violaceous in color, although they may evolve into nodules and ultimately ulcerate.
- **Lymph node involvement** can cause lymphedema. Internal disease can present with vague symptoms and can occur in the absence of mucocutaneous manifestations.
- **Gastrointestinal involvement** can cause abdominal pain or bleeding.
- **Pulmonary involvement** by KS may cause interstitial infiltrates or hemorrhagic effusions, resulting in cough and/or dyspnea.

Diagnostic Testing

Diagnosis is established by **biopsy of lesions;** bronchoscopy or esophagoduodenoscopy may be necessary for internal involvement. Serology for anti-HHV-8 antibodies is not central to the diagnosis.

TREATMENT

- It is important to note that KS is **not considered a curable malignancy.** The treatment decisions are based on the presence and extent of symptomatic and extracutaneous manifestations.
- **Optimization of HAART therapy** is the first line of therapy.
- **Local therapy** is used for bulky lesions or for cosmesis. Therapeutic options for local treatment include topical alitretinoin, intralesional chemotherapy with vinblastine, radiation therapy, laser therapy, and cryotherapy.
- Individuals with more advanced or progressive disease are treated with **systemic chemotherapy.** First-line chemotherapeutic drugs are liposomal anthracyclines such as doxorubicin and daunorubicin. Paclitaxel is a second-line agent. High-dose interferon-alpha therapy can be used for patients following immune reconstitution, but it is associated with significant side effects. Targeted therapy including VEGF inhibitors, KIT and PDGFR inhibitors, and mTOR inhibitors are being investigated in clinical trials.

PROGNOSIS

The AIDS Clinical Trials Group classifies patients with AIDS-related KS into good- and poor-risk groups based on tumor burden, CD4 counts, and the presence of systemic illness. However, in the post-HAART era, the CD4 count is less important.[5] Advanced age and associated AIDS-defining illnesses also affect the outcome of patients with KS.

HUMAN IMMUNODEFICIENCY VIRUS–RELATED LYMPHOMAS

GENERAL PRINCIPLES

Epidemiology

HIV-associated lymphomas constitute the second most common type of malignancy encountered in patients with HIV infection. Systemic NHL is the most common type, although the greatest increase in risk over the general population seems to be with primary central nervous system lymphoma (PCNSL). Approximately 10% HIV patients develop NHL. It appears to be more common in males than in females. Introduction of HAART significantly decreases the incidence of a subset of NHL, such as immunoblastic lymphoma and PCNSL.[6]

Pathophysiology

Various pathogenic mechanisms are attributed to development of lymphoma in HIV, including HIV-induced immunosuppression, chronic antigenic stimulation, genetic abnormalities, cytokine dysregulation, dendritic cell impairment, and viral infections associated with Epstein–Barr virus (EBV) and HHV-8.[7]

NON-HODGKIN LYMPHOMA

GENERAL PRINCIPLES

HIV-related NHLs are a heterogeneous group of tumors. More than 95% of the tumors are derived from B cells. Notable differences between HIV-related lymphoma and NHL in the general population include propensity for advanced disease, presence of B symptoms, extranodal disease including bone marrow involvement, leptomeningeal disease, and disease in unusual locations.

- **Diffuse large B-cell lymphoma** (DLBCL) is the most common HIV-related lymphoma. It is divided into centroblastic and immunoblastic types. The immunoblastic type is more characteristic of HIV infection and is more frequently associated with EBV infection (90%) compared to the centroblastic type (30%). Overexpression of Bcl-6, a proto-oncogene product, is usually associated with centroblastic and not immunoblastic DLBCL.
- **Burkitt lymphoma** accounts for 30% of HIV-related lymphoma. Thirty to forty percent of HIV-related Burkitt lymphomas in Western countries are associated with EBV infection, and c-MYC activation is involved in all cases.
- **PCNSL** represents a distinct extranodal presentation of DLBCL in HIV infection. It is usually of the immunoblastic type and is associated with severe immunosuppression (CD4 count <50) and universal EBV infection. Its involvement is usually confined to the craniospinal axis, without any systemic involvement. Its prognosis is extremely poor.
- **Primary effusion lymphoma** represents <5% of HIV-related lymphomas. It is associated with HHV-8 infection and frequent coinfection with EBV. It is an aggressive tumor and morphologically varies from the immunoblastic to the anaplastic type. It is of B cell origin but does not express B cell antigens.

- **Plasmablastic lymphoma** is a subtype that typically involves the oral cavity and jaw. It is highly associated with EBV infection and lacks HHV-8 infection. The tumor consists of large plasmablast cells with the morphological features of immunoblasts, but the immunophenotypic features of plasma cells.

DIAGNOSIS

- Since many other HIV-associated diseases, including various infections, can mimic the clinical and imaging features of lymphoma, biopsy is typically needed for diagnosis. The staging workup includes CT of the chest, abdomen, and pelvis and bone marrow evaluation. Because CNS involvement is common, MRI of the brain and lumbar puncture for cerebrospinal fluid (CSF) analysis should be considered for all patients with HIV-related lymphoma.
- The workup of a brain mass requires special consideration. CNS imaging cannot reliably differentiate between CNS lymphoma and toxoplasmosis. A solitary lesion is more likely to be lymphoma. If brain biopsy is hazardous, PCR for CSF EBV DNA is 80% sensitive and almost 100% specific for PCNSL and, hence, could substitute for a diagnostic biopsy.

TREATMENT

- With the use of HAART and anticipated immune restoration, standard-dose chemotherapy is the standard of care in patients with HIV-related NHL. Concurrent HAART and chemotherapy regimens CHOP (cyclophosphamide, vincristine, doxorubicin, and prednisone) or CDE (cyclophosphamide, doxorubicin, and etoposide), or dose-adjusted EPOCH (etoposide, prednisone, doxorubicin, cyclophosphamide, and vincristine) without highly active antiretroviral therapy (HARRT) have proven to be effective and tolerable.
- If HAART is used with chemotherapy, zidovudine should be avoided due to an increased risk of myelosuppression. Also, caution should be exercised with didanosine, stavudine, and zalcitabine, which may potentiate vincristine-induced neuropathy.
- The role of rituximab in AIDS-related lymphoma remains unclear. Rituximab should not be given to DLBCL patients with CD4 <50 due to high risk of infection.
- Prophylactic intrathecal methotrexate may be delivered at the time of initial CSF analysis to reduce the risk of leptomeningeal disease, particularly in patients with Burkitt lymphoma, Burkitt-like lymphoma histology, bone marrow, paranasal or paraspinal involvement, or EBV virus coinfection.
- PCNSL is treated with high-dose methotrexate chemotherapy and/or whole-brain irradiation.
- Select patients with relapsed or refractory lymphoma can be considered for high-dose chemotherapy with stem cell support.

PROGNOSIS

Poor prognostic factors include low CD4 counts (<100), elevated lactate dehydrogenase, poor performance status, presence of extranodal disease, prior AIDS-defining illness, advanced stage, and aggressive histology of lymphoma.

HODGKIN LYMPHOMA

Clinical features of HIV-associated Hodgkin lymphoma include a high frequency of B symptoms, advanced-stage disease, a higher incidence of bone marrow involvement, and universal EBV coinfection. Histological subtypes most often seen are mixed cellularity and lymphocyte depleted. Although chemotherapy outcomes are improving in the post-HAART era, the prognosis is significantly worse than that for HIV-negative patients. Timing of HAART therapy again remains inconclusive. Chemotherapy regimens that have been studied include ABVD (doxorubicin, bleomycin, vinblastine, and dacarbazine), BEACOPP (bleomycin, etoposide, doxorubicin, cyclophosphamide, vincristine, procarbazine, and prednisone), and the Stanford V regimen (doxorubicin, vinblastine, mechlorethamine, etoposide, vincristine, bleomycin, prednisone), and involved field radiation for initial bulky disease.

CERVICAL CANCER

- HIV infection is a strong risk factor for cervical cancer independent of the usual demographic and behavioral risk factors for cervical cancer. HIV-positive women have significantly increased rates of cervical intraepithelial neoplasia compared to HIV-negative individuals, and the incidence of cervical intraepithelial neoplasia increases with the severity of immunosuppression. However, there has been no convincing evidence to show increased invasive cervical neoplasm in HIV-infected individuals compared to HIV-negative women. HIV-positive patients are more likely to be infected with the oncogenic human papilloma virus (HPV) strains 16, 18, and 31 and, also, with multiple HPV subtypes compared to HIV-negative individuals. HPV infection is more persistent in HIV-positive patients and correlates with the severity of immunosuppression.[8]
- The **Centers for Disease Control recommends two Pap smears at a 6-month interval for any woman newly diagnosed with HIV.** If both are negative, a Pap smear should be repeated annually.
- HIV-positive patients with cervical cancer have more intractable disease and have a higher relapse rate compared to the HIV-negative group. Restoring immune function with HAART may improve the treatment outcome.

OTHER CANCERS

In large database studies of linked HIV and cancer registries, several other cancers have been shown to be increased in incidence compared to that in the general population: invasive anal carcinoma (an HPV-associated illness), multiple myeloma, leukemia, lung cancer, and malignancies of the oral cavity, lip, esophagus, stomach, liver, pancreas, larynx, heart, vulva, vagina, kidney, and soft tissues. Multiple myeloma in HIV-infected individuals occurs at a younger age and has a more aggressive clinical picture. The most common epithelial neoplasms seen in the general population—breast cancer, colon cancer, and prostate cancer—do not appear to occur more frequently in HIV-infected patients. In contrast to the adult malignancies, the clinical pathology and optimal therapy of AIDS-related malignancies in children are unclear.

REFERENCES

1. Engels EA, Pfeiffer RM, Goedert JJ, et al. Trends in cancer risk among people with AIDS in the United States 1980–2002. *AIDS.* 2006;20:1645–1654.
2. Cheung MC, Pantanowitz L, Dezube BJ. AIDS-related malignancies: emerging challenges in the era of highly active antiretroviral therapy. *Oncologist.* 2005;10:412–426.
3. Barbaro G, Barbarini G. HIV infection and cancer in the era of highly active antiretroviral therapy (review). *Oncol Rep.* 2007;17:1121–1126.
4. Mesri EA, Cesarman E, Boshoff C. Kaposi's sarcoma and its associated herpesvirus. *Nat Rev Cancer.* 2010;10:707–719.
5. Stebbing J, Sanitt A, Nelson M, et al. A prognostic index for AIDS-associated Kaposi's sarcoma in the era of highly active antiretroviral therapy. *Lancet.* 2006;367:1495–1502.
6. Lim ST, Levine AM. Recent advances in acquired immunodeficiency syndrome (AIDS)-related lymphoma. *CA Cancer J Clin.* 2005;55:229–241, 260–221, 264.
7. Pagano JS. Viruses and lymphomas. *N Engl J Med.* 2002;347:78–79.
8. Ferenczy A, Coutlee F, Franco E, et al. Human papillomavirus and HIV coinfection and the risk of neoplasias of the lower genital tract: a review of recent developments. *CMAJ.* 2003; 169:431–434.

Cancer of Unknown Primary

33

Gayathri Nagaraj

GENERAL PRINCIPLES

Definition

- Cancer of unknown primary (CUP) is defined as biopsy-proven metastatic cancer where the site of origin of the primary tumor is not identified after standard evaluation, including a thorough history and physical examination, imaging studies, laboratory data and detailed pathologic evaluation.
- Cancer of unknown primary includes a heterogeneous group of patients characterized by an aggressive clinical course and that is less responsive to chemotherapy. The search for the primary site of cancer has been increasingly facilitated by the advancement in diagnostic modalities. Historically, the median survival for this group of patients ranged from 6 to 10 months in clinical trials, however life expectancy has been noted to be as low as 2 to 3 months in unselected patient populations.[1,2] There are, however specific subgroups of patients with CUP who have treatment-responsive disease and may be able to achieve long-term disease-free survival with appropriate management. The workup of a patient with an unknown primary tumor should focus on identifying the patients with these treatable conditions. An exhaustive search for the primary tumor after adds little to the overall management of the patient, as the primary tumor site is located in <20% of patients before death and up to 70% of cases remain undiagnosed even after autopsy.[3]

Classification

Based on the light microscopy findings, they are classified into the below five major subtypes: moderate to well-differentiated adenocarcinoma (~60% of cases), poorly differentiated carcinoma with or without features of adenocarcinoma (~30%), neuroendocrine carcinoma (~1%), poorly differentiated or undifferentiated malignant neoplasm (~5%), and squamous cell carcinoma (~5%) as outlined in Table 33-1. The poorly differentiated tumors can include neuroendocrine tumors, lymphomas, germ cell tumors, melanomas, sarcomas, embryonal malignancies or may remain unspecified even after complete pathologic evaluation.[4,5]

Epidemiology

The exact incidence of CUP tumors is unknown, as they are often not reported accurately in tumor registries. The SEER database and international registries demonstrates that the estimated incidence from of CUP accounts for ~5% of all initial cancer diagnoses.[4] It is generally a disease of the middle-aged, with the median age at diagnosis being 60 years and is slightly more frequent in males.[1]

TABLE 33-1	CLASSIFICATION BASED ON LIGHT MICROSCOPY FINDINGS OF THE METASTATIC TUMOR[4]

1. Moderate to well-differentiated adenocarcinoma (~60% of cases)
2. Poorly differentiated carcinoma with or without features of adenocarcinoma (~30%)
3. Squamous cell carcinoma (~5%)
4. Poorly differentiated or undifferentiated malignant neoplasm (~5%)
5. Neuroendocrine carcinoma (~1%)

Etiology

The extreme heterogeneity within this group of patients precludes any specific identifiable etiologic or associated risk factors that may contribute to its pathogenesis.

Pathophysiology

CUP is a heterogeneous group of tumors. The molecular basis of this entity has not been elucidated. They are known to possess a unique set of clinical characteristics apart from the obvious absence of primary tumor such as: early dissemination, unpredictable metastatic pattern, aggressive disease and overall poor prognosis. The absence of the primary site of tumor is likely attributed to the slow growth pattern of the primary tumor or involution of the tumor at its primary site.

DIAGNOSIS

Extensive workup in the evaluation of patient with CUP identifies the primary tumor ~20% to 30% of patients ante mortem and autopsy studies remains inconclusive in majority of patients.

Clinical Presentation

A thorough history and physical examination is warranted in every patient with newly diagnosed cancer of unknown primary. Patients typically present with symptoms of widely metastatic disease and often have multiple symptoms at presentation. While pain is the most common presenting symptom, other common symptoms include weight loss, anorexia, fatigue, new mass, lymphadenopathy, central nervous system abnormalities, and bone pain or fracture. A careful physical examination may point towards additional sites of metastatic disease, but these are often not helpful to identify the site of primary involvement. In a series of 657 patients studied at M.D. Anderson Cancer Center, lymph nodes were the most frequently involved site of metastasis, while other major sites of involvement included liver, bone, lung, pleura, and brain.[6] Cervical adenopathy can be a manifestation of primary lung, breast, or head and neck cancer, as well as lymphoma. Lung and pancreatic cancers were most frequently identified in an autopsy series as the primary tumor site in patients with CUP, followed by other gastrointestinal and gynecological malignancies.[3] It is important to keep in mind that CUP tumors can metastasize to any site and the pattern of metastasis, while sometimes suggestive of an underlying primary tumor, does not confirm the diagnosis.

Diagnostic Testing

Standard diagnostic testing includes chest x-ray, blood chemistries and blood counts, standard imaging with CT scan and pathologic evaluation of the tumor. Tumor markers, mammogram, additional imaging studies including PET scan, testicular ultrasound or breast MRI and endoscopic evaluation depend on the site of the metastasis and features noted on pathology that are discussed below. The appropriate workup of an occult primary tumor after baseline evaluation with standard diagnostic tools includes identification of specific clinicopathologic subsets with favorable prognosis.

- **Diagnostic pathology.** An accurate pathologic evaluation of tumor specimen is paramount to the diagnostic evaluation of patents with CUP. An adequate tumor sample is cornerstone to obtaining valuable information from light microscopy, immunohistochemical staining and other sophisticated testing including genetic/molecular studies and electron microscopic evaluation in some cases.
    - **Light microscopy.** This technique provides basic information with regards to the morphology and level of differentiation of the tumor. It rarely provides information necessary to identify the origin of the metastasis. Some special staining techniques may help to rule out sarcomas and lymphomas, however these histochemical techniques have limited utility and are less sensitive and specific than their immunohistochemistry counterparts.
    - **Immunohistochemistry** (IHC). This technique is widely available and is often useful in identification of the primary origin of malignancy. Immunohistochemistry uses a panel of monoclonal and polyclonal antibodies to various cell components including enzymes, structural components of cells, hormone receptors, oncofetal antigens and other substances identified by the immunoperoxidase technique. Important staining characteristics of some of the common malignancies are shown in Table 33-2. Among the tumors identified as adenocarcinomas, staining for the cytokeratin CK7 and CK20 is the most common first step. CK7+/CK20– tumors include lung (adenocarcinoma), biliary tract and pancreas, ovary (nonmucinous), endometrium, thyroid, cervical and breast cancer, while CK7–/CK20+ tumors include gastrointestinal, ovary (mucinous) and Merkel cell carcinoma. CK7+/CK20+ tumors include urothelial, biliary tract and pancreas and ovary (mucinous). CK7–/CK20– tumors are head and neck, liver, lung (squamous and small cell) prostate and kidney.
    - **Electron microscopy** (EM). EM is not widely available and is expensive, but it may contribute to the diagnosis in rare cases, especially in the evaluation of poorly differentiated tumors. For example, secretory granules can be seen in neuroendocrine tumors, Weibel–Palade bodies in angiosarcomas, premelanosomes in melanomas and prekeratin filaments and desmosomes in squamous cell carcinoma. Electron microscopy is recommended in the evaluation of poorly differentiated neoplasm in young adults when the IHC is inconclusive.
    - **Cytogenetics and molecular diagnostics.** Cytogenetic analysis is an evolving field and may also be useful in certain situations. Isochromosome 12p and 12q are seen in germ cell tumors, translocation t(11;22) is seen in Ewing sarcoma and primitive neuroectodermal tumors, while t(8;14) translocation can be seen in some lymphoid malignancies, especially Burkitt's lymphoma. Overexpression of c-myc, ras, c-erbB2, EGFR and VEFG among others are demonstrated by IHC in various frequencies in different studies, although the exact role of this diagnostic evaluation is not completely clear at this time.

TABLE 33-2 IMMUNOHISTOCHEMISTRY CHARACTERISTICS OF COMMON TUMORS

Tumor	Immunoperoxidase Staining
Carcinoma	CK (CK7 and 20 variable), EMA+
Lymphoma	CLA, EMA (+/–)
Sarcoma	Vimentin, desmin, factor VIII antigen
Melanoma	S-100, HMB-45, Vimentin, NSE
Neuroendocrine	Chromogranin, synaptophysin, CK, EMA, NSE
Germ cell	CK, EMA, β-HCG, AFP
Prostate	PSA, CK7(–), CK20(–), EMA
Breast	CK7(+), CK20(–), EMA, ER, PR, HER2, gross cystic fluid protein 15+
Thyroid	Thyroglobulin (follicular), CK, EMA, calcitonin (medullary)
Colorectal	CK7(–), CK20(+)
Lung cancer	TTF-1(+), Surf-A and Surf-B(+)
Adenocarcinoma of lungs	CK7(+), CK20(–), TTF-1(–)
Other non-small-cell lung cancer	TTF-1(+), chromogranin, NSE
Small-cell lung cancer	
Pancreas	CK7(+), CA 19–9(+)

CK, cytokeratin; EMA, epithelial membrane antigen; CLA, common leukocyte antigen; HMB, human melanoma black; NSE, neuron-specific enolase; ER, estrogen receptor; PR, progesterone receptor; HER2, human epidermal growth factor receptor 2; TTF-1, thyroid transcription factor 1; β-HCG, human chorionic gonadotropin; AFP, alpha feto protein; PSA, prostate specific antigen.[3–5]

- **Gene expression profiling.** High throughput molecular profiling technologies are rapidly accumulating data on expression of multiple genes in several human tumors. By identifying the pattern of "typical gene expression profile" for each tumor with the help of these advanced techniques, it is becoming increasingly possible to molecularly assign a primary tumor of origin in patients with CUP. The overall accuracy from 12 studies using several tumor samples is in the range of 75% to 85%.[7,8] It has to emphasize that while a primary site of the metastatic tumor can be molecularly assigned, it is not yet clear if these tumors will have the same biology and response to therapy as their metastatic counterpart with known primary. The prognostic and predictive value of this diagnostic tool is presently unclear and needs to be validated in prospective trials. It is not considered a part of standard workup for CUP at this time.

Laboratories

In addition to routine evaluation with standard chemistry and blood counts, tumor markers are additional laboratory testing that may be warranted in certain clinical situations to identify specific treatable CUPs.

- **Tumor markers.** Some of these clinical situations include β-HCG and AFP in young men with CUP to identify extra-gonadal germ cell tumors, PSA in men to identify metastatic prostate cancer, serum thyroglobulin in rare patients with bone metastasis to identify occult thyroid cancer and serum CA 15–3 and CA125 can be helpful in women with isolated axillary lymph node enlargement or peritoneal papillary adenocarcinomatosis. Routine evaluation of commonly used epithelial tumor markers, such as CEA, CA19–9, and CA125 are nonspecific and do not provide any additional diagnostic value in identifying the primary tumor and most often nonspecific elevation in multiple tumor markers may be noted in patients with CUP.

Imaging

The importance of CT scan is well established in the workup and staging of patients with newly diagnosed malignancy. Mammography and/or ultrasound of the breast are recommended in clinically suspicious cases of breast cancer. MRI of the breast is a very sensitive test to evaluate clinically occult breast cancers and can be requested in suspected cases when mammography and ultrasound are not diagnostic. The use of fluorodeoxyglucose (FDG)-PET scans done in conjunction with a noncontrast CT study is used sometimes to provide better anatomic localization. Small studies suggest that PET/CT may be more sensitive than traditional imaging studies in locating a primary tumor, but larger follow-up studies have yet to be reported. For now, clinical judgment governs the use of PET/CT in the workup of CUP, and clinicians should consider this imaging test if the results would significantly change further management.

Diagnostic Procedures

- **Endoscopy.** The decision regarding the need for endoscopy is based on the clinical presentation of the patient with CUP. Upper airway evaluation by ENT with an endoscope is recommended for patients with isolated cervical lymph node involvement. Bronchoscopy and gastrointestinal endoscopies are indicated in patients with pulmonary or abdominal signs and symptoms respectively. Proctoscopy and/or colposcopy are recommended for patients presenting with inguinal lymph node involvement.

TREATMENT

Historically patients with CUP are known to have a poor outcome. The identification of subset of patients with favorable features who enjoy a longer disease-free survival is an important step in the management of patients with CUP. These patients with favorable features have a distinct clinicopathologic characteristics and their management is outlined separately. For patients with lack of favorable characteristics, palliative approach with combination chemotherapy is the cornerstone of management. It is important to establish the goals of care and assess their candidacy for chemotherapy in patients with unfavorable features. The general principles of management are shown in Table 33-3 and the paragraphs below summarize the management based on histology.

- **Well-differentiated or moderately differentiated adenocarcinoma.** Well-differentiated or moderately differentiated adenocarcinoma is the most frequent type of CUP, accounting for 60% of cases. These patients are typically elderly, with multiple sites of metastasis and their presentation depends on the sites of involvement. Immunohistochemistry is of limited value in this group of patients, although identification of ER/PR status or PSA is valuable for treatment and

TABLE 33-3 SIMPLIFIED APPROACH TO MANAGEMENT OF PATIENTS WITH CANCER OF UNKNOWN PRIMARY SITE[3]

1. **Diagnosis of metastatic carcinoma**
2. **Initial search for primary site.** A thorough workup includes a complete history and physical examination, laboratory data, tumor markers, thorough pathologic evaluation, diagnostic radiology information and other specific tests as necessary.
3. **Exclude potentially treatable or curable tumors.** With the help of additional immunohistochemistry, molecular testing or electron microscopy and other specific tests based on clinical suspicion.
4. **Characterize the specific clinicopathologic entities.**
5. **Treatment planning.** Appropriate loco-regional and/or systemic therapy with curative/treatable intent in the favorable subgroup of patients and palliative intent with combination chemotherapy for selected patients in the unfavorable subsets.

prognosis. Few patients in this group fit into a favorable treatment subset. Most patients have a poor prognosis and are mainly treated with palliative intent. Patients with a good performance status should be considered candidates for systemic therapy and/or clinical trials. Multiple chemotherapy regimens have been evaluated in these patients with the aim of stabilizing their disease. The combination chemotherapy regimens listed under NCCN guidelines based on available data from clinical trials as is shown in Table 33-4.

TABLE 33-4 PRINCIPLES OF CHEMOTHERAPY: CANCER OF UNKNOWN PRIMARY NCCN GUIDELINES[9]

Adenocarcinoma

Paclitaxel 200 mg/m^2 IV day 1
Carboplatin AUC = 6 day 1, repeat cycle every 3 wk
Paclitaxel 200 mg/m^2 IV day 1
Carboplatin AUC = 6
Etoposide 50 mg/d alternating with 100 mg/d PO day 1–10, repeat cycle every 3 wk
Docetaxel 65 mg/m^2 IV day 1
Carboplatin AUC = 6 day 1, repeat cycle every 3 wk
Gemcitabine 1250 mg/m^2 IV day 1 and 8
Cisplatin 100 mg/m^2 IV day 1, repeat cycle every 3 wk
Gemcitabine 1000 mg/m^2 IV day 1 and 8
Docetaxel 75 mg/m^2 IV day 8, repeat cycle every 3 wk

Squamous cell carcinoma

Paclitaxel 175 mg/m^2 IV day 1
Cisplatin 100 mg/m^2 IV day 2
5-FU 500 mg/m^2/d continuous infusion over 120 h, repeat every 3 wk
Docetaxel 75 mg/m^2 IV day 1
Cisplatin 75 mg/m^2 IV day 1
5-FU 750 mg/m^2/d continuous infusion days 1 to 5, repeat cycle every 3 wk

- **Poorly differentiated carcinoma with or without features of adenocarcinoma.** This group accounts for about ~30% of CUP cases. The majority of the patients have a poorly differentiated carcinoma histology, while a third have some features of adenocarcinoma differentiation. In comparison to patients with moderately or well-differentiated adenocarcinoma, these patients tend to be younger, have more rapidly progressive symptoms, and have peripheral lymph nodes, and mediastinal or retroperitoneal involvement. Favorable subsets with specific therapeutic implications have to be excluded from this group of patients. The prognosis and treatment for the remaining patients with unfavorable features are similar to the ones with well-differentiated adenocarcinoma group. Recent clinical trials by investigators at the Minnie Pearl Cancer Research Network incorporating several newer agents including targeted therapy have noted further improvement in outcome.[4]
- **Squamous cell carcinoma.** Squamous cell carcinoma accounts for 5% of all cases of CUP. Majority of patients in this subgroup fall into specific clinical syndromes and are largely treatable, hence appropriate diagnostic workup should be undertaken. Management of patients with squamous cell carcinoma involving the cervical, supraclavicular and inguinal lymph nodes are outlined below. Patients with squamous cell carcinoma involving other areas should be evaluated for occult lung primary with CT scan and bronchoscopy. Other sites of origin of tumor include head and neck, esophagus, cervix, anus, rectum, and bladder. Patients should be evaluated for additional sites when indicated, as some adenocarcinoma can undergo squamous differentiation and immunohistochemistry may be helpful in these situations. Table 33-4 outlines the chemotherapy regimens listed under the NCCN guidelines for squamous cell carcinoma of unknown primary.
- **Poorly differentiated neoplasm.** Poorly differentiated neoplasm account for ~5% of CUP. Detailed pathologic evaluation is very important in this subgroup, as treatment may differ radically based on the results. Many of these tumors can be characterized as atypical lymphomas, neuroendocrine tumors, or germ cell tumors by careful pathologic testing. If a specific diagnosis cannot be made, then poorly differentiated neoplasms are treated the same as poorly differentiated adenocarcinoma. It is again important to exclude important treatable clinical scenarios, for example if a male patient aged <50 years old presents with a poorly differentiated neoplasm (especially with mediastinal or retroperitoneal mass), particular attention should be paid to exclude the diagnosis of an atypical germ cell tumor.
- **Neuroendocrine carcinoma.** Neuroendocrine carcinoma of unknown primary site accounts for a minority of the CUP patients. Some are well differentiated or low grade with features typical of carcinoid, or islet cell tumors and have metastatic involvement of the liver or bone. They can be associated with syndromes such as Zollinger-Ellison and carcinoid from secretion of bioactive amines. In some of these patients, a primary site can be found in the small intestine, rectum, pancreas, or bronchus on further evaluation. These tumors are generally indolent and their treatment recommendation is per the standard guidelines for metastatic carcinoid or islet cell malignancies with known primary site. The other types of neuroendocrine tumors include those with aggressive behavior either with neuroendocrine histology or lack of distinctive neuroendocrine features on light microscopy. The neuroendocrine features in this later group are only recognized on detailed pathologic evaluation. The

treatment recommendation for small-cell carcinoma of unknown primary is combination chemotherapy as recommended for small-cell lung cancer. Patients with poorly differentiated neuroendocrine carcinoma of unknown primary site are still a highly treatable subgroup and a trial of combination chemotherapy with platinum-based regimen is recommended.

SPECIAL CONSIDERATIONS

Below are the distinct clinicopathologic entities that require special attention, as these represent subgroup of patients with specific therapy recommendation and relatively better outcomes given their treatable and/or curable situations.

- **Extragonadal germ cell tumor presenting as poorly differentiated carcinoma/ malignancy with midline distribution.** Extragonadal germ cell tumors should be suspected in men aged <50 years old with midline tumors, either mediastinal or retroperitoneal tumors, and a relatively short duration of symptoms. Tumor markers (AFP and β-hCG) should be checked and treatment should be formulated. For example, poor prognosis germ cell tumors are treated with platinum-based regimens. High overall response rates of more than 50% with 15% to 25% complete responses and 10% to 15% long-term disease-free survival rates have been noted in this subgroup.[3]
- **Women with peritoneal carcinomatosis.** Women may present with peritoneal carcinomatosis with histologic features suggestive of ovarian adenocarcinoma, such as psammoma bodies and papillary structure, in the absence of primary tumor even after abdominal exploration. Patients often have elevated CA-125 levels and they rarely metastasize outside of the peritoneal cavity. These women should be treated as stage III ovarian cancer with surgical cytoreduction followed by adjuvant chemotherapy with a platinum based regimen. Approximately 11% to 25% of patients are noted to have long-term survival with this management.[3]
- **Women with adenocarcinoma involving axillary lymph nodes.** Breast cancer should be suspected in this group of patients. Breast exam and mammography should be performed, as well as staining for estrogen and progesterone receptors and HER2 status. Breast MRI can also be used if initial studies are unrevealing. In this group of patients with negative exam and imaging, occult breast primary, usually measuring less than 2 cm in diameter has been found in 44% to 80% of mastectomy specimens.[4] Patients should be evaluated for other metastatic involvement, and if evaluation is negative, they should be treated for stage II or III breast cancer. The treatment should include lymph node clearance with primary breast surgery and/or breast irradiation. Patients should receive adjuvant systemic treatment based on their age, lymph node status, ER/PR status, and HER2 status. If patients are found to have additional metastatic disease, they may have metastatic breast cancer and may benefit from therapy for metastatic breast cancer.
- **Men with suspected prostate cancer.** All men with metastatic adenocarcinoma with unknown primary should have their PSA levels checked. Their tumors can also be stained for PSA. Patients with elevated PSA should undergo hormonal treatment for prostate cancer even if the clinical features are atypical, as many will have significant palliation of their symptoms along with prolonged disease control.

- **Patients with a single metastatic lesion.** On occasion, only one site of metastatic disease is found even after complete evaluation and they represent a favorable prognostic group. Treatment should include aggressive local therapy of the metastatic lesion with surgical resection or radiation or a combination of both modalities. The role of systemic treatment is not yet defined in these patients, but can be considered for patients with good performance status and poor differentiation, especially in the context of clinical trials.
- **Squamous cell carcinoma involving cervical and supraclavicular lymph nodes.** Primary head and neck cancer should be suspected in patients with squamous cell carcinoma involving upper and middle cervical lymph nodes. These patients are usually elderly with history of tobacco and alcohol abuse. CT scan to evaluate the head and neck region is important to define the extent of the disease and identify the primary site. Careful direct and endoscopic evaluation of these areas is also indicated to complete the workup. The treatment recommendation is similar to the loco-regional management for locally advanced head and neck cancer with radical neck dissection, local radiation or a combined modality approach. About 30% to 40% of these patients achieve long-term disease free survival with this local therapy.[4] Systemic chemotherapy administered concurrently with radiation or in the adjuvant setting can also be considered in patients with unknown primary in a similar fashion as indicated for head and neck cancers with known primary. In patients with lower cervical and supraclavicular lymph node involvement, a search for a primary lung tumor has to be undertaken. Local treatment to the neck is recommended when the primary site remains unidentified.
- **Squamous cell carcinoma involving inguinal lymph nodes.** In patients with inguinal lymph node involvement, careful physical examination of the perineum and anorectal region should be undertaken to reveal a primary site. Anoscopy in all and pelvic examination in females should be part of the evaluation. If no primary site is identified, patients should undergo inguinal lymph node dissection with or without radiation therapy, especially if extensive disease is identified. Systemic chemotherapy can be considered in the adjuvant or neoadjuvant setting.
- **Gestational choriocarcinoma.** Metastatic gestational choriocarcinoma should be suspected in young women with poorly differentiated carcinoma and pulmonary nodules. A recent history of pregnancy, spontaneous abortion, or missed menses may be elicited. Imaging of the abdomen may show enlarged uterus and an elevated β-hCG is often helpful in making the diagnosis. These patients carry a high cure rate with single agent methotrexate.

MONITORING/FOLLOW-UP

There are no definite guidelines for monitoring and follow-up given the overall poor outcomes and short life expectancy in this patient population. Patients who fall into specific subgroup as mentioned earlier should follow the guidelines similar to the primary malignancy. While patients receiving palliative chemotherapy should follow the treatment schedule, the symptomatic patients should receive supportive management as often as needed.

OUTCOME/PROGNOSIS

This is a heterogeneous group with median survival of 6 to 10 months.[1] Features such as lymph node involvement, pathologic diagnosis of carcinoma, squamous carcinoma, and neuroendocrine carcinoma confer a survival advantage, while male sex, pathologic diagnosis of adenocarcinoma, increasing number of involved organ sites and visceral involvement including liver, lung, bone, pleura, or brain are associated with poor survival.[6] Although the outcome overall is poor, it is worth mentioning again the importance identifying the patients that belong to the favorable subgroups who can be cured or treated with very encouraging long-term outcomes. The decision to treat the rest of patients in the unfavorable subgroup must be individualized and based on performance status and the patient's desire to proceed.

REFERENCES

1. Pavlidis N, Fizazi K. Carcinoma of unknown primary (CUP). *Crit Rev Oncol Hematol.* 2009;69:271–278.
2. van de Wouw AJ, Janssen-Heijnen ML, Coebergh JW, et al. Epidemiology of unknown primary tumours; incidence and population-based survival of 1285 patients in Southeast Netherlands, 1984–1992. *Eur J Cancer.* 2002;38:409–413.
3. Pavlidis N, Briasoulis E, Hainsworth J, et al. Diagnostic and therapeutic management of cancer of an unknown primary. *Eur J Cancer.* 2003;39:1990–2005.
4. Greco FA, Hainsworth JD. Cancer of unknown primary site. In: DeVita VT Jr., Hellman S, and Rosenberg SA, eds. *Cancer: Principles and Practice of Oncology.* 8th ed. Philadelphia: Lippincott Williams & Wilkins; 2008:2363–2387.
5. Hainsworth JD, Greco FA. Treatment of patients with cancer of an unknown primary site. *N Engl J Med.* 1993;329:257–263.
6. Abbruzzese JL, Abbruzzese MC, Hess KR, et al. Unknown primary carcinoma: natural history and prognostic factors in 657 consecutive patients. *J Clin Oncol.* 1994;12:1272–1280.
7. Pentheroudakis G, Greco FA, Pavlidis N. Molecular assignment of tissue of origin in cancer of unknown primary may not predict response to therapy or outcome: a systematic literature review. *Cancer Treat Rev.* 2009;35:221–227.
8. Pentheroudakis G, Golfinopoulos V, Pavlidis N. Switching benchmarks in cancer of unknown primary: from autopsy to microarray. *Eur J Cancer.* 2007;43:2026–2036.
9. NCCN clinical practice guidelines in oncology. National Comprehensive Cancer Network. Last accessed: 4/22/2011 <http://www.nccn.org/professionals/physician_gls/f_guidelines.asp.>

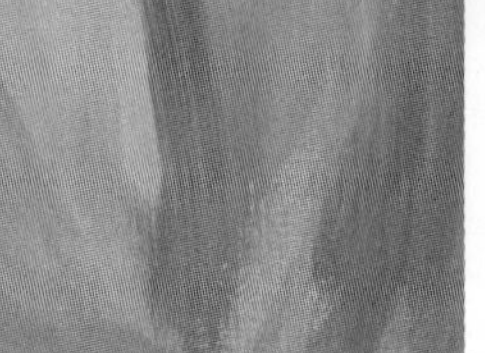

Supportive Care in Oncology

34

Brian A. Van Tine

GENERAL PRINCIPLES

Supportive care addresses the physical, mental, and spiritual needs of the cancer patient. Physical symptoms can arise from the cancer itself, the side effects of therapy, medications, or comorbid medical conditions. This chapter focuses on symptom control as an important element of oncology practice, including pain management, nausea and vomiting, mucositis, diarrhea, anorexia, and dyspnea. It also addresses the emotional issues of depression, anxiety, and delirium, and presents an approach to addressing spiritual needs of the cancer patient.

MANAGEMENT BY PHYSICAL SYMPTOM

PAIN MANAGEMENT

GENERAL PRINCIPLES

Pain is a prevalent complaint in cancer patients, occurring in 50% to 70% of all patients with cancer. More than one half of cancer patients experience moderate to severe pain, and 50% to 80% of cancer patients are not satisfied with their pain relief. The undertreatment of cancer pain can be attributed to multiple barriers, including physician, patient, and societal factors. A physician must remember that each person's pain is different and must be treated as such.[1]

Definition

Pain is always subjective. The International Association for the Study of Pain defines pain as "an unpleasant sensory and emotional experience associated with actual or potential tissue damage, or described in terms of such damage. Each individual learns the application of the word through experiences related to injury early in life." Acute pain may be associated with physical signs, including tachycardia, hypertension, hyperventilation, facial grimacing, and verbalizations. However, patients with chronic pain may not exhibit any of these overt physical signs and may not "appear in pain." It is important to remember that pain is always subjective, and the patient's self-reporting is a key element to an accurate pain assessment.[1]

DIAGNOSIS

- The first step in the management of pain depends on a comprehensive pain assessment gathered through history, physical exam, and review of laboratory and radiology studies. Important pain characteristics to elicit from the patient should be descriptions of the pain with regard to **onset, duration, intensity,**

quality, and **exacerbating or relieving factors.** The physician can use each of these characteristics to identify potential etiologies and institute the appropriate pain management plan.

- Simple tools can reliably aid in the measurement of pain. The most common clinical assessment tools are verbal rating scales and visual analog scales. A verbal rating scale uses words to describe pain such as none, mild, moderate, severe, or excruciating. A visual analog scale uses a line with or without verbal clues or numbers and asks patients to place their pain rating on this scale. The specific scale used to measure pain is less important than the consistent use of a scale over time. For illiterate or pediatric patients, a visual analog scale can be used with pictures to describe the levels of pain as a better pain assessment tool.

TREATMENT[1–4]

- The World Health Organization (WHO) recommends the use of an analgesic ladder in the approach to the selection of opioids to treat cancer pain. Analgesic selection should be guided by the severity of cancer pain. Patients with mild to moderate pain are usually started on acetaminophen or nonsteroidal anti-inflammatory drugs (NSAIDs). Patients with moderate to severe pain, or those who had insufficient relief after a trial of acetaminophen or NSAIDs, are treated with an opioid used for moderate pain, such as codeine, hydrocodone, dihydrocodeine, and oxycodone. This opioid may be combined with acetaminophen or an NSAID or an alternative adjuvant drug (tricyclic antidepressant, anticonvulsant, or topical anesthetic). Many of the drugs used for moderate to severe cancer pain are available in the United States as a combination of the opioid and acetaminophen or aspirin (ASA). The drug can be titrated until the maximum safe dose of acetaminophen (4 g/d) or ASA is reached.
- Patients with severe pain, including those who fail to reach adequate pain relief with drugs from the second step on the WHO ladder should receive an opioid that is useful in the treatment of severe cancer pain. The drugs useful in the treatment of severe cancer pain include morphine, hydromorphone, fentanyl, oxycodone, and methadone. These opioids may also be combined with acetaminophen or an NSAID or an adjuvant drug when needed. Patients can experience a variation of analgesia and side effects between the different opioids. A clinician may need to rotate among the various opioids to identify the drugs that have the correct balance between pain control and side effects. These **drugs should be titrated to analgesic effect or intolerable side effects.** There is no maximum dose limitation on the opioid medication itself.
- In the treatment of cancer pain, it is **important to distinguish between acute and chronic pain,** as the goals of treatment are slightly different. Acute pain is a linear event; the pain starts, and, with relief of the offending event, the pain stops. Chronic pain is cyclical in nature, repeating itself over time. For acute pain, the goal of treatment is pain relief. To accomplish pain relief, the drugs administered should have a rapid onset of action, with the desired duration of action (e.g., 2 to 4 hours). These drugs are given as needed. Common side effects, such as sedation, are usually acceptable and well tolerated by the patient. An example of an acute pain scenario is the patient who falls and suffers a hip fracture at the site of a previous bone metastasis. The patient is treated with

short-acting IV narcotics until surgery can be performed to stabilize the fracture.

- **Chronic pain management** has a different focus. The overall goal is pain prevention and the avoidance of undesirable side effects, such as sedation. The analgesic regimen should include long-acting narcotics administered on a regular schedule and should be individualized for the patient based on side effects. Patients with chronic pain also need to have the understanding of how to manage acute exacerbations with short-acting, rapid-onset analgesics, most commonly referred to as breakthrough pain relief. Many cancer patients have chronic pain. Chronic pain is ineffectively managed when the clinician focuses on acute control of the pain in this setting.

Medications[1–4]

- Opioid therapy can provide effective pain relief to the majority of patients with cancer pain. Opioids can be classified as pure agonists or agonist antagonists, based on their interactions with opioid receptors in the body. The drugs that are included in the agonist–antagonist subclass include butorphanol (Stadol), nalbuphine (Nubain), pentazocine (Talwin), and buprenorphine (Buprenex). Drugs in this subclass have a ceiling effect for analgesia and may reverse the effects of pure agonists. For these reasons, use of the mixed agonist–antagonist subclass is not recommended in the treatment of cancer pain.
- When managing chronic pain, it is important to remember that there are wide variations in dose requirements. This variation is not based on the size or age of the patient or the amount of disease present. The analgesic dose required to keep a patient out of pain cannot be predicted, but rather, must be determined by educated trial and error. The following are guidelines for opioid use in chronic pain patients.
    - **Start with one drug at the lowest effective dose.** Titrate the drug to pain relief or intolerable side effects. If the patient is unable to tolerate one narcotic due to undesirable side effects, switch to an alternative agent.
    - **Use around-the-clock dosing schedules** to avoid peaks and valleys in serum analgesic levels.
    - Sustained or long-acting release preparations of narcotics are very useful in this population. When converting between modes of administration or drugs, calculate the equianalgesic dosages to avoid undermedicating a patient. See Table 34-1.
    - **Breakthrough pain medications should be the same or a similar drug used for long-acting pain relief.** The minimum effective breakthrough pain medication dose should be equivalent to 12.5% of the patient's total daily narcotic requirements, or 25% of a single BID dose.
    - Keep the regimen as simple as possible. Avoid mixing a variety of analgesic regimens.
    - **Always start a bowel regimen when placing a patient on narcotics,** as constipation is a side effect of all narcotics.
    - **Educate the patient and family about dosing and side effects.** Discuss and reassure the patient and family about addiction, tolerance, and physical dependence.

TABLE 34-1 **EQUIVALENT OPIOID DOSES**

	PO (mg)	SC/IV (mg)
Morphine	30	10
Hydromorphone	7.5	1.5
Methadone	20	10
Codeine	200	NA
Oxycodone	20	NA
Fentanyl	NA	0.05–0.1

NA, not available.

- **Morphine** is the drug of choice for moderate to severe cancer pain. It has a wide range of doses available and flexible methods of delivery. Morphine is available as sustained-release, immediate-release, liquid/sublingual, and parenteral preparations. The sustained-release tablets may be given per rectum or sublingually in patients unable to swallow. **Oxycodone** is available orally as immediate- and sustained-release preparations. **Fentanyl** is available in the parenteral route, as well as the fentanyl (Duragesic) patch for patients unable to swallow or who cannot tolerate morphine or oxycodone. The patches are applied to the chest wall or back and changed every 48 to 72 hours. The onset of action in these long-acting preparations is 12 hours. When starting a patient on long-acting agents, the clinician needs to provide the patient with immediate-relief preparations for use in the interim, until the long-acting narcotic can achieve adequate serum levels for analgesia.
- **Meperidine (Demerol) should be avoided in the treatment of chronic pain.** Meperidine has the very short half-life of 2 to 3 hours. This is ineffective in the management of chronic pain. Meperidine has a toxic metabolite, normeperidine, which is a weaker analgesic but a potent CNS stimulant. Normeperidine has a half-life of ≥25 to 30 hours in the setting of renal failure. This can rapidly lead to accumulation of the drug when used for more than 48 to 72 hours. CNS toxicity can include irritability, tremors, myoclonus, agitation, and seizures. When CNS toxicity occurs, it is important to stop the drug. Naloxone (Narcan) should not be administered, as the effects of normeperidine are not reversed with naloxone and can precipitate worsening CNS toxicity.
- **Propoxyphene (Darvon-N) is another narcotic agent that is ineffective in the treatment of chronic pain.** Despite its widespread use, the drug has no more analgesic properties than ASA (650 mg). Propoxyphene has the long half-life of 6 to 12 hours. It also has a toxic metabolite, norpropoxyphene, with a half-life of 30 to 36 hours. Norpropoxyphene has been associated with pulmonary edema, cardiotoxicity, and cardiac arrest.
- IM injections should be avoided for the management of cancer pain. The use of IM injections is painful, and absorption is unreliable. The onset of action can be 30 to 60 minutes, and this is not acceptable in the acute pain setting. IV or transmucosal (sublingual or rectal) routes are much more efficacious at getting rapid onset of action in the acute pain setting.

- The perception that the administration of opioid analgesics for chronic pain management causes addiction is prevalent and is a barrier to adequate pain control. Confusion about the differences among addiction, tolerance, and physical dependence is in part responsible.
  - **Addiction** is a pattern of drug abuse characterized by drug craving and overwhelming behaviors that are used to obtain a drug.
  - **Tolerance** is a state in which escalating doses of opioids are needed to achieve pain control as the drug effectiveness reduces over time. Tolerance occurs with all of the side effects of narcotics, with the exception of constipation. It is important to educate patients and family members that tolerance too many of the common side effects, such as itching or sedation, will develop, and that the drug should not be abruptly discontinued.
  - **Physical dependence** is the onset of signs and symptoms of withdrawal with abrupt discontinuation of the opioid. Abrupt withdrawal may result in tachycardia, hypertension, diaphoresis, nausea, vomiting, abdominal pain, psychosis, and hallucinations. This is not the same as addiction. Physical dependence and addiction are not synonymous. When stopping chronic opioid medications, the dose should be reduced in increments of 20% every 2 to 3 days to avoid the risk of withdrawal symptoms. Finally, it should be remembered that patients experiencing inadequately controlled pain may engage in what appears to be drug-seeking behavior, which is easy to confuse with addiction.
- **Adjuvant analgesics** can be important in the treatment of cancer pain. Adjuvant analgesics include antidepressants, anticonvulsants, corticosteroids, and local anesthetics. Within the antidepressants, tricyclics are the most effective as an adjunctive therapy for neuropathic pain. Common side effects from the tricyclics include orthostatic hypotension, sedation, urinary retention, confusion, and sexual dysfunction. Doses of the tricyclic antidepressants should be started low and titrated for analgesia. Anticonvulsants are also helpful adjunctive therapies in the treatment of neuropathic pain syndromes. These drugs include carbamazepine (Tegretol), phenytoin (Dilantin), gabapentin (Neurontin), and pregabalin (Lyrica). The usual initiating dose of gabapentin is 100 mg TID titrated up to a maximum of 3600 mg/d. Side effects of these drugs can be self-limiting, including sedation, confusion, and dizziness.
- **Corticosteroids** can be useful in the management of bone metastases, nerve compression, elevated intracranial pressure, and obstruction of a hollow viscus. Local anesthetics, such as nerve blocks, lidocaine patches, and eutectic mixture of local anesthetics (EMLA) cream, can aid in the treatment of cancer pain. In extreme cases, IV administration of anesthetics can be used in conjunction with IV or intraspinal narcotics to allow the clinician to administer lower doses of narcotics and spare the patient the complications of sedation seen with high doses of narcotics.
- **Bisphosphonates** (pamidronate, zoledronic acid) and calcitonin have been used to treat pain from bony metastases. Clinical trials have failed to demonstrate clear evidence for the ability of bisphosphonates to deliver an analgesic benefit over placebo. Calcitonin provides no benefit in metastatic bone pain over placebo, but some studies suggest that it may reduce the intensity and frequency of neuropathic pain.

CONSTIPATION[5]

GENERAL PRINCIPLES

Most constipation in cancer comes from opioid pain management, but the differential diagnosis of constipation is broad.

DIAGNOSIS

- Before assuming that all constipation is pain medicine related in the cancer patient, one must remember to consider bowel obstruction, spinal cord compression, hypercalcemia, hypokalemia, diabetes mellitus, hypothyroidism, timing of chemotherapy, uremia, etc., as these must be treated differently. Other possible considerations are different classes of drugs, such as: antacids, anticholinergics, antidepressants, calcium channel blockers, cholestyramine, clonidine, diuretics, levodopa, NSAIDs, psychotropics, and sympathomimetics.
- During opioid treatment, constipation should be expected. Prophylactic measures should always be initiated with the start of opioid therapy. Constipation occurs with all opioids, and pharmacologic tolerance rarely develops. Symptoms from constipation may become so severe that patients may decide to discontinue pain medications. This is preventable with the use of an aggressive laxative regimen.

TREATMENT[5]

- Dietary interventions are almost never sufficient to prevent constipation. Combinations of agents are often necessary. Clinicians should also avoid the use of bulk-forming agents in the absence of a motility agent, especially in debilitated or anorectic patients. When using these agents, it should be remembered that stool softeners and bulking agents do little to relieve constipation but may make stools more comfortable to pass. Their sole use will only lead to constipation with soft stools, and another agent is necessary for adequate treatment. Also, it should be remembered that the onset of abdominal pain or nausea in a patient taking opioids may be due to unrecognized constipation.
- Laxatives can be classified into three categories: stimulant, osmotic, and detergent agents (Table 34-2). **Stimulant laxatives** irritate the bowel, leading to increased peristaltic activity. **Osmotic laxatives** draw water into the bowel lumen and increase the moisture content of the stool. In addition, they add to overall stool volume. **Detergent laxatives** facilitate the dissolution of fat in water and increase the water content of stool. Laxatives can be titrated to a maximal therapeutic dose. Clinicians should try to simplify the bowel regimen, as this will improve patient compliance. Combinations of stimulant and detergent laxatives such as docusate/senna (Senokot-S) are ideal for preventing opioid-induced constipation.
- **Prokinetic agents** such as metoclopramide (Reglan) can increase peristaltic activity and facilitate stool movement. This agent can be used in combination with other laxative agents. Lubricant stimulants and large-volume enemas can also be used but are not recommended for daily use and prophylaxis of

TABLE 34-2 LAXATIVES

Stimulant laxatives	
Senna	2 tablets bid, titrated to effect (up to 8/d)
Bisacodyl (Dulcolax)	5 to 15 mg PO or 10 mg PR qhs
Osmotic laxatives	
Lactulose	20 g/30 mL PO every 4 to 6 h, titrated to effect (or every 2 h in severe constipation)
Sorbitol	30 mL PO every 4 to 6 h, titrated to effect
Milk of magnesia	15 to 30 mL/d or twice daily
Magnesium citrate	300-mL bottle per day, bid, scheduled or prn
Detergent laxatives	
Docusate sodium or calcium	100 mg PO per day or twice daily
Phosphosoda enema	PRN

opioid-related constipation. The use of these agents is effective while titrating other laxatives to ensure that the patient is having regular bowel movements.

- Often patients present with constipation from narcotics of the order of days to weeks in duration. It is important to identify this immediately and treat it aggressively. One can use enemas or suppositories per rectum, or oral regimens such as lactulose, 20 g every 2 hours, until the bowels move. Patients should be instructed to inform their physician if they do not have a bowel movement within any 48-hour time period while they are on narcotics to avoid potentially life-threatening complications.

DIARRHEA[5]

GENERAL PRINCIPLES

Diarrhea can be defined as stools that are looser than normal and that may be increased in number over baseline. The definition is based on the frequency, volume, and consistency of stools. In cancer patients, getting up to go to the bathroom multiple times day and night can be exhausting. If persistent, diarrhea can lead to dehydration and electrolyte abnormalities that can lead to the need for a hospital admission.

DIAGNOSIS

Potential causes of diarrhea in the cancer patient can include infections, malabsorption, gastrointestinal bleeding, medications, chemotherapy (particularly 5-FU), radiation to the abdomen or pelvis, and overflow incontinence. It is important to remember that herbals such as ginkgo biloba, ginseng, and licorice may also cause diarrhea.

TREATMENT

- Patients should be instructed on the establishment of normal bowel habits. Any change from the normal baseline should be reported to the physician to avoid severe dehydration or electrolyte imbalances. Patients should be counseled on the avoidance of foods containing lactose or other gas-forming foods that can increase abdominal cramping and pain. Another general approach to diarrhea is to increase the bulk of the stools with the addition of psyllium, bran, or pectin. However, sometimes bulk-forming agents can worsen abdominal cramping and bloating.

- For the medical management of transient or mild diarrhea, the use of attapulgite (Kaopectate) or bismuth salts (Pepto-Bismol) can be useful. Care should be taken to rule out infection by checking *Clostridium difficile* toxin before using antiperistaltic medications in the setting of recent antibiotic use. Potential infectious workup may include checking for fecal leukocytes, ova, and parasites and stool culture. For more persistent and severe diarrhea, agents that slow down peristalsis are more useful, including the following:
  - **Loperamide** (Imodium), 2 to 4 mg PO every 6 hours (maximum, 8 tablets/day)
  - **Diphenoxylate/atropine** (Lomotil), 2.5 to 5 mg PO every 6 hours (maximum, 8 tablets/day)
  - **Tincture of opium,** 0.7 mL PO every 4 hours and titrated as needed (Belladonna can be added as an antispasmodic agent.)
  - **Octreotide** (Dandostatin LAR Depot), 10 to 20 mg IM every 4 weeks
- For persistent, severe secretory diarrhea, the patient should be admitted for parenteral fluid support and the initiation of octreotide.
  - **Octreotide** (Sandostatin), 50 to 500 μg SC/IV every 8 to 12 hours. Begin at 50 μg SC/IV, then titrated up 100 μg per dose every 48 hours to a maximum of 500 μg SC every 8 hours, with titration based on response; may also be given as a continuous IV infusion, 10 to 80 μg/h.

NAUSEA AND VOMITING[5,6]

GENERAL PRINCIPLES

Nausea and vomiting are commonly associated with advanced malignancies as a direct result of the disease or as side effects of chemotherapy or other medications. There are multiple potential causes of nausea and vomiting in the cancer patient. Different etiologies for nausea and vomiting may require different interventions for control of the symptoms.

DIAGNOSIS

- The three most common forms of chemotherapy-associated nausea are **acute,** which begins within 1 to 2 hours of chemotherapy; **delayed,** which occurs 24 hours to 5 days after chemotherapy; and **anticipatory,** which is a conditioned response from prior occurrences of chemotherapy.
- A thorough assessment of nausea and vomiting is important to gain an understanding of potential etiologies and to allow for an appropriate choice of antiemetics. A common mnemonic for potential etiologies is the "11 M's of emesis": metastases, meningeal irritation, movement, mental (anxiety), medications, mucosal irritation, mechanical obstruction, motility, metabolic, microbes,

and myocardial (ischemia, congestive heart failure). Identification of the source of nausea and vomiting dictates treatment.

TREATMENT

- For **prevention of chemotherapy-associated acute nausea,** the three classes of drugs with the highest efficacy are corticosteroids (dexamethasone), 5-HT_3 receptor antagonists (dolasetron, granisetron, ondansetron, palonosetron), and the neurokinin-1 (NK1) receptor antagonist aprepitant (Emend). Treatment recommendations for acute nausea and vomiting are dependent of the emetogenic potential of the chemotherapy.
  - For low-emetogenic therapies, dexamethasone or metoclopramide (a dopamine antagonist) is used. For moderately emetogenic therapies, a 5-HT_3 is combined with dexamethasone.
  - For highly emetogenic chemotherapies, such as platinum-based regimens, aprepitant is combined with a 5-HT_3 and dexamethasone.
  - For delayed nausea, either single-agent dexamethasone or dexamethasone plus metoclopramide is recommended. If the combination treatment does not work, aprepitant should be considered.
  - Anticipatory emesis is a conditioned response from prior cycles of chemotherapy. Patients benefit from benzodiazepines and behavioral therapy (hypnosis, desensitization, relaxation, etc.). The best way to prevent anticipatory emesis is good control of acute and delayed emesis in prior cycles of chemotherapy.
- **Nausea and vomiting from a bowel obstruction** can be a challenge to treat, especially when surgery is not an option. **Octreotide** has been shown to effectively inhibit the secretion of fluid into the intestinal lumen and decrease bloating and abdominal pain, as well as nausea and vomiting. It may be started by continuous infusion or intermittent SC injection at a dose of 100 μg every 8 to 12 hours and titrated every 24 to 48 hours for effect.
- **Dopamine antagonists** are one of the most frequently used antiemetics. These medications have the potential to cause sedation and extrapyramidal symptoms. Medication options include the following.
  - Haloperidol (Haldol), PO, IV, SC
  - Prochlorperazine (Compazine), PO, PR, IV
  - Droperidol (Inapsine), IV
  - Promethazine (Phenergan), PO
  - Perphenazine (Trilafon), PO, IV
  - Trimethobenzamide (Tigan), PO, PR
  - Metoclopramide (Reglan), PO, IV
- **Histamine antagonists** may also cause sedation and can have a beneficial effect in some patients. The antihistamines also have the added benefit of anticholinergic properties, which can also be beneficial in patients with dual etiologies of nausea. These drugs include the following:
  - Diphenhydramine (Benadryl), PO, IV
  - Meclizine (Antivert), PO
  - Hydroxyzine (Atarax), PO, IV
- **Scopolamine** is an anticholinergic agent that is useful in treating nausea induced by the vestibular apparatus. It can also be used adjunctively with other antiemetics in empiric therapy. Scopolamine can be given as an IV or SC

scheduled or continuous infusion but is also conveniently available as a transdermal patch.

- **Serotonin antagonists** have been effective in the treatment of chemotherapy-associated nausea and vomiting. They are also useful for refractory nausea but are typically tried when other medications have failed. The medications available are as follows:
  - Ondansetron (Zofran), PO, IV
  - Granisetron (Kytril), PO, IV
  - Dolasetron (Anzemet), PO, IV
  - Palonosetron (Aloxi), IV
- The NK1 receptor antagonist **aprepitant** (Emend) has become first-line therapy on day 1 for highly emetogenic chemotherapies.
- The use of **dronabinol** (Marinol) and **benzodiazepines** is beneficial in some patients, but the mechanism of action remains unclear. Benzodiazepines (i.e., lorazepam [Ativan] at a 1-mg dose) often are useful in conjunction with other classes of antiemetics and may have a synergistic effect.

MUCOSITIS[5]

GENERAL PRINCIPLES

Mucositis refers to painful inflammation and ulceration of the oral mucosa. Mucositis can result from chemotherapy or radiation therapy. Chemotherapeutic agents that are associated commonly with mucositis include bleomycin, cytarabine, doxorubicin, melphalan, methotrexate, etoposide, and 5-FU. Radiation to the head and neck may also cause mucositis. Patient factors that can contribute to worsening symptoms include poor-fitting oral prostheses, periodontal disease, and overall poor oral hygiene. Patients should undergo repair of ill-fitting prostheses, tooth extraction, and repair of periodontal disease before the initiation of chemotherapy. In the event that repair cannot be done before chemotherapy, the physician should make a referral to an oral surgeon once the patient's peripheral blood counts have returned to baseline.

DIAGNOSIS

A **mucositis grading system** established by the National Cancer Institute allows the physician to assess mucositis severity in terms of both pain and the patient's ability to continue to eat or drink, graded on a scale from 0 to 4. A score of 0 is given when there is no evidence of mucositis. When a patient develops nonpainful erythema or ulcers, but is able to eat or drink, a score of 1 is given. A score of 2 is given when there are mildly to moderately painful erythema or ulcers, but the patient is still able to eat or drink without difficulty. This may require intermittent analgesia. Severe erythema, painful ulcers that cause interference with eating and drinking requiring constant analgesia, scores a 3. Finally, a score of 4 is given when the severity of symptoms requires parenteral analgesia and/or nutritional support.

TREATMENT

A standardized approach to the prevention and treatment of mucositis is essential to quality care in the oncology patient. The prophylactic measures usually used include

mouth rinses with sodium chloride, sodium bicarbonate, chlorhexidine (Peridex) or calcium phosphate (Caphosol). Regimens commonly used for the treatment of mucositis and the associated pain include a **local anesthetic** such as lidocaine, **magnesium-based antacids** (Maalox, Mylanta), **diphenhydramine** (Benadryl), and an **antifungal** such as nystatin (Mycostatin) or Mycelex. These agents are used either alone or at equal concentrations in a mouthwash. The patient can use the mouthwash up to five times per day for relief. In the treatment of severe mucositis, narcotics may need to be used in addition to the agents mentioned earlier.

ANOREXIA AND CACHEXIA[7]

GENERAL PRINCIPLES

Anorexia and cachexia frequently occur with advanced malignancies and are characterized by a loss of muscle mass and adipose tissue. The increased catabolism of cancer and the anorexia that accompanies it result in increased muscle protein breakdown and lipolysis. These symptoms typically represent progression of disease and are not reversible with parenteral or enteral nutrition. Anorexia and cachexia are significant causes of distress to the patient and their family members.

DIAGNOSIS

Weight loss of more than 5%, decreased appetite and deceased food intake are the hallmarks of cancer related anorexia and cachexia. The specific etiologies of these symptoms are not well understood. The clinician should always assess for other potential etiologies underlying the loss of appetite and weight such as dysphagia, odynophagia, infections, and side effects of medications.

TREATMENT

There are several approaches to the general management of anorexia and cachexia.

- Patients should be offered their favorite foods and nutritional supplements if the patients enjoy them. Any **dietary restrictions should be eliminated.** Portion sizes can be reduced, and food should be made to look appetizing. Foods that have potent odors should be avoided.
- There is a variety of pharmacologic approaches for improving appetite. **Corticosteroids** have an appetite-stimulating effect, as well as effects on the patient's mood and energy level. Dexamethasone (Decadron) at doses of ≤4 mg/d is recommended. Dexamethasone is preferred because of the relative lack of mineralocorticoid effects, but any steroid will be efficacious such as Prednisone 20 mg/d. Steroids are considered only for short-term treatment, as they lose their efficacy over days to weeks. If longer treatment is anticipated, **megestrol** (Megace) has also been shown to improve appetite in cancer patients. There is a large variation in the effective dose of megestrol between individual patients. One should begin with 200 mg PO every 6 to 8 hours and titrate up to 400 to 800 mg/d or Megace ES, 650 mg PO daily. The **cannabinoids,** such as dronabinol (Marinol), have been shown to promote weight gain in cancer patients.

- It should be understood that clinical studies have demonstrated no impact on overall survival or improvement in quality of life when anorexia and cachexia are pharmacologically managed. Thus, treatment of anorexia and weight loss is done primarily because anorexia is distressing to the patients and their families.

DYSPNEA[7]

GENERAL PRINCIPLES

Dyspnea can be one of the most frightening symptoms to patients and their family members. Some patients with severe tachypnea will not complain of dyspnea, while others who are not tachypneic report severe dyspnea. For the majority of patients, relief of dyspnea can be achieved with simple interventions.

DIAGNOSIS

Respiratory rate, oxygen saturation, and blood gas levels often do not correlate with the patient's subjective report. The clinician must accept the patient's self-report and try to identify and/or correct the underlying etiology of the symptom. In patients with known advanced disease, the burden of investigating the etiology of the dyspnea must be weighed against the limited potential benefit from therapeutic interventions.

TREATMENT

There are three widely used medical approaches for symptomatic breathlessness: supplemental oxygen, opioids, and anxiolytics.

- A therapeutic trial of **supplemental oxygen** may be beneficial; it has been suggested that there is a placebo effect in nonhypoxemic patients. In addition, the cool air moving across the patient's face from the supplemental oxygen can also have a calming effect and help to relieve the feelings of air hunger. Studies have reported that stimulation of the trigeminal nerve with oxygen can cause a central inhibitory effect and relieve dyspnea. A fan in the room can also help achieve this effect.
- **Opioids** can provide relief in dyspnea without any measurable effect on respiratory rate or blood gas measurements. The precise mechanism by which opioids exert this effect is not known. In an opioid-naïve patient, doses lower than those used to achieve analgesia may be effective. Doses of hydrocodone, 5 mg PO every 4 hours, or codeine, 30 mg PO every 2 hours, can be beneficial in these patients. Other opioids can be useful and administered IV for urgent situations or when the PO route is not available. Patients can be maintained on a fixed schedule of opioid IV every 4 to 6 hours. An additional dose of a short-acting opioid, equivalent to 25% to 50% of the amount of baseline opioid taken every 4 hours can be used hourly for intermittent periods of worsening dyspnea. Sublingual morphine can also be helpful in the terminal dyspneic patient.
- Dyspnea may cause severe anxiety. Some patients with dyspnea may need more effective treatment for their anxiety. **Benzodiazepines** can be used in addition to opioids and other nondrug therapies to reduce dyspnea. The clinician should begin with low doses and titrate for desired effects. Sublingual lorazepam has been shown to be quite effective if there is no IV access.

ANEMIA[8]

GENERAL PRINCIPLES

Anemia in cancer patients may be due to the effects of their underlying malignancy (particularly when there is bone marrow involvement) and/or treatment. The basic mechanisms involved are decreased erythropoiesis, impaired iron metabolism, and decreased survival time for RBCs. In addition, erythropoietin production may be impaired.

DIAGNOSIS

Diagnosis is made by CBC, with a hemoglobin and hematocrit that are less than normal.

TREATMENT

Current treatment approaches are aimed at treating the underlying malignancy and boosting red cell mass. Transfusions offer only transient effects and have side effects such as transfusion reactions, iron overload, volume overload, and cardiac congestion. It is recommended that transfusions be administered only to those patients who are suffering from symptoms of anemia with hemoglobin <8 g/dL. Recombinant **erythropoietin** has been shown to reduce transfusion requirements and improve outcomes in terms of quality of life and response to treatment. ESAs have also been associated with tumor growth and shorter overall survival. Strict guidelines for the use of ESAs of erythropoiesis-stimulating agents (ESAs) have been published by the FDA and can be viewed at http://www.fda.gov/Drugs/DrugSafety/PostmarketDrugSafety InformationforPatientsandProviders/ucm200297.htm. ESAs can now only be prescribed by registered users for cancer patients.

EMOTIONAL SYMPTOM MANAGEMENT[9]

GENERAL PRINCIPLES

Depression occurs in approximately half of cancer patients, though it is often underdiagnosed and undertreated. Specific problems facing these patients include pain, medication side effects, and changes in functional status.

DIAGNOSIS

Typical features of major depression may be present, such as depressed mood for at least 2 weeks, feelings of guilt or worthlessness, inability to concentrate, decreased energy, preoccupation with death or suicide, anhedonia, and changes in eating or sleeping habits. In the cancer patient, one must be aware that drugs such as prednisone, dexamethasone, procarbazine, vincristine, and vinblastine can also cause depression like symptoms. Loss of appetite, fatigue, or insomnia may be secondary to chemotherapy, the cancer itself, or pain, making it difficult to diagnose depression.

Excessive guilt, low self-esteem, the wish to die, and hopelessness are most diagnostic of depression in the cancer patient. One must be careful to screen for suicidal ideation, as the incidence of suicide is higher in both men and women with cancer.

TREATMENT

- Depression should be screened for and treated in all cancer patients. In addition to counseling by oncologic psychologists, medications can by useful in the treatment of depression.
- **Antidepressants** may require up to 6 weeks before symptoms are alleviated. The selective serotonin reuptake inhibitors (e.g., citalopram, 20 to 80 mg PO daily), bupropion SR (200 to 400 mg PO daily), and mirtazapine (usual dosage range, 30 to 45 mg PO daily; mirtazapine has sedating effects but may aid those with insomnia) are all reasonable first-line agents. Tricyclic antidepressants have the ability to treat depression and potentiate the effects of opioids on neuropathic pain. Imipramine, amitriptyline, and doxepin are started at 25 mg PO at bedtime, then titrated up 25 to 50 mg every 24 to 48 hours until the desired effect is achieved.
- The **psychostimulants** methylphenidate, dextroamphetamine, and modafinil are an alternative for depressed patients with cancer (e.g., methylphenidate, 5 mg PO at 9:00 a.m. and noon daily). They begin to work within a short period of time, provide relief from the sedating effects of opioids, and give the patient improved energy. Tolerance can develop to stimulants, and dosages may have to be adjusted over time.

ANXIETY[9]

DIAGNOSIS

The diagnosis and recognition of anxiety can be challenging. Patients often complain of physical and somatic manifestations of anxiety. The patient's subjective level of distress from fear, isolation, estrangement, or other common stressors is often the impetus for treatment.

TREATMENT

Anxiety is usually treated with benzodiazepines, neuroleptics, antihistamines, or nonpharmacologic psychotherapies. Benzodiazepines are first-line therapy for the treatment of anxiety disorders.

- Lorazepam, 0.5 to 2.0 mg PO, IV, or IM, every 3 to 6 hours
- Alprazolam, 0.25 to 1.0 mg PO, every 6 to 8 hours
- Diazepam, 2.5 to 10 mg PO, PR, IM, or IV every 3 to 6 hours
- Clonazepam, 1 to 2 mg PO, every 8 to 12 hours

Other anxiolytics include the following.

- Haloperidol (0.5 to 5 mg PO, IV, or SC every 2 to 12 hours), if there is concern about respiratory depression
- Thioridazine (10 to 25 mg PO tid), if insomnia and agitation are also present

- Hydroxyzine (25 to 50 mg every 4 to 6 hours PO, IV, or SC), which has mild anxiolytic, sedative, and analgesic properties
- Buspirone (10 mg PO tid), a nonbenzodiazepine anxiolytic that is useful in patients with chronic anxiety or anxiety related to adjustment disorders

Nonpharmacologic interventions for anxiety and distress include supportive psychotherapy and behavioral interventions used alone or in combination, relaxation, guided imagery, and hypnosis.

DELIRIUM[9]

GENERAL PRINCIPLES

Delirium is common in advanced cancer and is strongly associated with mortality. The differential diagnosis for delirium in the cancer patient includes dehydration, hypo- and hypernatremia, hypocalcemia, uremia, liver failure, drugs (opiates, radiation, chemotherapeutics, benzodiazepines, tricyclic antidepressants, etc.), brain metastases, paraneoplastic syndrome, and infection.

DIAGNOSIS

One must identify the underlying cause so that supportive therapies can be given. Many scales exist for the diagnosis of delirium, including the Mini Mental Status Exam and Memorial Delirium Assessment Scale, and these should be used to both diagnose and follow delirium.

TREATMENT

If supportive techniques do not work, treatment with neuroleptics or sedative medications can be tried.

- Haloperidol (Haldol), 0.5 to 1 mg every 1 to 2 hours PO, IV, or SC is the first drug of choice for treatment of delirium and is usually effective for agitation, paranoia, and fear.
- Zyprexa, 5 to 10 mg PO, sublingually, is another possible first-line agent, as it can be given under the tongue.
- Lorazepam, 0.5 to 1.0 mg PO or IV, plus haloperidol (but not lorazepam alone) can be tried next.
- Chlorpromazine can be used if no response to antipsychotics is observed within 24 to 48 hours, as it is much more sedating.

INSOMNIA[7]

DIAGNOSIS

Insomnia, or inability to sleep, is often a result of pain, medications, anxiety, or a mood disorder. Poor sleep can be distressing in the cancer patient, as it can make pain, anxiety, and delirium worse. Proper sleep hygiene and adequate management of pain and other symptoms are beneficial.

TREATMENT

Benzodiazepines (e.g., lorazepam, 0.5 to 2 mg PO qhs) or antidepressants with sedating effects (e.g., trazodone, 50 mg PO qhs, or amitriptyline, 25 to 50 mg PO qhs) may be used in conjunction with the nonpharmacologic measures. Newer agents such as Ambien/Ambien CR (5 to 10 mg/6.25 to 12.5 mg PO qpm), Lunesta (2 to 3 mg PO qpm), and Rozerem (8 mg PO qpm) can be tried. One should be careful when treating insomnia in terminally ill patients, as these can be hypnotic drugs. For some patients, improved cognition may be achieved by discontinuing the medications without an effect on insomnia.

ADDRESSING SPIRITUAL CARE[10]

- When a person has a malignancy, suffering occurs at many levels. Religion or spiritual belief can be a source of great strength or considerable pain to a patient. Some find new faith during a cancer experience, while others find great turmoil. Spiritual care for the oncology patient can be either uncomfortable for the physician or, if the physician is overzealous, uncomfortable for the patient. Many doctors and nurses are appropriately uneasy when it comes to talking about religion because they fear they might be imposing their religious beliefs on others. The role of the physician is to advocate and try to connect a patient with chaplains, the patient's own religious community, or nonreligious groups that might help to provide solace.
- The role of the **oncologic chaplain** can greatly aid in the spiritual journey of a patient, both as an inpatient and as an outpatient. Chaplains can help identify patients in spiritual distress and address the religious or spiritual issues raised by their illness. Those who have never had strong religious beliefs may not feel an urge to turn to religion, but as trained listeners, chaplains can help patients identify core beliefs, recognize coping skills, and, potentially, help patients to find sources of strength within or beyond themselves.
- Chaplains also help families identify spiritual resources to enhance their coping with the level of distress during a loved one's illness. Often, chaplains are privy to information that may not be provided to the medical professional. This can, with permission, be shared for the benefit of the patient and improvement of care. Therefore, it is appropriate to involve chaplaincy in a patient's care. It is not necessary to ask whether a patient would like a chaplain, as the patient may feel undue pressure based on distorted understandings of a professional chaplain's role. A trained chaplain showing up at the bedside can lead to positive outcomes, even if the patient is enabled to say, "No, thank you" to spiritual care. Chaplains work to help people in crisis find a measure of control in the midst of what can feel like chaos.

REFERENCES

1. National Comprehensive Cancer Network. Cancer pain treatment guidelines for patients. Version I, 2011. Adult cancer pain. In: National Comprehensive Cancer Network Practice Guidelines in Oncology, 2011:1. Last accessed: 2/14/2011 <http://www.nccn.org/professionals/physician_gls/pdf/pain.pdf>.
2. Pharo GH, Zhou L. Pharmacologic management of cancer pain. *J Am Osteopath Assoc.* 2005; 105(11 Suppl 5):S21–S28.

3. Levy MH. Drug therapy: pharmacologic treatment of cancer pain. *N Engl J Med.* 1996; 335:1124–1132.
4. Bonica JJ, Ventafridda V, Twycross RG. Cancer pain. In: Bonica JJ, ed. *The Management of Pain.* 2nd ed. Philadelphia: Lea & Febiger; 1990:400–460.
5. Ludwig H, Zojer N. Supportive care. *Ann Oncol.* 2007;18(Suppl 1):i37–i44.
6. National Comprehensive Cancer Network. Antiemesis. Version 3, June 2011. In: National Comprehensive Cancer Network Practice Guidelines in Oncology. Last accessed 2/14/2011 <http://www.nccn.org/professionals/physician_gls/pdf/antiemesis.pdf>.
7. National Comprehensive Cancer Network. Palliative Care. Version 3, June 2011. In: National Comprehensive Cancer Network Practice Guidelines in Oncology. Last accessed 4/03/2011 <http://www.nccn.org/professionals/physician_gls/pdf/palliative.pdf>.
8. National Comprehensive Cancer Network. Cancer- and Chemotherapy-Induced Anemia, Version 2, 2011. In: National Comprehensive Cancer Network Practice Guidelines in Oncology, 2011. Last accessed 4/03/2011 <http://guidelines.nccn.org/epc-guideline/guideline/id/EDDAC6A8-9CDE-B334-F2EB-B9C9062EB883?jumpTo=false#;history=1_EDDAC6A8-9CDE-B334-F2EB-B9C9062EB883_empty_-1>.
9. National Comprehensive Cancer Network. Distress Management. Version I, 2011. Adult cancer pain. In: National Comprehensive Cancer Network Practice Guidelines in Oncology, 2011:1. Last accessed 4/3/2011 <http://www.nccn.org/professionals/physician_gls/pdf/distress.pdf>.
10. Berger J. Identifying spiritual landscapes among oncology patients. *Chaplaincy Today.* 1998; 4(2):15–21.

Oncologic Emergencies

35

Michael Ansstas

INTRODUCTION

- True oncologic emergencies are relatively infrequent. However, physicians who treat cancer patients are often called on to rule out an oncologic emergency. To diagnose and appropriately treat an oncologic emergency, physicians must have a working knowledge of the distinct presentation, appropriate diagnostic testing, and management of a wide array of complications that are often unique to cancer patients. These complications primarily result from pressure or obstruction by space-occupying lesions, metabolic abnormalities, or cytopenias.

MALIGNANT PERICARDIAL EFFUSION AND TAMPONADE

GENERAL PRINCIPLES

- Malignancy is a frequent cause of pericardial disease including pericardial effusion, cardiac tamponade, and constrictive pericarditis. An autopsy series of 3314 patients found that cardiac metastases occur in 10% of patients dying of cancer.[1] However, many of these cases were not clinically significant. Malignant pericardial disease is generally a manifestation of an advanced malignancy.
- The most common malignancies associated with pericardial involvement are lung cancer, breast cancer, and lymphoma.

Pathophysiology

- Breast and lung tumors generally spread locally to cause pericardial disease. Lymphomas involving the mediastinum can involve the pericardium, whereas leukemias can infiltrate the myocardium, resulting in a pericardial effusion. Tumors in the pericardial space can cause bleeding and create a more rapidly accumulating effusion than in an exudative or transudative process. Patients with acute promyelocytic leukemia treated with all-trans retinoic acid can develop a treatment-related pericardial effusion.

DIAGNOSIS

Clinical Presentation

- Patients with small, slowly expanding effusions may present with subtle nonspecific complaints such as weakness, fatigue, and dyspnea. If a large effusion accumulates rapidly, patients can develop cardiac tamponade and hemodynamic collapse.

- On evaluation, patients with **tamponade** exhibit signs of hypotension, tachycardia, jugular venous distention, and dulled heart tones. Another sign indicative of tamponade is pulsus paradoxus. The difference in systolic pressures at which the Korotkoff sounds are heard between inspiration and expiration quantifies the pulsus paradoxus, which is normally no more than 10 mm Hg. Classically, Ewart's sign (dullness at the left infrascapular area due to bronchial compression by a large effusion) may be seen, but it is rarely observed in practice.[2]

Differential Diagnosis

- The differential diagnosis of pericardial disease in a patient with malignancy also includes nonmalignant causes, such as radiation-induced effusion, hypothyroidism, autoimmune disorders, infection, drug induced, uremia, and idiopathic pericardial disease.
- Other pathologic entities may present with similar symptoms in the cancer patient.
  - Cardiotoxicity leading to **congestive heart failure** can result from chemotherapy (such as anthracyclines, mitoxantrone, ifosfamide, and cyclophosphamide) or biologics (such as the monoclonal antibody trastuzumab). 5-Fluorouracil (5-FU), a commonly used antimetabolite, is associated with acute cardiotoxicity that can lead to cardiac arrhythmia, myocardial ischemia, and, rarely, cardiogenic shock. Radiation therapy can also cause cardiomyopathy in the absence of pericardial disease (especially in the setting of mediastinal radiation for non-Hodgkin or Hodgkin lymphoma and left breast radiation for breast cancer). One must always consider other causes of cardiovascular emergencies in the cancer patient, such as coronary artery disease, heart failure, and infectious endocarditis.

Diagnostic Testing

Patients with suspected pericardial disease should have an immediate chest radiograph and electrocardiogram (ECG).

- On **chest x-ray**, in the presence of a large effusion, the cardiac silhouette is enlarged in a globular, symmetric fashion. Chest x-ray may also reveal signs of pulmonary congestion and/or pleural effusions.
- **ECG** commonly shows sinus tachycardia and may reveal reduced voltage or, with very large effusions, electrical alternans.
- **Transthoracic echocardiography** is the diagnostic test of choice and should be ordered emergently whenever the diagnosis of tamponade is suspected. It will diagnose the effusion and indicate the degree of hemodynamic compromise. Early signs of tamponade on echo include right atrial and ventricular collapse.
- **CT scan** is also sensitive for diagnosing an effusion. It can detect as little as 50 mL of pericardial fluid and, similar to an echocardiogram, can give an idea of intracardiac masses.
- **MRI** also can provide direct imaging of the pericardium. Both of these tests can give some clues as to the nature of the fluid (bloody, serous, chylous), but they rarely provide clinically useful information.

TREATMENT

- With severe hemodynamic compromise, emergent **pericardiocentesis** by a percutaneous, subxiphoid approach should be performed. Giving a **rapid IV fluid bolus and inotropics** can be temporizing measures to support the patient until echocardiographic guidance is available.
- Complications with "blind" approach include ventricular perforation, arrhythmias, and pneumothoraxes, and range from 5% to 20%. Complications are less likely (about 2%) when echocardiography is used to delineate the size and location of the fluid with respect to normal cardiac structures.[3]
- A pericardial drain or a pericardial window may be necessary. To prevent recurrence, sclerosing agents such as thiotepa are available but are often less effective and have more risks than placing a **surgical pericardial window.** A surgical pericardial window is generally the definitive treatment for a clinically significant pericardial effusion.
- Radiation therapy can be used to manage pericardial effusions secondary to radiosensitive tumors, such as leukemia and lymphoma. Small asymptomatic effusions may be observed without therapy.

SUPERIOR VENA CAVA SYNDROME

GENERAL PRINCIPLES

Definition

Superior vena cava syndrome (SVCS) is the result of **obstruction of the** SVC, by either external compression or internal thrombosis.

Etiology

- **Lung cancer (non-small-cell lung cancer followed by small-cell lung cancer)** and **lymphoma** are the most common causes (~85%), although SVCS has been reported in breast cancer and other malignancies of the chest as well.[4] These less common malignancies of the chest include germ cell tumors, thymoma, and mesothelioma.
- **Thrombosis of the** SVC in patients with central venous catheters is an increasingly common cause of SVCS. Other nonmalignant causes of SVCS include granulomatous infections, goiter, aortic aneurysms, and fibrosing mediastinitis.

DIAGNOSIS

Clinical Presentation

- Patients typically present with swelling of the neck, face, and upper extremities. Jugular venous distention, cyanosis, and facial plethora may also be present.
- Shortness of breath, dizziness, and rarely obtundation from cerebral edema are possible if the onset is rapid. Very rarely, the process causes laryngeal edema and compromise of the upper airway.
- Vocal cord paralysis and Horner syndrome are also possible if neural structures are invaded. With slowly progressive obstruction, collateral flow has time to develop, and symptoms related to vascular obstruction may be subtle.

Diagnostic Testing

- **Chest radiography** may show a widened superior mediastinum and pleural effusions.
- **CT scan** of the chest with IV contrast is the diagnostic test of choice. CT findings are notable for reduced or absent opacification of central venous structures with prominent collateral venous circulation. There is no advantage of MRI over CT.
- A diagnosis of the mass should be attempted before treatment is begun if the tissue type of tumor is unknown. Sputum cytology, biopsy of lymph nodes, bronchoscopy, thoracentesis (if a pleural effusion is present), mediastinoscopy, or thoracotomy can be diagnostic. The workup generally progresses first through less invasive diagnostic testing (e.g., sputum cytology) before more invasive tests are performed (e.g., mediastinoscopy).

TREATMENT

- Supportive measures including a low-salt diet, head elevation, and oxygen can be temporizing.
- **Diuretics** and **corticosteroids** (e.g., dexamethasone, 4 mg IV every 6 hours) have traditionally been used for treatment at presentation. Although corticosteroids are likely only helpful in SVCS caused by lymphoma, diuretics have not been shown to be helpful at all. If compression is not life-threatening, then a tissue diagnosis should be made before beginning treatment.
- **Radiation therapy** is useful for non-small-cell lung carcinoma and other metastatic solid tumors.[5]
- **Chemotherapy** is more useful in small-cell lung cancer and lymphoma owing to their exquisite chemosensitivity, but small trials suggest that chemotherapy may be as effective as radiation therapy in treating SVCS secondary to non-small-cell lung cancer, which is relatively chemoinsensitive.
- SVCS resulting from catheter-related thrombus is treated by anticoagulation and, in limited cases, fibrinolysis. For emergent cases in which a prompt response is needed, experienced centers can perform angioplasty and stent placement. These approaches have largely replaced open surgical intervention, which is now generally done only when the surgical resection of the tumor is of benefit.

PROGNOSIS

Multiple studies suggest that patients with SVCS do not have shortened survival compared to similarly staged patients with the same underlying malignancy and no history of SVCS.

ACUTE TUMOR LYSIS SYNDROME

GENERAL PRINCIPLES

- Acute tumor lysis syndrome (ATLS) represents a myriad of metabolic and electrolyte abnormalities that results from the release of intracellular products by rapidly dividing tumor cells prior to therapy or from the **lysis** of sensitive tumor cells **during therapy**. ATLS usually occurs in the setting of therapy of rapidly

TABLE 35-1 RISK FACTORS FOR TUMOR LYSIS SYNDROME

Patients at risk for acute tumor lysis syndrome

Tumor type
- High-grade non-Hodgkin lymphoma (for example: Burkitt lymphoma)
- Acute leukemia (AML or ALL)
- Rapidly-growing solid tumors (small cell lung cancer)

Extent of disease
- Bulky tumors
- Elevated lactate dehydrogenase
- Elevated WBC count

Underlying renal dysfunction/oliguria

Elevated pretreatment uric acid

Adapted from DeVita VT, Rosenberg SA, Hellman S, eds. *Cancer: Principles and Practice of Oncology.* 7th ed. Philadelphia: Lippincott, Williams & Wilkins; 2005:2292–2294.

growing, hematologic malignancies, classically acute lymphoblastic leukemia and high-grade non-Hodgkin lymphoma (e.g., Burkitt lymphoma). Rarely, ATLS has been described after the treatment of solid tumors such as breast cancer. The size of the tumor, rate of tumor growth, and sensitivity of the tumor cells to chemotherapy determine the risk of development of ATLS (Table 35-1).

DIAGNOSIS

Clinical Presentation

ATLS is characterized by the following **electrolyte derangements:** hyperuricemia, hyperkalemia, hyperphosphatemia, and hypocalcemia. These electrolyte abnormalities place patients at risk for cardiac arrhythmias and seizures. Acute renal failure and uremia can develop from precipitation of uric acid and calcium phosphate crystals in the renal tubules (Table 35-2).

TABLE 35-2 CAIRO–BISHOP DEFINITION OF ACUTE TUMOR LYSIS SYNDROME

Laboratory tumor lysis syndrome
- Uric acid >8 mg/dL or 25% increase from baseline
- Potassium >6 mEq/L or 25% increase from baseline
- Phosphorus >4.49 mg/dL or 25% increase from baseline
- Calcium <7 mg/dL or 25% decrease from baseline

Clinical tumor lysis syndrome
- Creatinine >1.5 times the upper limit of normal (adjusted for age)
- Cardiac arrhythmia or sudden death
- Seizure

Adapted from Cairo MS, Bishop M. Tumour lysis syndrome: new therapeutic strategies and classification. *Br J Haematol.* 2004;127:3–11.

TREATMENT

The best management of ATLS includes identifying patients at risk for ATLS and taking preventive measures.

- **IV hydration** should occur 24 to 48 hours before initiation of chemotherapy (3 $L/m^2/d$) and during therapy. Consider using IV furosemide (Lasix) to improve urine flow rate if it is $<$100 $mL/m^2/d$. Electrolytes including phosphorus, calcium, and magnesium; uric acid; blood urea nitrogen; and creatinine should be measured three times a day in patients at risk for ATLS.
- **Hyperkalemia** should be treated with standard therapy: glucose and insulin (acutely), sodium–potassium exchange resins (Kayexalate), and IV calcium if ECG changes are noted.
- **Hyperuricemia** can be controlled with allopurinol (maximum 800 mg/d PO or 600 mg/d IV in adults) and/or rasburicase. Uric acid is relatively insoluble and can precipitate in renal tubules, causing acute renal failure. Allopurinol decreases the production of uric acid by inhibiting the enzyme, xanthine oxidase, which converts xanthine and hypoxanthine to uric acid. Allopurinol must be dose-reduced in patients with renal failure. Also, allopurinol inhibits the degradation of 6-mercaptopurine and azathioprine so these drugs must be dose-reduced if the patient is taking allopurinol. Allopurinol does not decrease the amount of uric acid already present. Thus, **one must initiate allopurinol before chemotherapy in patients with preexisting hyperuricemia or in those at high risk for ATLS.**
- **Rasburicase** is a recombinant form of the enzyme, urate oxidase, which is derived from yeast and not found in humans. Urate oxidase breaks down uric acid to form allantoin. Allantoin is much more soluble in the urine than uric acid and can thus be renally excreted. Rasburicase is **contraindicated in patients with glucose-6-phosphate dehydrogenase deficiency,** as it can cause hemolysis. Other side effects of rasburicase include methemoglobinemia, bronchospasm, and anaphylaxis. The dosing of rasburicase is still not defined, but many institutions use 0.15 to 0.2 mg/kg for one dose and repeat doses only if hyperuricemia is still present.[6] Rasburicase has not yet been rigorously tested in randomized, controlled trials in adults; however, case reports and pediatric data have demonstrated its efficacy. Rasburicase is now generally the standard of care for pediatric and adult patients with ATLS, while allopurinol remains the standard prophylactic therapy.
- **Alkalinization of the urine** to increase uric acid excretion can also be considered in the treatment of hyperuricemia. However, there is no clear evidence that it improves outcomes.
- **IV calcium should not be administered for hypocalcemia unless the patient is symptomatic or hyperphosphatemia is corrected.** Symptoms of hypocalcemia include muscular (cramps, spasms, and tetany), cardiac (arrhythmias and hypotension), and neurologic (confusion or seizures) abnormalities. A positive Chvostek or Trousseau sign is indicative of symptomatic hypokalemia. With a high serum phosphate level, IV calcium repletion may result in metastatic calcification and renal failure.
- In the setting of **hyperphosphatemia,** mild cases may be managed with PO antacids (phosphate binders), but **dialysis** may be necessary in patients with poor renal function or metabolic abnormalities not corrected by conservative measures.

HYPERCALCEMIA OF MALIGNANCY

GENERAL PRINCIPLES

Hypercalcemia is the most common paraneoplastic syndrome, seen in 10% to 20% of patients with cancer. Malignancies of the lung, breast, head/neck, and kidney, as well as multiple myeloma, are most often associated with hypercalcemia.[7]

Etiology

Most commonly, a tumor causes hypercalcemia by producing ectopic parathormone-related protein (PTHrP), which stimulates osteoclasts to cause bone resorption as well as causing renal tubular calcium retention. Less commonly, tumor in bone can have a direct osteolytic activity through local cytokines. Rarely, lymphomas can produce ectopic activated vitamin D to cause hypercalcemia.

DIAGNOSIS

Clinical Presentation

Presentation is often nonspecific. Common symptoms include fatigue, anorexia, constipation, polydipsia, polyuria, nausea, vomiting, lethargy, and apathy. Nephrolithiasis is possible. In severe cases, mental status alterations, seizures, and coma can be seen. Hypercalcemia can cause renal parenchymal damage and nephrogenic diabetes insipidus. Hypercalcemia produces a brisk diuresis, and patients are often severely volume depleted. Most clinicians will remember the symptoms of hypercalcemia from the mnemonic: "stones, bones, abdominal groans, and psychic moans."

Diagnostic Testing

Management includes obtaining an **ionized calcium level** (or an albumin level to correct for the hypoalbuminemia that is frequently seen in cancer patients). Serum **intact parathormone (PTH) levels** should be checked to rule out primary hyperparathyroidism. Intact PTH levels are suppressed in the hypercalcemia of malignancy. There is generally no need to check a PTHrP, as the diagnosis of malignant hypercalcemia is often made by history alone. Other causes of hypercalcemia such as thiazide diuretics, granulomatous disease, and vitamin D intoxication can also be ruled out by history alone. A **serum phosphate level** must be checked, as hypercalcemia often leads to clinically significant hypophosphatemia.

TREATMENT

- The acute treatment of hypercalcemia begins with **IV fluids** (4 to 8 L). Normal saline is started at 200 to 500 mL/h and decreased after the volume deficit is corrected. At least 3 to 4 L should be given in the first 24 hours, and a positive fluid balance of at least 2 L should be achieved. Further saline diuresis (100 to 200 mL/h) will aid in calcium excretion. Serum electrolytes, including potassium, phosphate and magnesium, should be measured every 6 to 12 hours and corrected accordingly. Oral phosphate repletion is standard if the serum phosphate level is low and the patient has normal renal function. With IV phosphate repletion, there is the risk of calcium phosphate precipitation and renal failure. Its use should be reserved for serious cases of hypophosphatemia managed by experienced physicians. **Furosemide** can lead to greater calcium loss through the urine; however, its use is **contraindicated until the patient is euvolemic,** and it is generally not necessary.

- Other than IV fluids, the mainstay of the treatment of hypercalcemia is a **bisphosphonate.** Two bisphosphonates are FDA approved for the treatment of hypercalcemia of malignancy: **pamidronate** (Aredia; 60 to 90 mg IV over 2 hours) and **zoledronic acid** (Zometa; 4 mg IV over 15 minutes).
  - Bisphosphonates work by inhibiting bone resorption by osteoclasts.
  - Side effects include flulike symptoms and fever, as well as renal failure (rarely). These drugs must be used with extreme caution in patients with underlying renal insufficiency and generally avoided in patients with significant renal impairment (creatinine clearance, <30 mL/min). Also, the dose of bisphosphonates will often need to be reduced in patients with renal insufficiency. Rarely, patients treated with bisphosphonates develop osteonecrosis of the jaw. The onset of action of the bisphosphonates is at between 2 and 4 days, with the peak effect generally between day 4 and day 7.
- **Salmon calcitonin** (4 international units/kg) is usually administered intramuscularly or subcutaneously every 12 hours; doses can be increased up to 6 to 8 IU/kg every 6 hours. Nasal application of calcitonin is not efficacious for treatment of hypercalcemia. Calcitonin is safe and relatively nontoxic. It lowers the serum calcium concentration by a maximum of 1 to 2 mg/dL beginning within 4 to 6 hours. Thus, it is useful in combination with hydration for the initial management of severe hypercalcemia. The **efficacy of calcitonin is limited to the first 48 hours,** even with repeated doses, indicating the development of tachyphylaxis, perhaps due to receptor downregulation. Because of its limited duration of effect, calcitonin is most beneficial in symptomatic patients with calcium >14 mg/L, when combined with hydration and bisphosphonates. Calcitonin and hydration provide a rapid reduction in serum calcium concentration, while a bisphosphonate provides a more sustained effect.
- **Glucocorticoids** (e.g., prednisone at an initial dose of 0.5 to 1 mg/kg/d) may be effective in hypercalcemia due to some hematologic malignancies and myeloma. Results may take up to 10 days and side effects from steroid treatment are common. In addition, dialysis is effective if other treatments fail. Other drugs that are rarely used (now mostly in hypercalcemia refractory to bisphosphonates) include calcitonin, gallium nitrate, and plicamycin (mithramycin). Of course, the definitive treatment of hypercalcemia is successful treatment of the underlying malignancy.

SYNDROME OF INAPPROPRIATE ANTIDIURESIS AND HYPONATREMIA

GENERAL PRINCIPLES

The syndrome of inappropriate antidiuresis (SIAD) was formerly known as the syndrome of inappropriate secretion of antidiuretic hormone (SIADH). It is now recognized that antidiuretic hormone (ADH)/vasopressin levels are commonly suppressed in patients with the syndrome, but affected patients have their homeostatic set-point for sodium set at a lower level than normal. SIAD is seen most commonly in small-cell lung cancer but can also be seen in many other malignancies including tumors of the upper gastrointestinal and genitourinary tract.

Etiology

In addition to SIAD directly related to the malignancy, drugs can also cause the inappropriate release of vasopressin or attenuate its action. Common drugs that can cause SIAD include morphine, vincristine sulfate, and cyclophosphamide. Pulmonary and central nervous system disease can also cause SIAD that is not related to an underlying malignancy.

DIAGNOSIS

Clinical Presentation

Patients with SIAD and hyponatremia may present with complaints of anorexia and nausea. With rapid and severe decline in serum sodium concentrations, they may also present with confusion, coma, and seizures. Look for **decreased serum osmolality** (<270 mOsm/L) and **urine that is not maximally dilute** (>100 mOsm/L). In addition to the previously mentioned findings, the diagnosis of SIAD requires the **absence of a hypervolemic state** (manifest by ascites, edema) and **absence of volume contraction,** along with **normal thyroid, renal, and adrenal function.**

TREATMENT

- **Acute management** includes IV normal saline or, in more severe cases, 3% sodium chloride (which should typically *only* be given with the assistance of someone skilled in its use, such as a nephrologist). Allow only 1 to 2 mEq/L/h of correction for the first 3 to 4 hours and ≤0.5 mEq/L/h thereafter to avoid *demyelination* syndromes (use even lower rates of correction for patients with **chronic hyponatremia** or hyponatremia of unknown duration—generally 0.5 to 1 mEq/L/h). To avoid potentially catastrophic demyelination, the overall rate of correction is limited to 8 to 10 mEq/L at 24 hours and less than 18 mEq at 48 hours.[8] **Furosemide** may add to free water loss when given with saline. **Demeclocycline** is an antibiotic that lowers urine osmolality and can be useful in long-term therapy, but renal toxicity limits its use.
- **Vasopressin-receptor antagonists** are a new option for the treatment of SIAD. The vasopressin receptor antagonists produce a selective water diuresis without affecting sodium and potassium excretion. Intravenous **conivaptan** (which is used in hospitalized patients) and oral tolvaptan are available and approved for use in patients with hyponatremia due to SIADH. The utility of **tolvaptan** therapy is limited by excessive thirst, prohibitive cost (at least in the United States), and the potential for overly rapid correction of the hyponatremia which has led to the necessity for hospitalization for the initiation of therapy.[9]

NEUTROPENIC FEVER

GENERAL PRINCIPLES

Neutropenic fever is one of the most common complications of chemotherapy. Risk of infection is slightly increased with granulocyte counts <1000/μL, markedly increased with granulocytes <500/μL, and highest with granulocyte counts

<100/μL. Eighty percent of infections in the neutropenic patient originate from the patient's own flora. As many neutropenic patients also have long-term vascular access in place, these are common sources as well. Likely microbes include both gram-positive (*Staphylococcus, Streptococcus*) and gram-negative aerobes (*Escherichia coli, Klebsiella pneumonia, Pseudomonas aeruginosa*).

Definition

Neutropenic fever is defined as a single **temperature** >**38.3°C** (or a temperature >38.0°C for >1 hour) in patients with an **absolute neutrophil count** <**500/μL** (or <1000/μL that is expected to decrease to <500/μL).

DIAGNOSIS

Clinical Presentation

Signs of infection, such as exudate, erythema, and warmth, may not be evident because of the reduced numbers of neutrophils. Pneumonias may only be evident by rales, as an infiltrate on chest x-ray may be lacking. Physical examination should focus on the skin, ocular fundus, sinuses, CNS, pelvis, and perirectal area.

Diagnostic Testing

Management includes **searching for a source of infection** by obtaining two sets of **blood cultures,** with one set from any indwelling intravascular catheter. **Sputum and urine cultures** are indicated, and **chest x-ray** should also be obtained. If diarrhea is present, a workup for infectious etiologies is indicated including stool culture and *Clostridium difficile* antigen testing. **Lumbar puncture is not indicated unless clinical signs of meningitis are present,** as neutropenia does not predispose to meningitis. In addition, lumbar puncture in the setting of thrombocytopenia can be dangerous.

TREATMENT

Medications

- **Antimicrobial therapy. Antimicrobial therapy SHOULD NOT wait the results of diagnostic tests,** as patients can die of gram-negative sepsis in a matter of hours after their first fever, despite appearing well at initial presentation.[10]
- **Empiric antimicrobial therapy in neutropenic fever**
    - Initial therapy is antipseudomonal beta-lactam ± aminoglycoside. A single agent such as cefepime (2 g IV every 8 hours in patients with normal renal function) may be used, depending on local sensitivities.
    - If the patient is still febrile after 3 days of treatment: add vancomycin (1 g IV every 12 hours in normal renal function or adjusted based on trough levels).
    - If the patient is still febrile after 5 to 7 days, antifungal coverage should be added. Caspofungin, Micafungin, voriconazole, and posaconazole are reasonable choices, depending on the clinical circumstances. Treatment with amphotericin B is usually limited to refractory infections or critically ill patients who have not responded to the above agents.

- The above are only general guidelines. If the patient is penicillin allergic, consider substituting a fourth-generation fluoroquinolone or aztreonam. If contraindications to aminoglycosides are present, substitute a fluoroquinolone or aztreonam. One should consider using vancomycin or linezolid as initial therapy in addition to the previously mentioned antibiotics if the patient is hypotensive, has severe mucositis, is colonized with methicillin-resistant *Staphylococcus aureus,* recent quinolone prophylaxis or has signs of obvious catheter infection.
- Antibacterial choice may vary depending on organisms and resistance patterns at particular hospitals or communities. Always consider other causes of fever in the febrile neutropenic, such as thrombosis.
- Antimicrobials should be continued until the neutrophil count rises above $500/mm^3$ for 2 days and the patient has been afebrile without evidence of infection for the same duration.
- The role of colony-stimulating factors in neutropenic fever is controversial, but administration should be considered in critically ill patients.

Other Non-Pharmacologic Therapies

- Other precautions, such as visitor screening, hand washing, and proper isolation measures, should be maintained during this period.

EPIDURAL SPINAL CORD COMPRESSION

GENERAL PRINCIPLES

Epidural spinal cord compression (ESCC), occurring in 5% of cancer patients, is one of the most common oncologic emergencies. The dural sac is compressed by tumor in the epidural space at the level of the spinal cord or cauda equine; neurologic deficits may result. ***If ESCC is caught early, when pain is the only symptom, the patient can be spared significant disability.***

Etiology

Any malignancy can produce epidural compression, with lung, breast, and prostate cancers being the most common, followed by lymphoma, myeloma, and sarcoma. The thoracic spine is the most common location, followed by the lumbosacral and then the cervical spine. Osteolytic lesions of the vertebral column cause most cases. Compression occurs either by direct extension from metastases in the vertebral bone or by tumor growth through the intervertebral foramina. On occasion, tumor can metastasize directly to the epidural space.

DIAGNOSIS

Clinical Presentation

- **Back pain** is the first symptom in 90% of patients. The pain localizes in the back, near the midline, and is frequently accompanied by referred or radicular pain. The pain, unlike the pain of a herniated disc, may be exacerbated by recumbency and improved by the upright position. Many patients are unaware that back pain is related to their underlying malignancy and do not seek treatment.

- **Weakness and sensory impairment** may follow from hours to months after the onset of pain. Regardless of the spinal compression site, weakness tends to begin in the proximal legs. The weakness can progress to **paraplegia** and occasionally develops abruptly without prior clinical signs. At presentation, about 80% of patients complain of weakness, usually affecting gait. About 50% of patients have sensory complaints at presentation. These complaints range from paresthesias to loss of sensation.
- **Autonomic dysfunction,** including impotence and bowel/bladder dysfunction, occurs late and is generally not the sole presenting symptom.

Diagnostic Testing

- **Whole-spine MRI is the diagnostic test of choice** for ESCC. **The entire spine should be imaged because of the high incidence of asymptomatic multilevel disease.**
- **CT myelography** is necessary for patients with contraindications for MRI. In published studies, CT myelography is as accurate as MRI, but MRI is noninvasive, safer, and better tolerated. One must also consider other causes of spinal cord dysfunction, such as myelopathy, intramedullary metastases, hematoma, and abscess.
- Lumbar puncture to search for additional causes should not be performed until spinal cord compression is excluded.

TREATMENT

- **Dexamethasone** is the indicated medical treatment of nearly all patients with ESCC. Treatment should begin immediately after the diagnosis is suspected and not be delayed until the results of imaging studies are available. The dose is controversial, but a common regimen is a 10-mg IV bolus followed by 4 mg IV every 6 hours (although this regimen is not supported by published evidence).
- Next, all patients should have an immediate **neurosurgical consultation.** Patchell and colleagues (2005) published a pivotal randomized study showing that initial operative treatment benefits a subgroup of patients with ESCC.[11] The general indications for surgery include spinal instability with bony compression, neurologic progression during or after radiation therapy, unknown primary site with surgical decompression and biopsy, and a single site of cord compression. The exclusion criteria of the published study were patients with paraplegia for >48 hours prior to study entry, multiple compressive lesions, preexisting neurologic conditions including brain metastases, and radiosensitive tumors (lymphoma, leukemia, multiple myeloma, and germ cell tumors).
- **Radiation therapy** is also indicated in nearly all patients with ESCC, either in lieu of surgery or after surgery. The most common regimen is 10 uninterrupted fractions of 3 Gy each.

OTHER NEUROLOGIC EMERGENCIES

- **Increased intracerebral pressure and cerebral herniation** (from brain metastases, hemorrhage, venous sinus thrombosis, meningitis, head trauma, infarction, or abscess). Again, immediate consultation with neurosurgery is often essential. The patient should be stabilized, and maneuvers to lower intracranial pressures such as hyperventilation and IV mannitol and/or dexamethasone should be attempted. A head CT scan can aid in determining whether surgery is indicated.

- **Status epilepticus** (from brain metastases, metabolic derangement, or neurotoxicity of cancer therapy). Ensuring an airway should be the first and foremost concern. Laboratory studies such as glucose, electrolytes, Ca, Mg, serum and urine toxicology screens, serum alcohol level, CBC, urinalysis, and any pertinent medication levels must be obtained. IV benzodiazepines, phenytoin, and barbiturates are used in the treatment of status epilepticus. If the patient does not have IV access, benzodiazepines are also available in rectal, IM, or intranasal formulations.
- **Intracerebral hemorrhage** (from metastatic tumor, thrombocytopenia, or leukostasis). Headache, vomiting, and mental status changes are symptoms of significantly increased intracranial pressure and hemorrhage. Workup should include imaging with a STAT noncontrast head CT scan and possibly a lumbar puncture (if CT is nondiagnostic). Therapy largely focuses on maintenance of adequate blood pressure, supportive care, correction of coagulopathy and thrombocytopenia, and surgical consultation when appropriate.

PATHOLOGIC FRACTURES

GENERAL PRINCIPLES

- Pathologic fractures are defined as fractures occurring in diseased bone.
- Breast, prostate, kidney, and lung are the most common carcinomas to metastasize to bone and potentially cause fracture. The majority of patients have multiple metastatic lesions.

DIAGNOSIS

Clinical Presentation

Symptoms include **new-onset bone pain** in patients with a history of a primary carcinoma.

TREATMENT

- In the management of the pathologic fracture, consider life expectancy, as **most fractures are best treated surgically** with internal fixation. IV narcotics and fracture immobilization are used to control pain and bleeding. Consultation with orthopedics is necessary. Hip and femur fractures will require traction, whereas casts or splints may be used for distal fractures. Radiographs of the region in at least two planes are needed. A bone scan may be obtained to locate occult lesions. Radiographs of involved bones may identify other areas of impending fracture. Both the pathologic fracture and impending fractures could thus be repaired during one surgery.
- **Bisphosphonates** have an expanding role in the prevention of further pathologic fracture, and treatment with pamidronate or zoledronic acid should be considered in patients with pathologic fracture.
- **Consultation with radiation oncology** is indicated to determine whether the patient could benefit from radiation therapy as well.

REFERENCES

1. Abraham KP, Reddy V, Gattuso P. Neoplasms metastatic to the heart: review of 3314 consecutive autopsies. *Am J Cardiovasc Pathol.* 1990;3:195–198.
2. Ewart W. Practical aids in the diagnosis of pericardial effusion, in connection with the question as to surgical treatment. *Br Med J.* 1896;1:717–721.
3. Hall JB, Schmidt GA, Wood LD, et al, eds. *Principles of Critical Care.* New York: McGraw Hill; 1997:1405–1410.
4. Wilson LD, Detterbeck FC, Yahalom J. Superior vena cava syndrome with malignant causes. *N Engl J Med.* 2007;356:1862–1869.
5. Escalante CP. Causes and management of superior vena cava syndrome. *Oncology.* 1993;7:61–68.
6. Pui CH, Mahmoud HH, Wiley JM, et al. Recombinant urate oxidase for the prophylaxis or treatment of hyperuricemia in patients with leukemia or lymphoma. *J Clin Oncol.* 2001;19:697–704.
7. Stewart AF. Hypercalcemia associated with cancer. *N Engl J Med.* 2005;352:373–379.
8. Ellison DH, Berl T. The syndrome of inappropriate antidiuresis. *N Engl J Med.* 2007; 356:2064–2072.
9. Schrier RW, Gross P, Gheorghiade M, et al. Tolvaptan, a selective oral vasopressin V_2 receptor antagonist, for hyponatremia. *N Engl J Med.* 2006;355:2099–2112.
10. Hughes WT, Armstrong D, Bodey GP, et al. Guidelines for the use of antimicrobial agents in neutropenic patients with cancer. *Clin Infect Dis.* 2002;34:730–751.
11. Patchell RA, Tibbs PA, Regine WF, et al. Direct decompressive surgical resection in the treatment of spinal cord compression caused by metastatic cancer: a randomized trial. *Lancet.* 2005;366:643–648.

Index

Page numbers followed by *f* refer to figures; page numbers followed by *t* refer to tables.